THE MODERN COUNTRY HOME

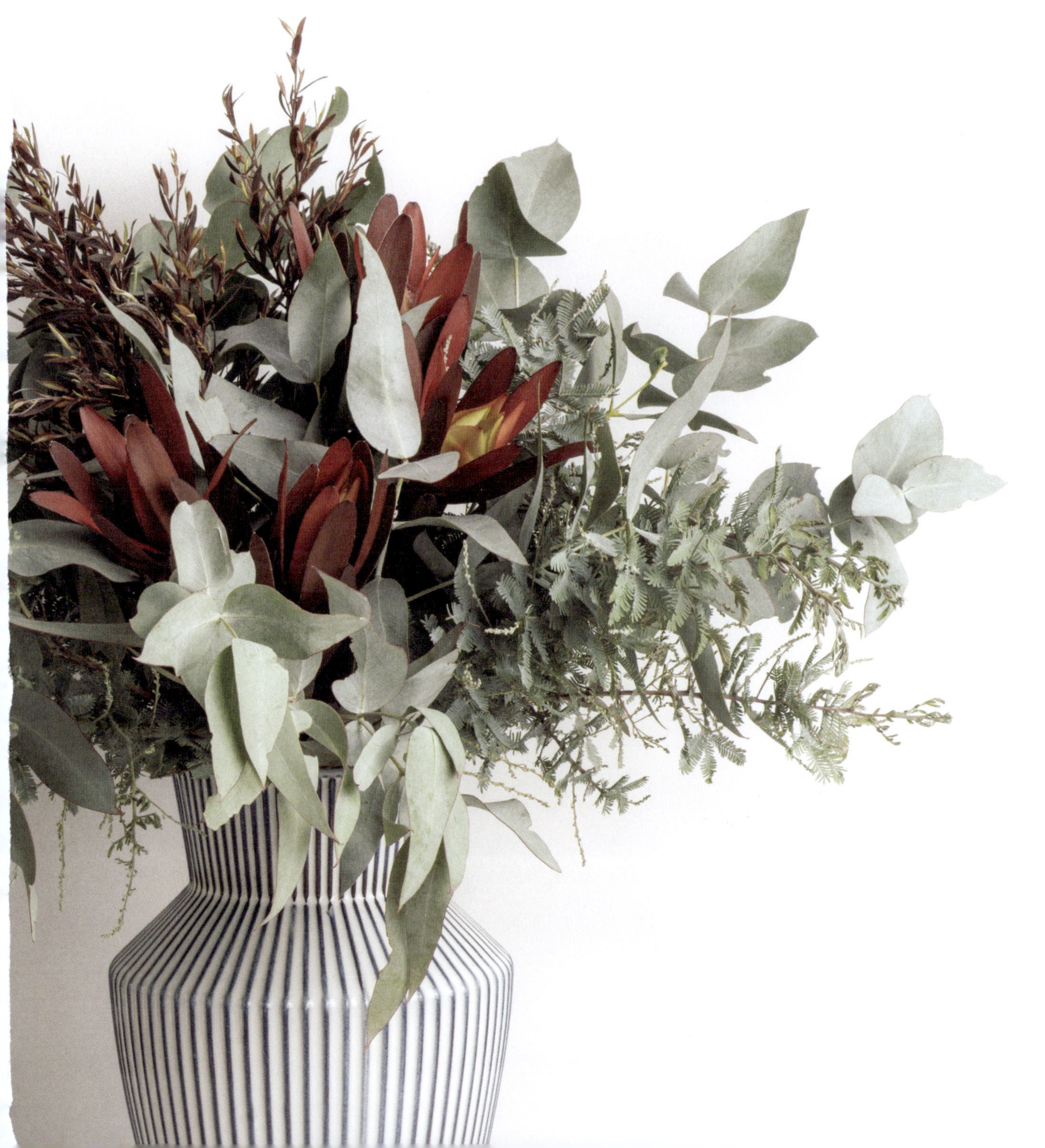

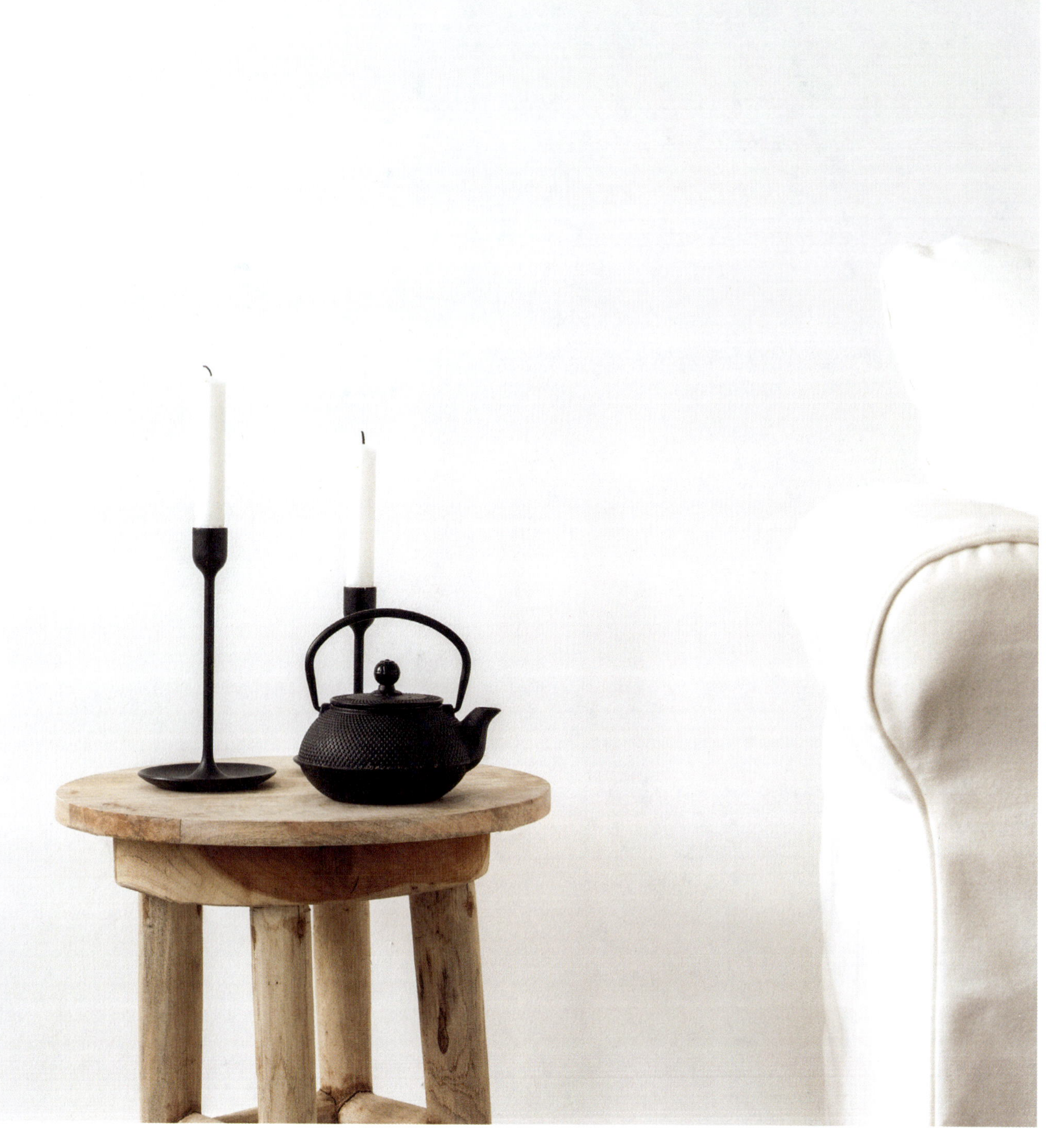

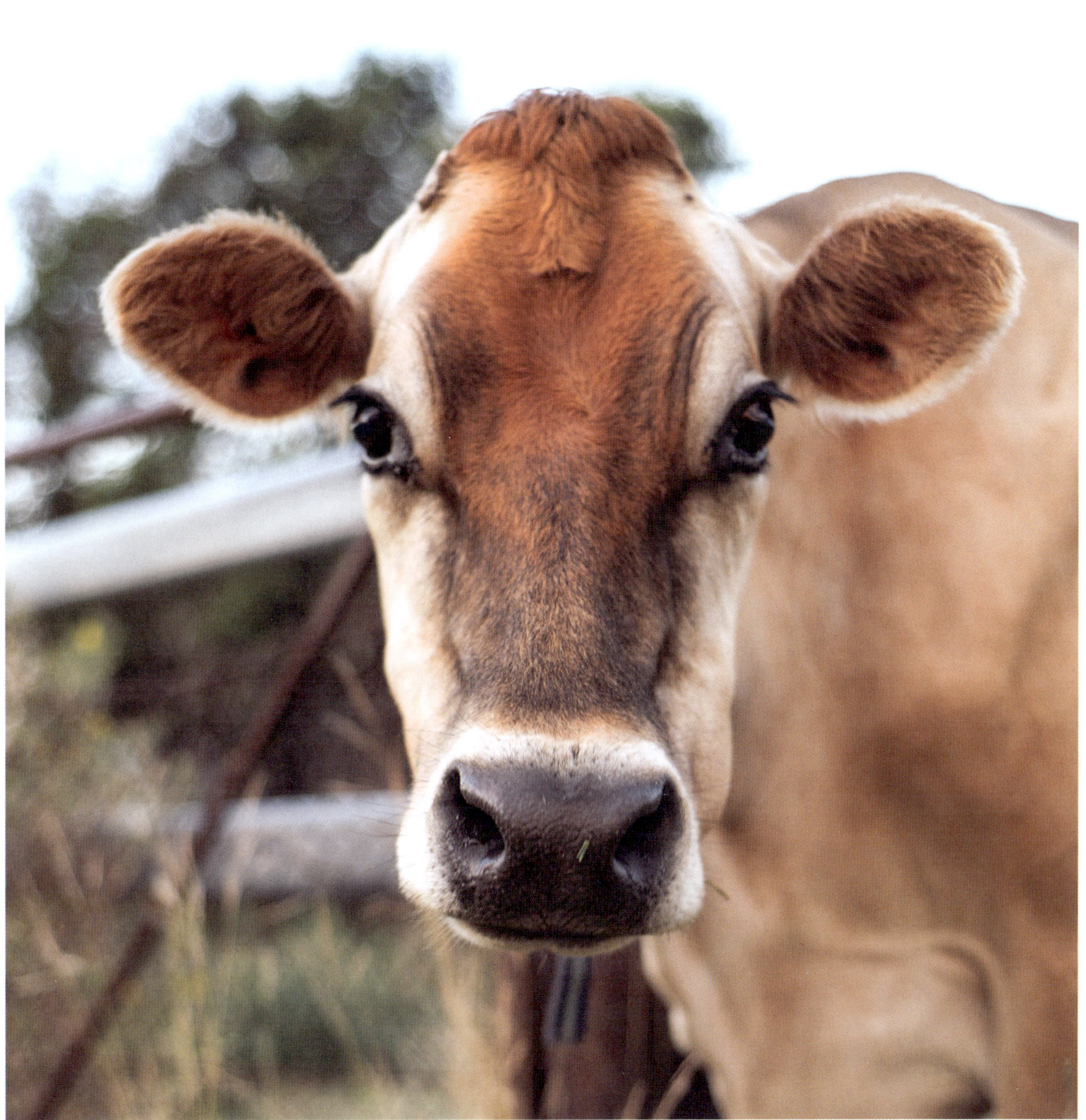

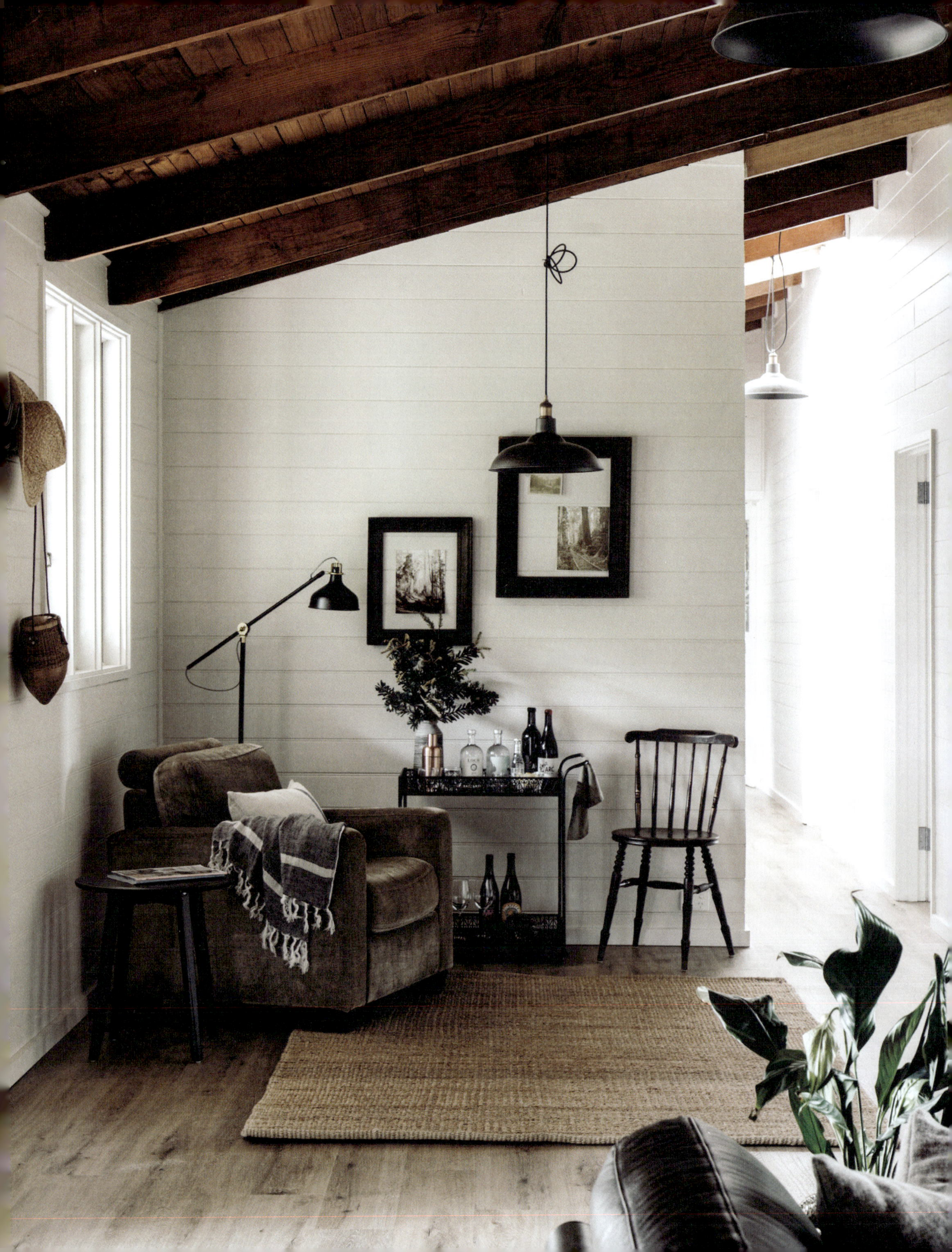

THE MODERN COUNTRY HOME

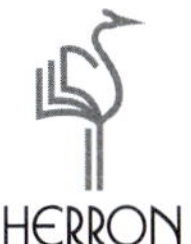

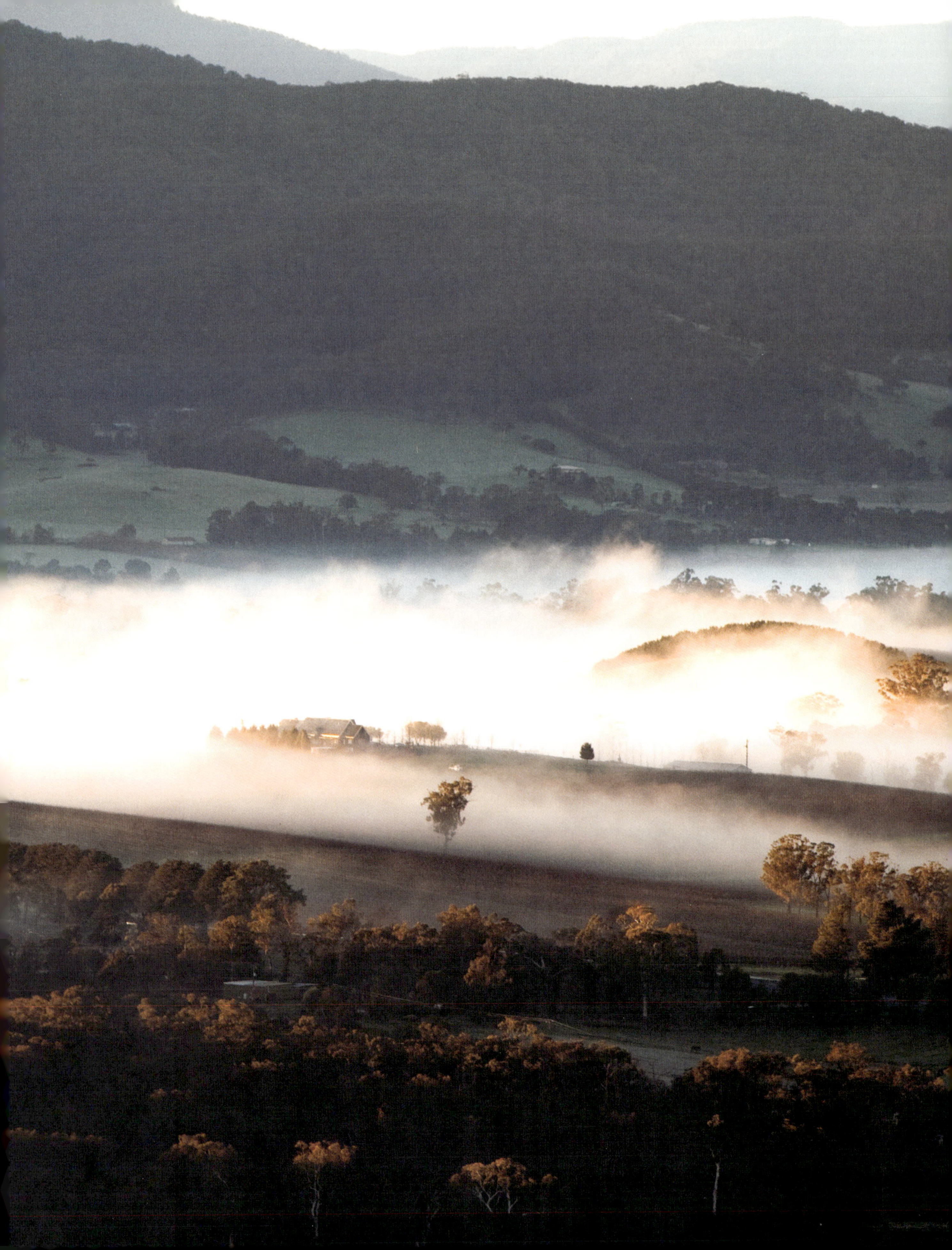

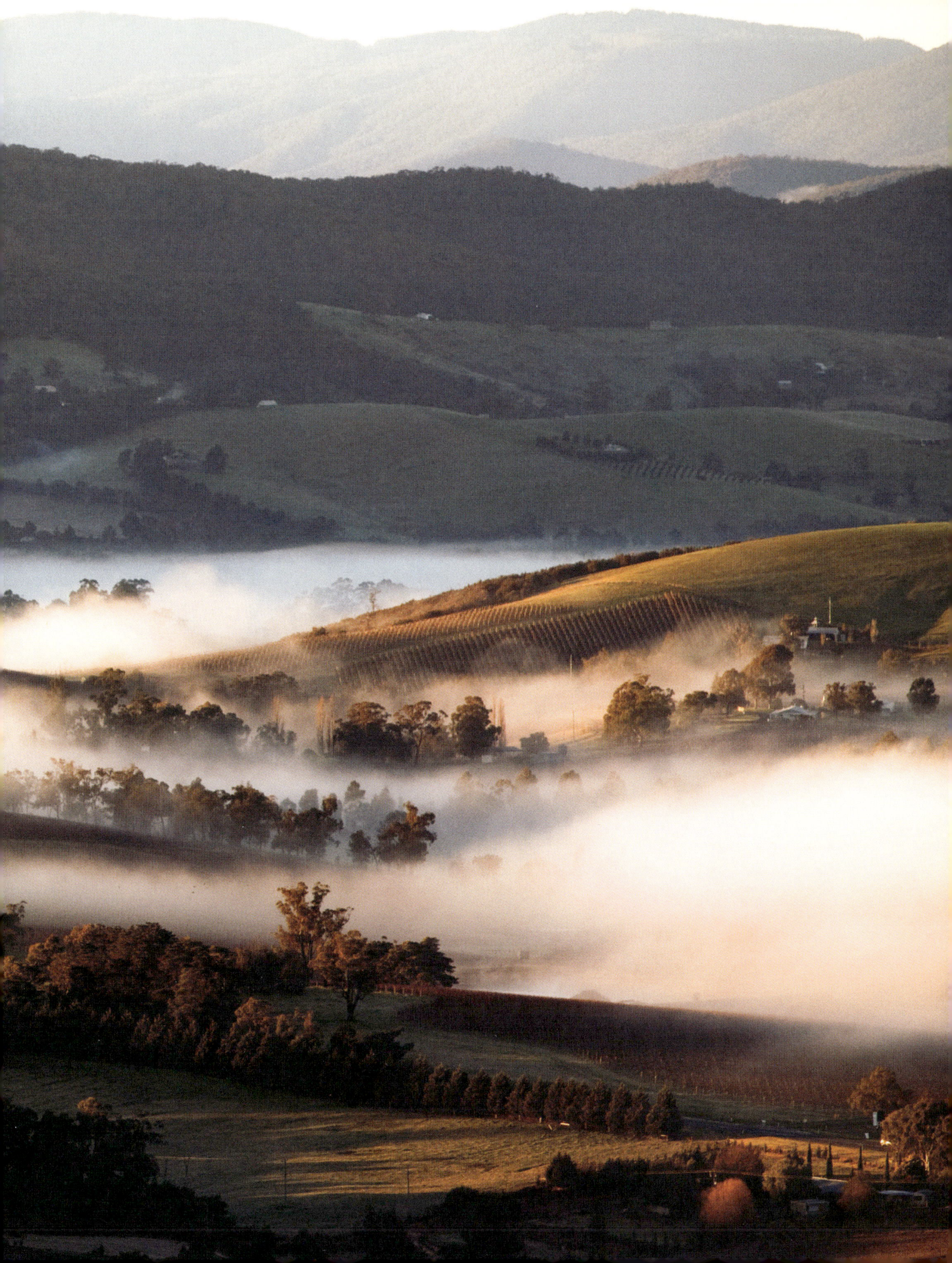

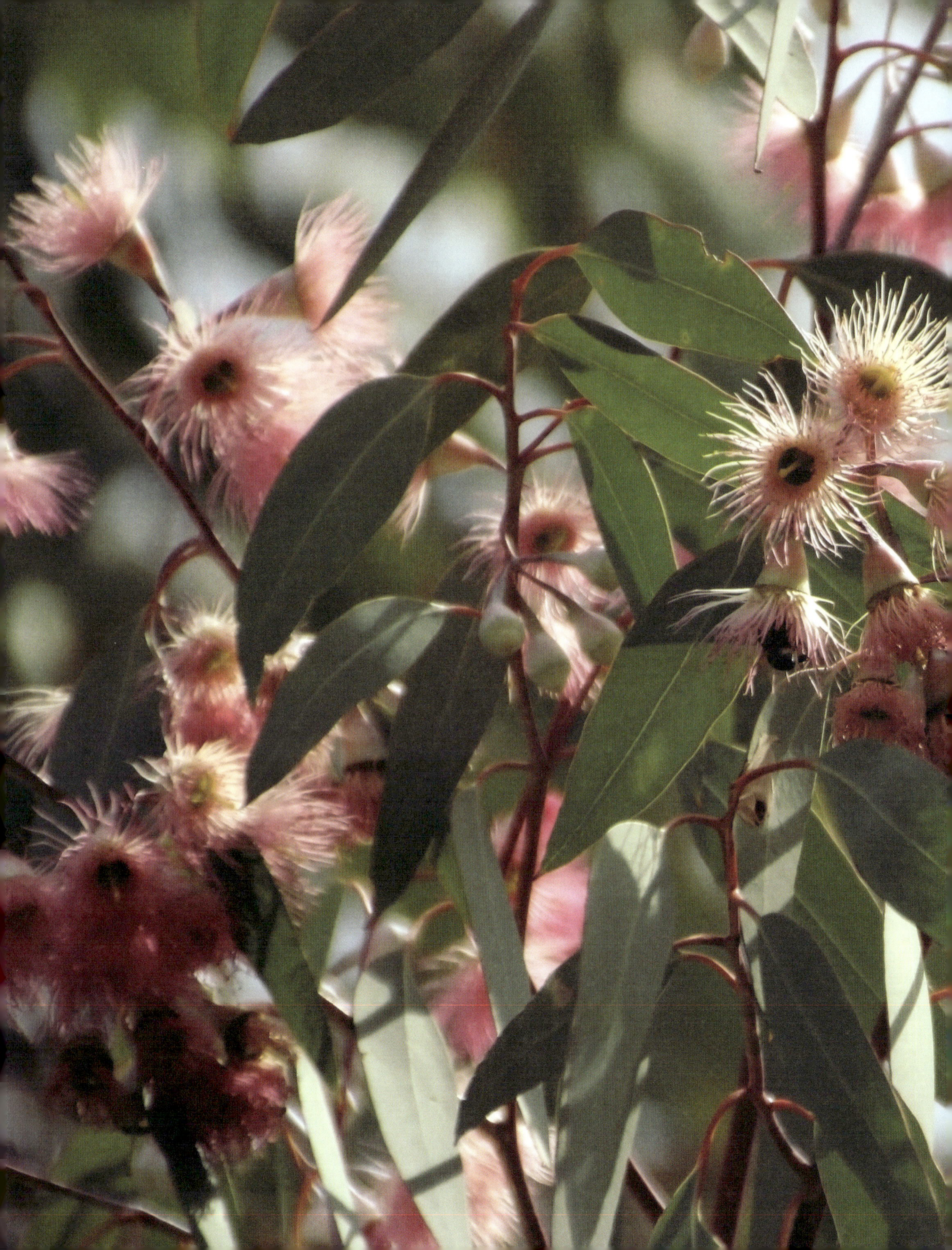

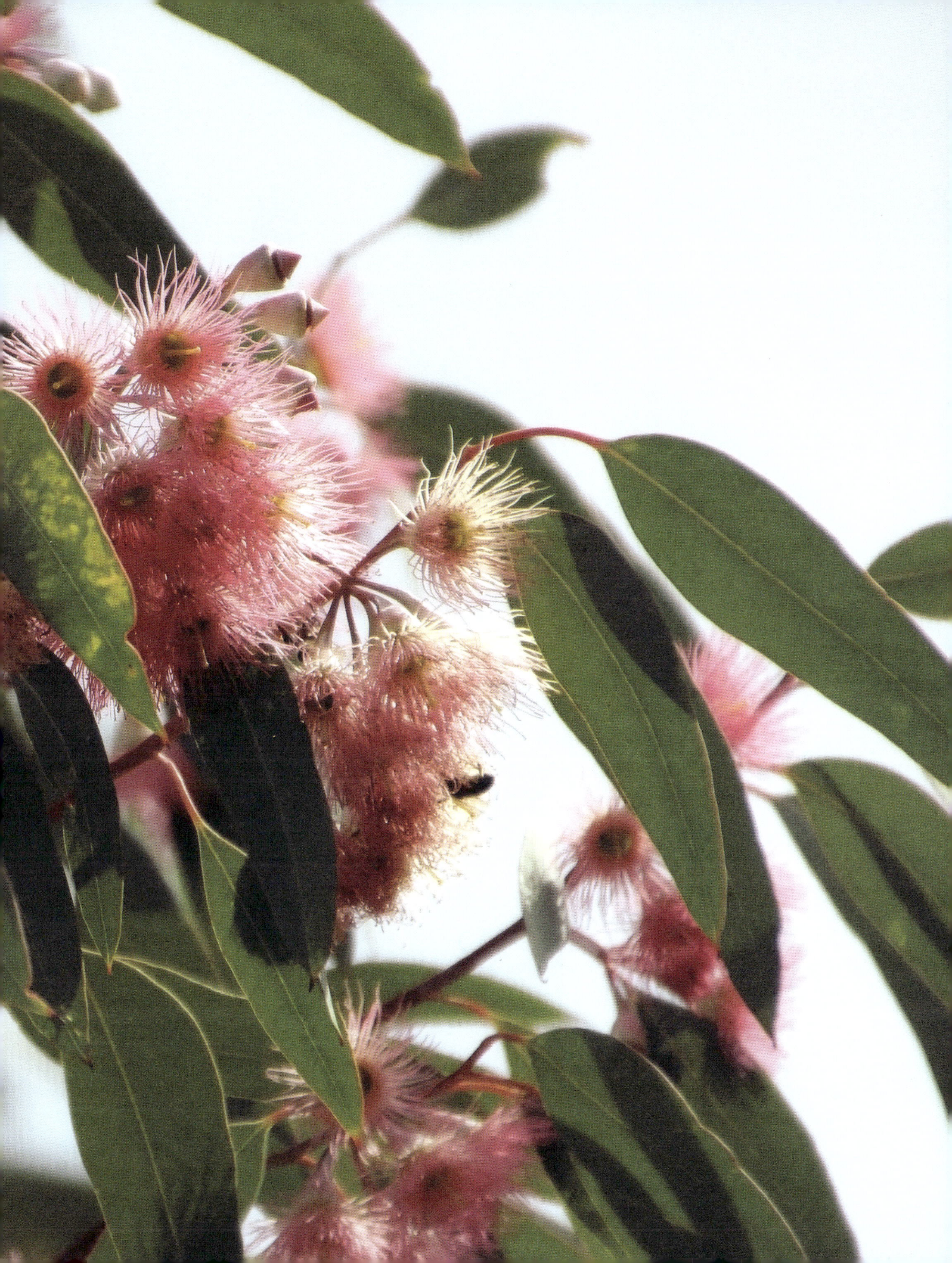

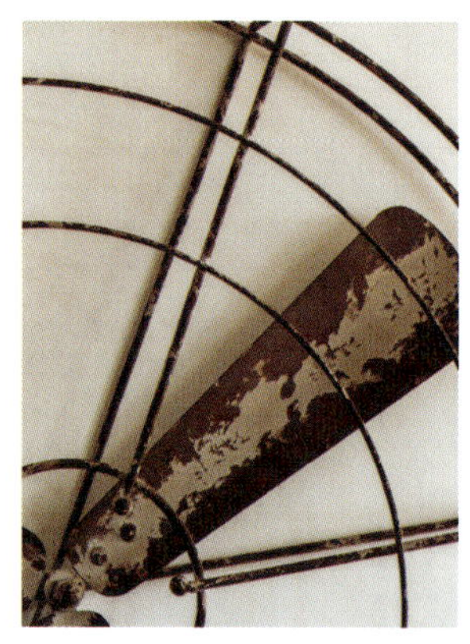

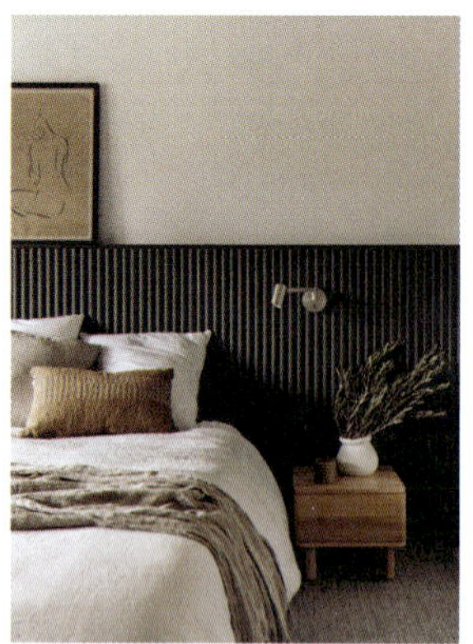

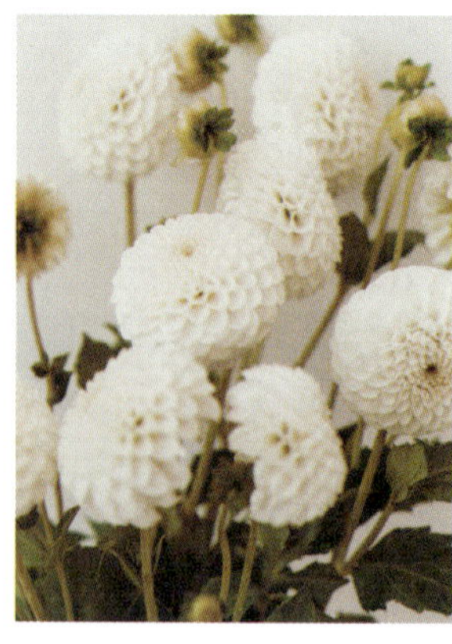

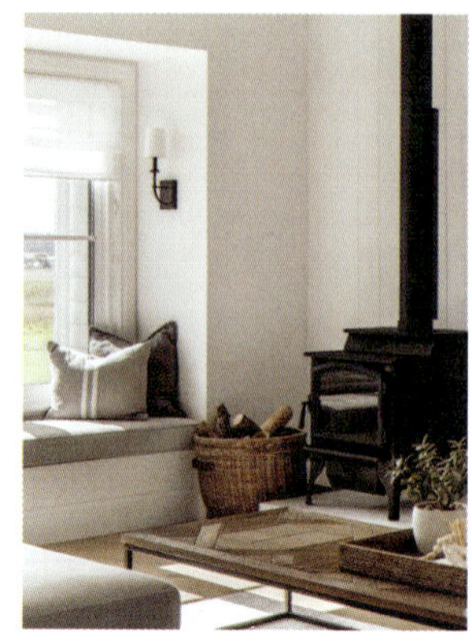

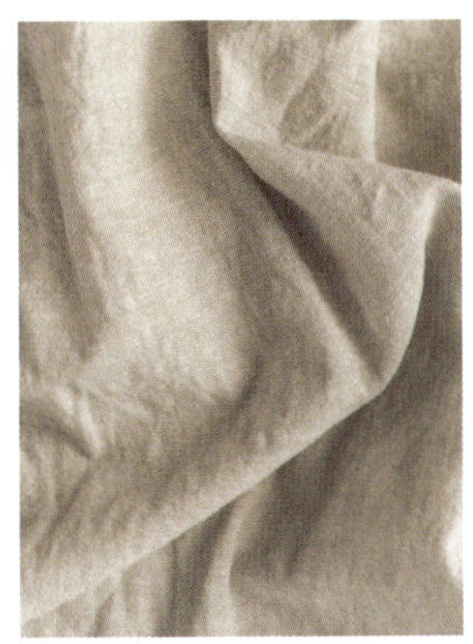

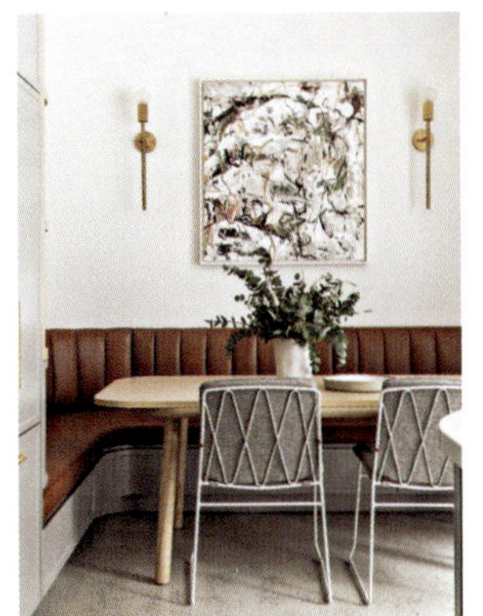

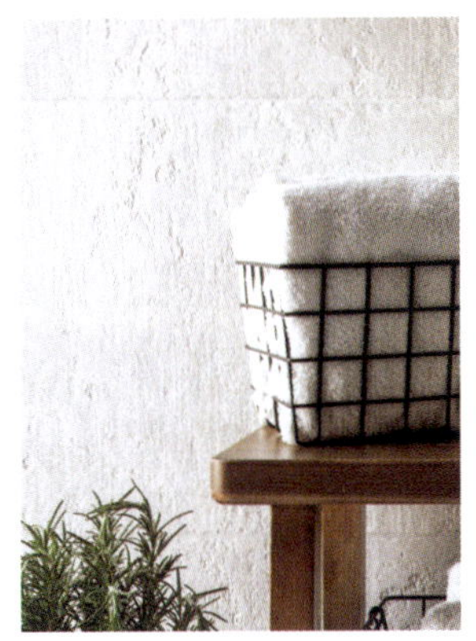

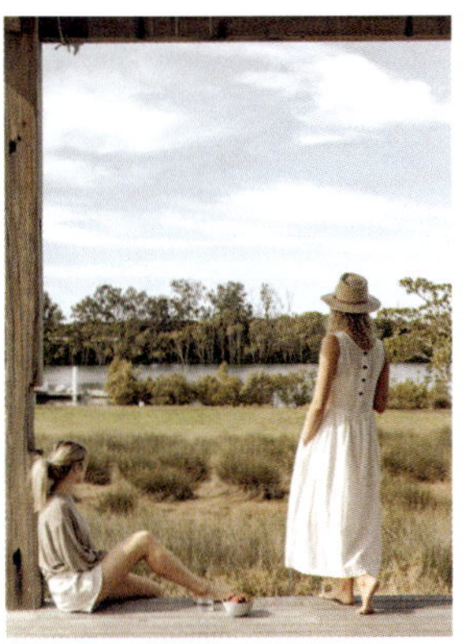

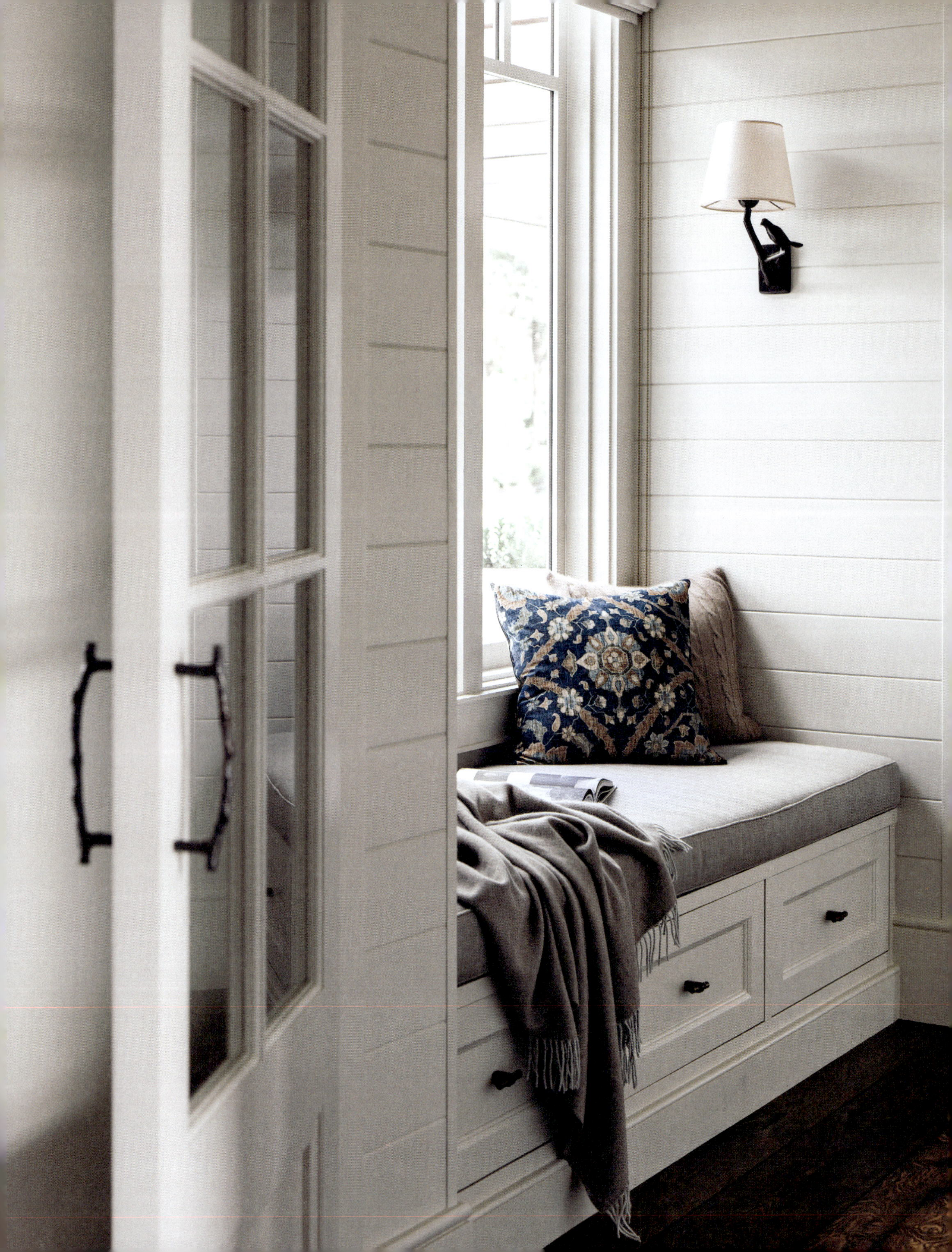

WELCOME

Immerse yourself in the beauty of modern Australian country home style, where contemporary interior design meets the tranquillity of nature and the sweet vibes of country living.

Standing sentry amid breathtaking farmland, tucked away in coastal hinterlands, the historic markers of small regional towns, or new homes nestled in an urban block: it might at first sight be hard to see what these diverse homes have in common. The answer is simple: they all share a focus on celebrating the sophistication and laid-back comfort that defines Australian country living.

From sun-drenched living rooms to the cosy charm of rustic kitchens, each space featured in this inspirational book has been thoughtfully crafted to deliver style with purpose.

Living spaces in the modern country style transcend functionality to become spaces of intimacy and beauty, thanks to a seamless integration of natural textures, hues and elements of decor.

Bedrooms ooze understated simplicity and charm, while bathrooms evoke spa-like tranquillity, and outdoor sanctuaries blur the lines between nature and nurture.

Discover the art of creating a home that not only inspires but also nurtures the soul – where every carefully crafted moment tells a personal story and speaks to the timeless elegance and cherished roots of country living.

As you flick through its pages, let this book inspire your interior-design plans, give grace to your coffee table, or serve as a reminder of the spectacular vistas of the Australian landscape and it's unique country lifestyle.

Essentials

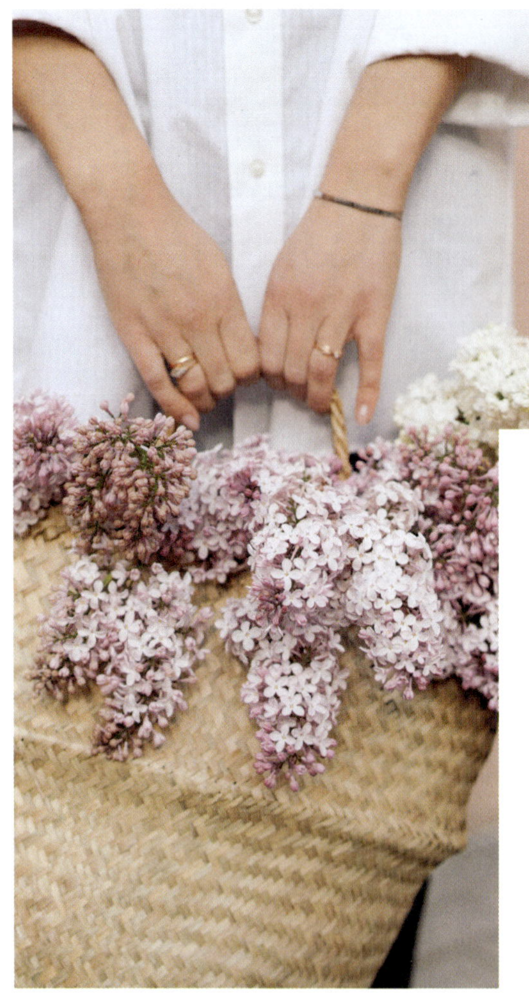

Refined with a touch of rustic

Functional and practical

Soft, muted colour palette

Warm, inviting and comfortable

Earthy materials, fibres, textures and colours

Reclaimed timber and tarnished metals

Flora and foliage as decor

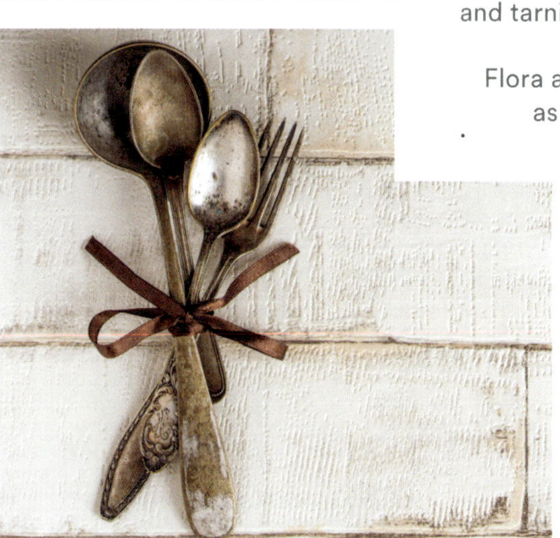

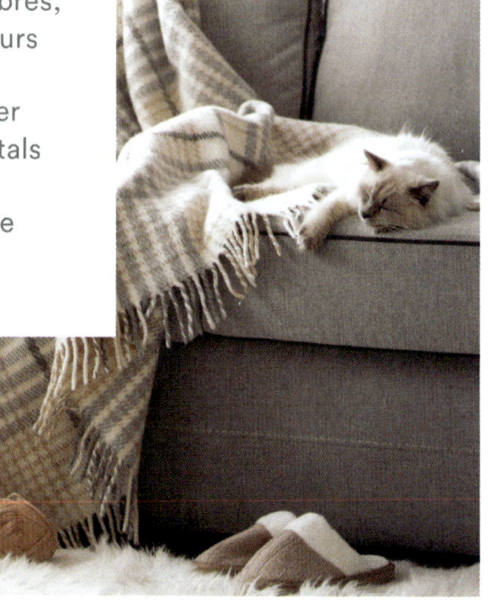

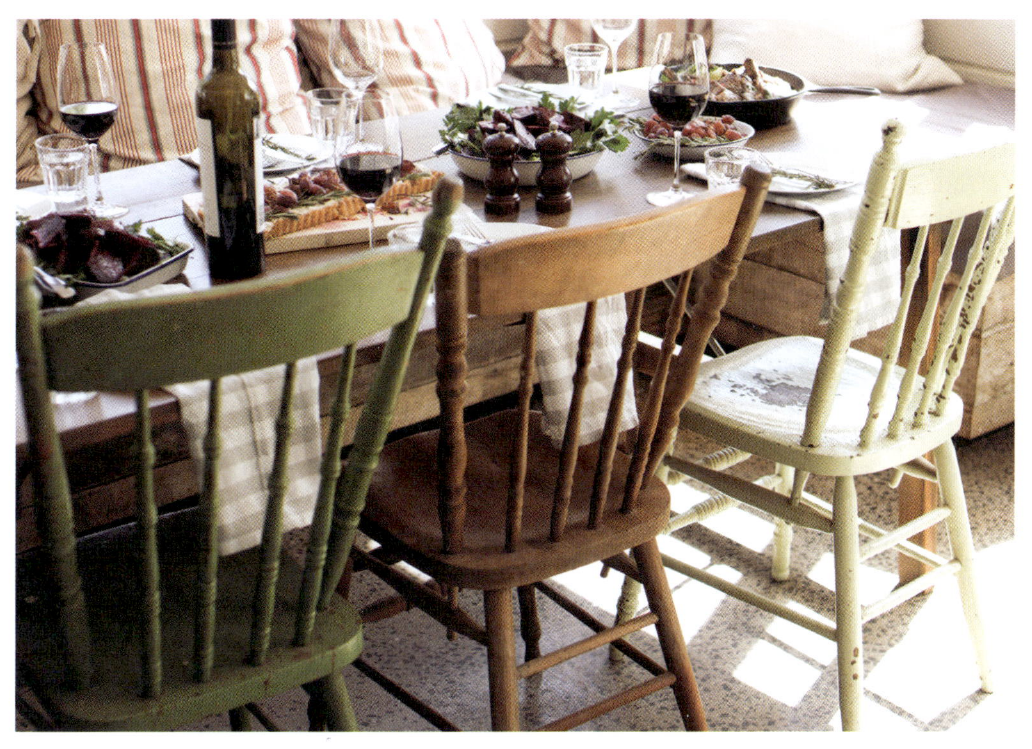

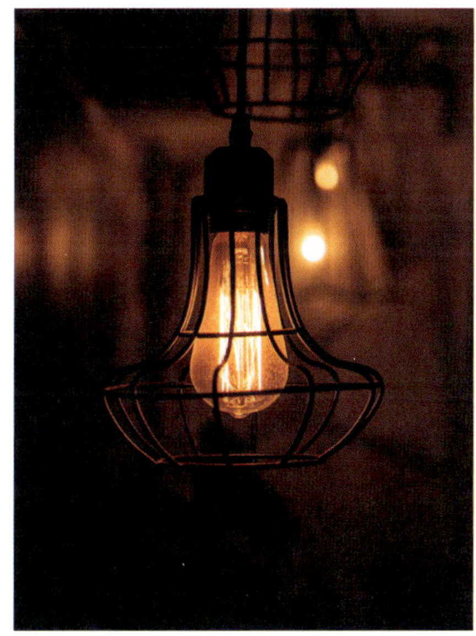

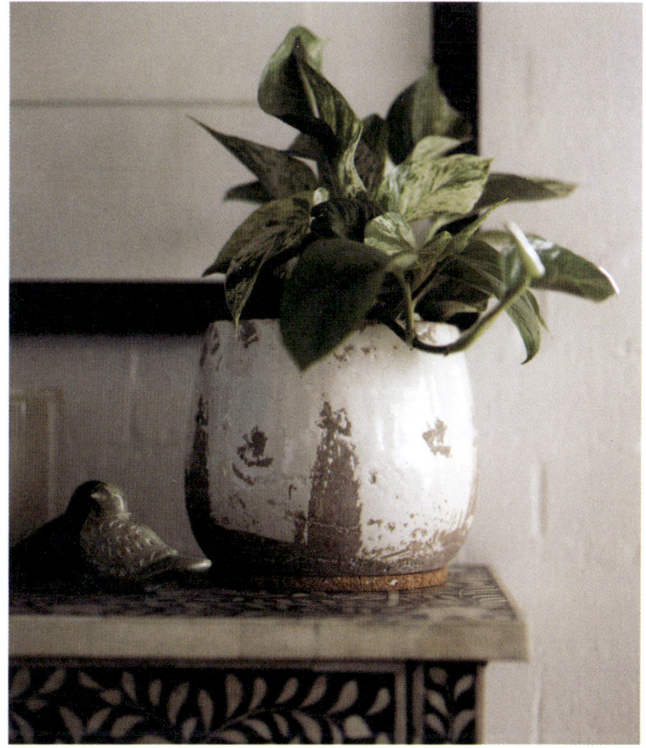

Essentials cont.

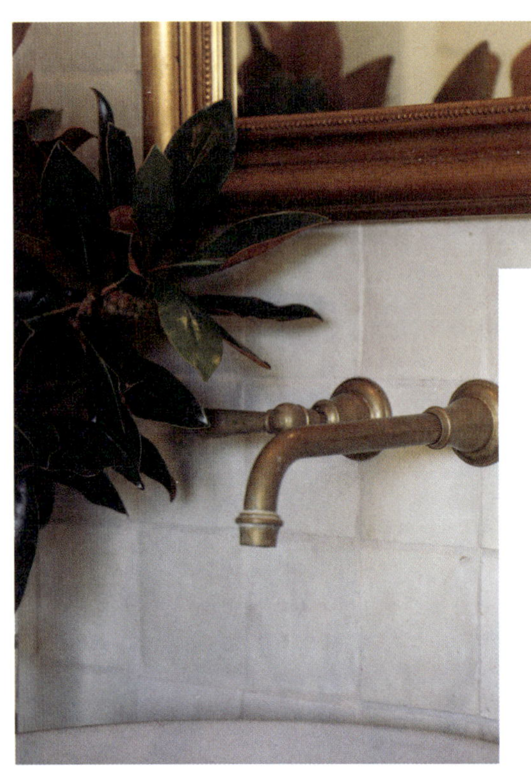

Celebrated imperfection

Nostalgic, vintage or handcrafted treasures

Open-plan living with a feature dining table

Feature fireplace

Stone or brick elements

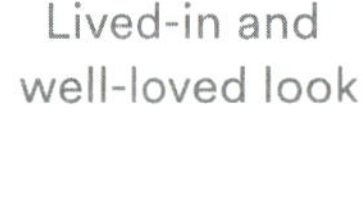

Items on display

Lived-in and well-loved look

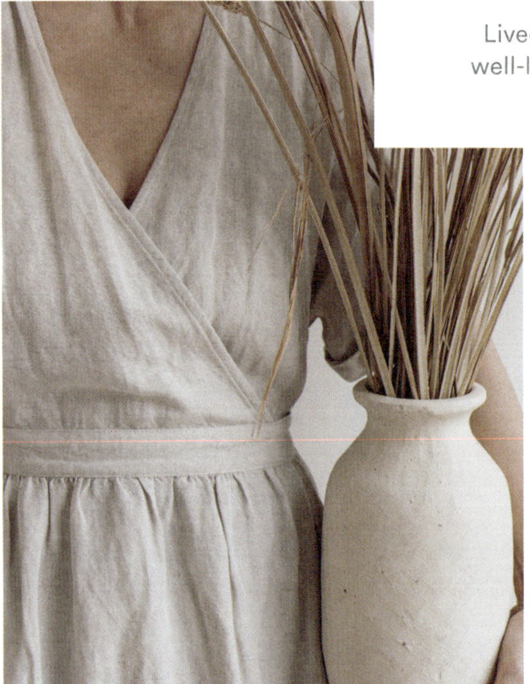

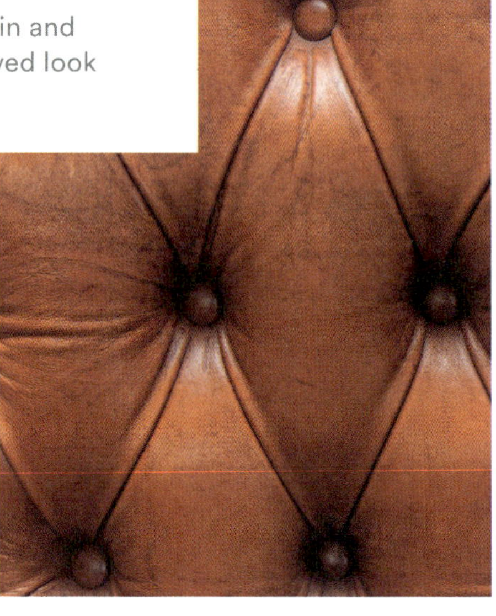

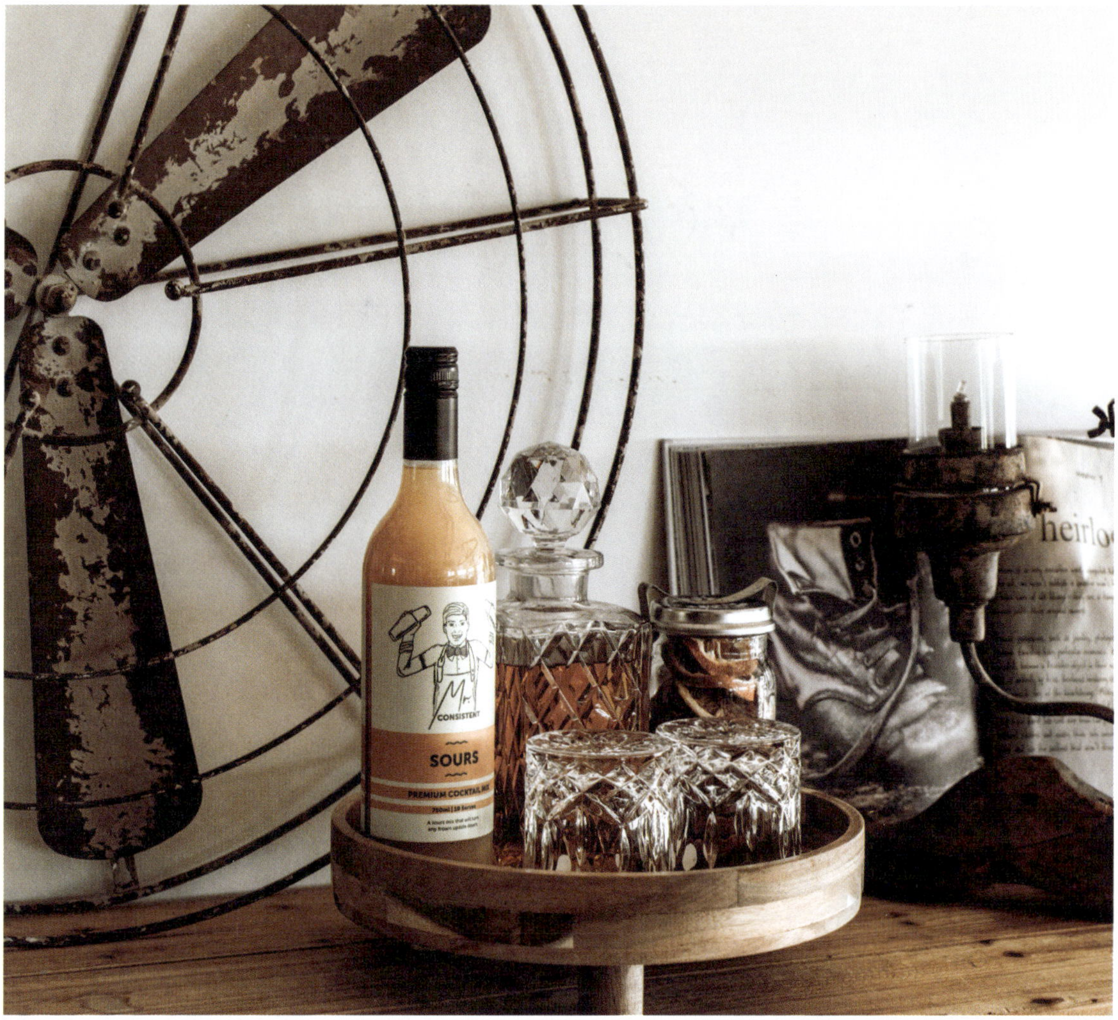

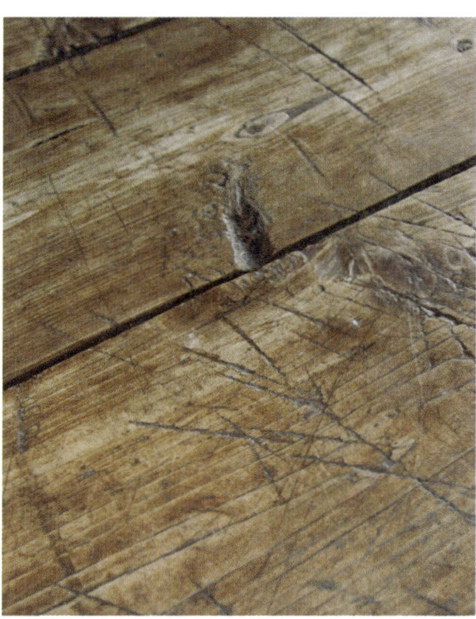

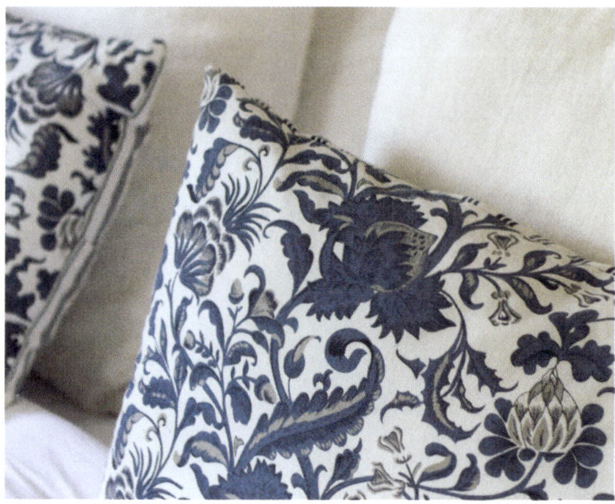

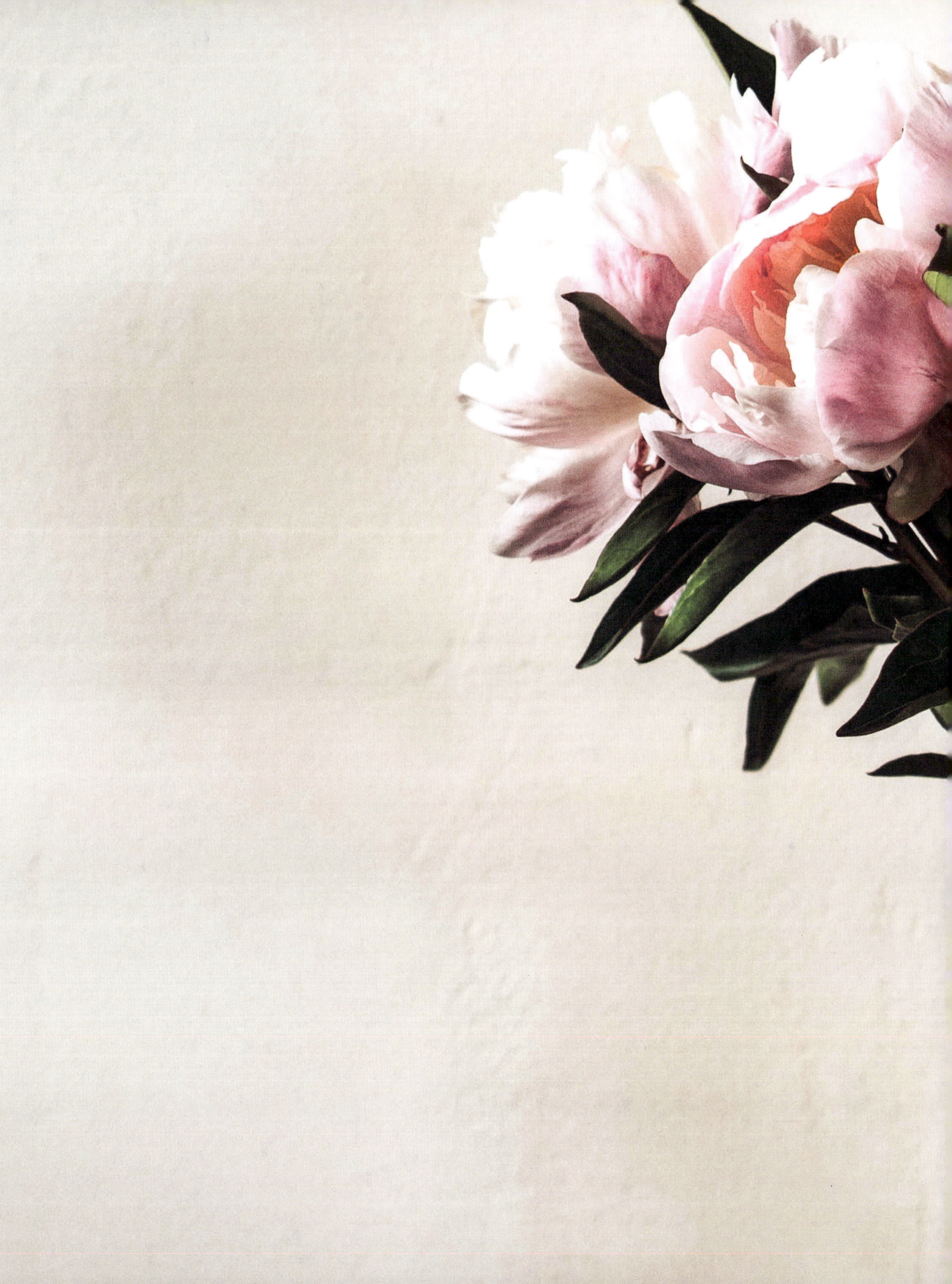

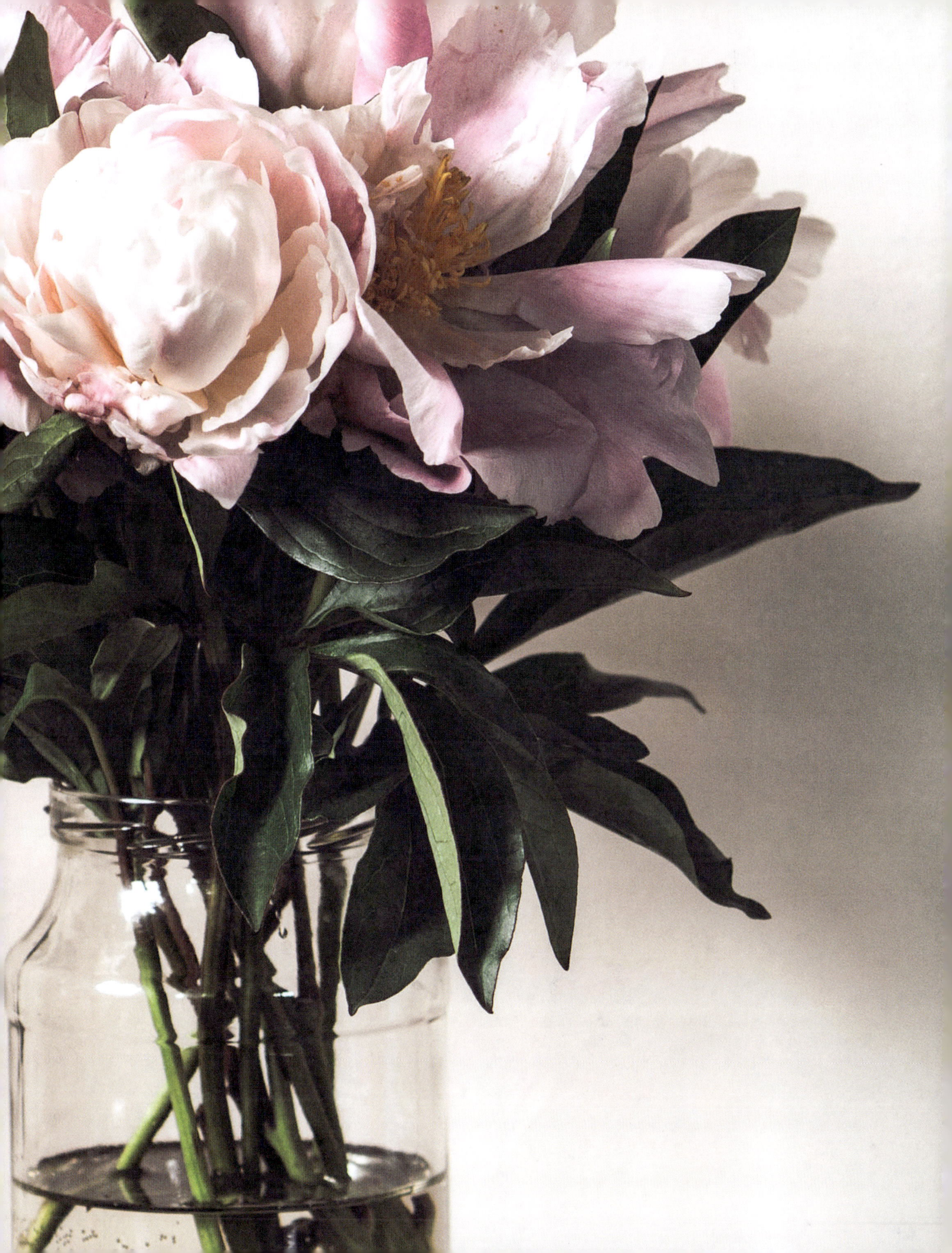

chapter one

mood

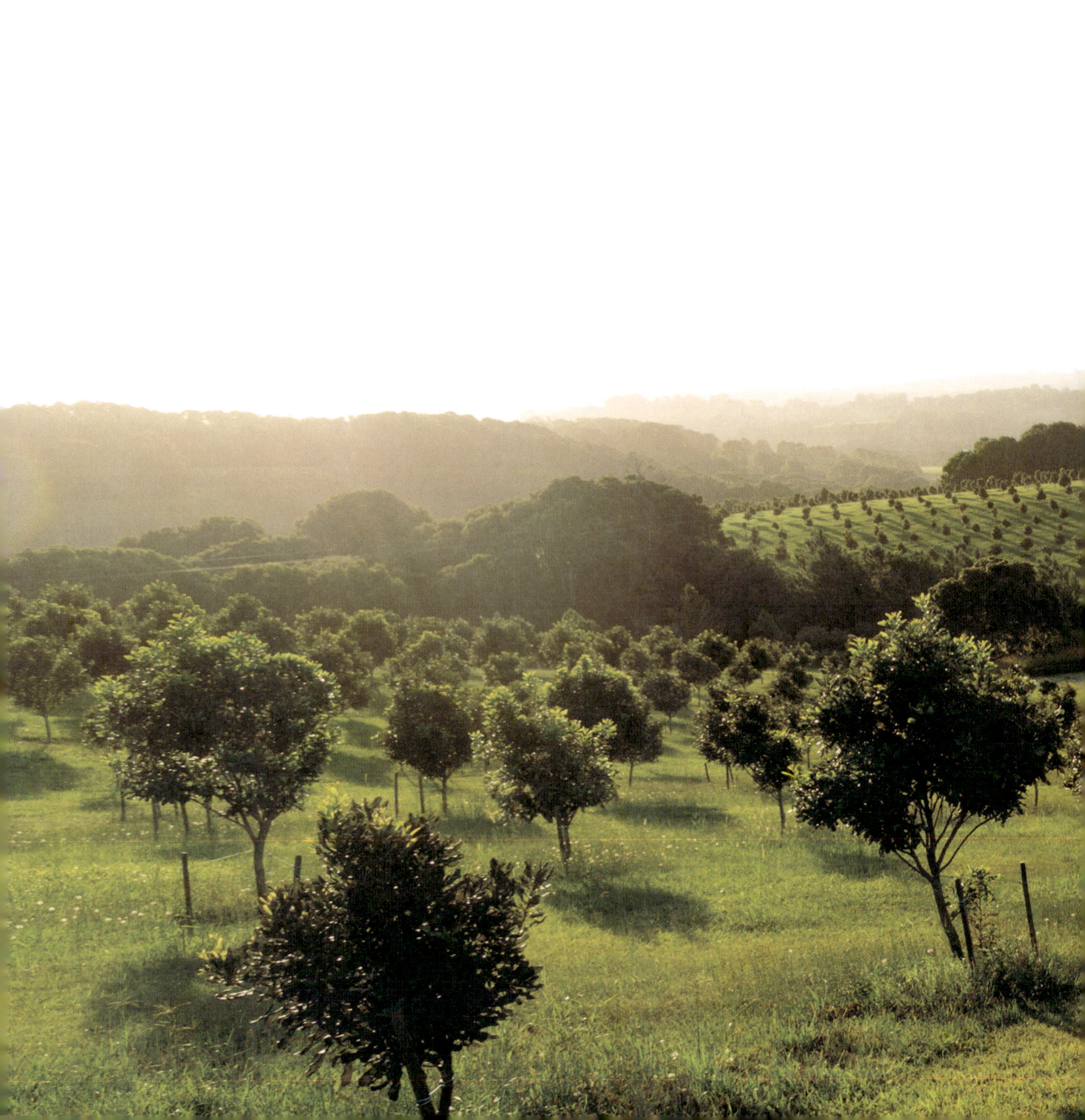

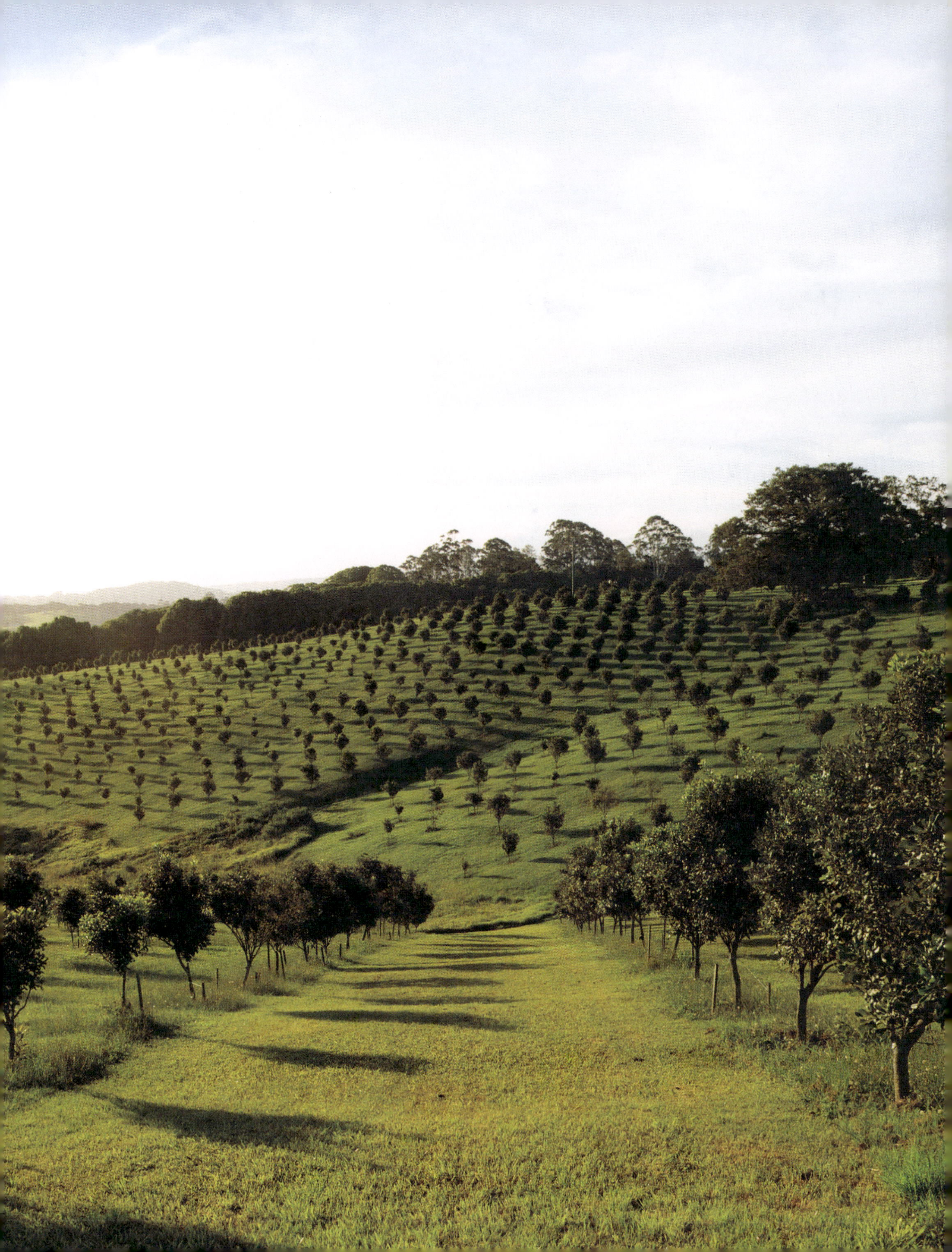

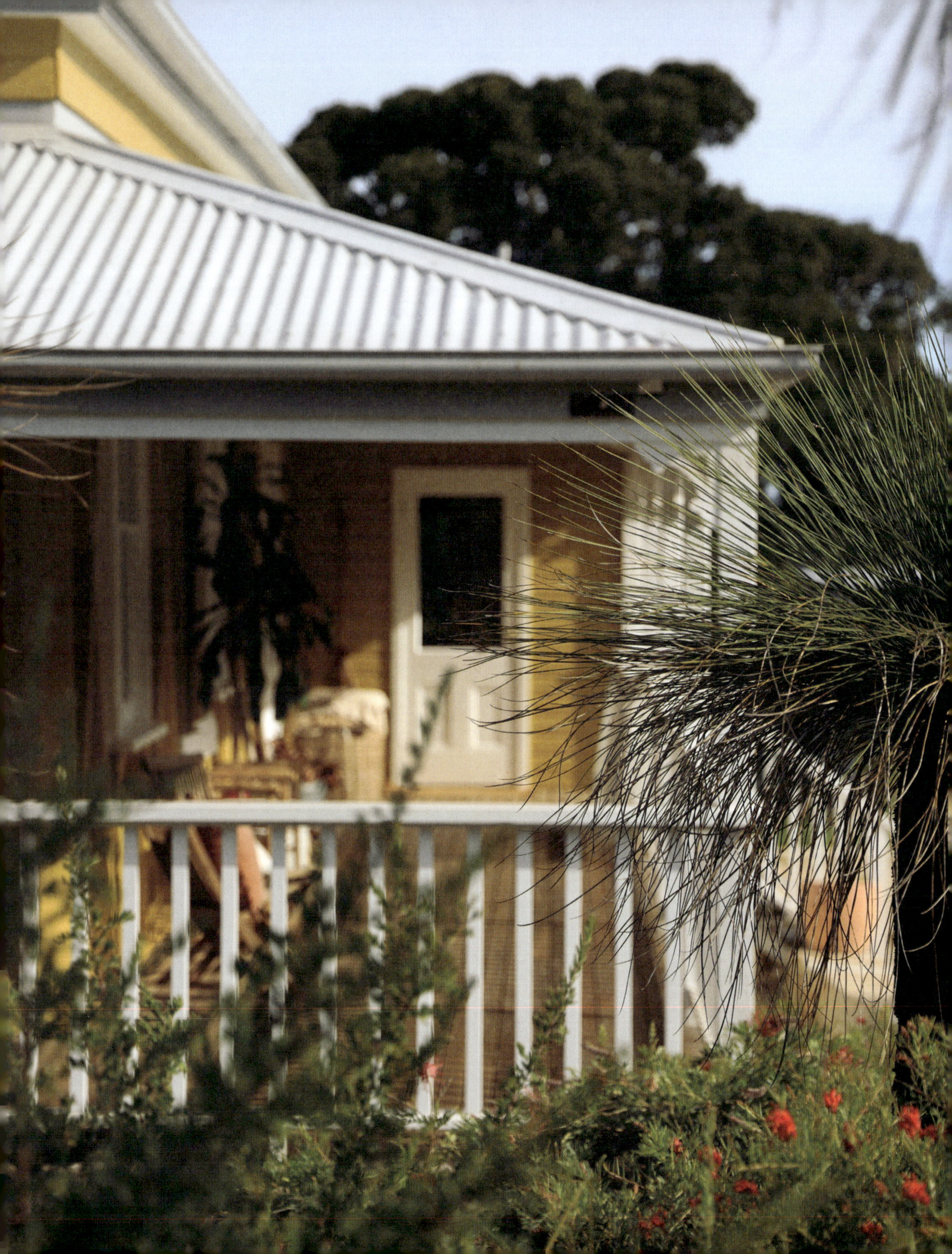

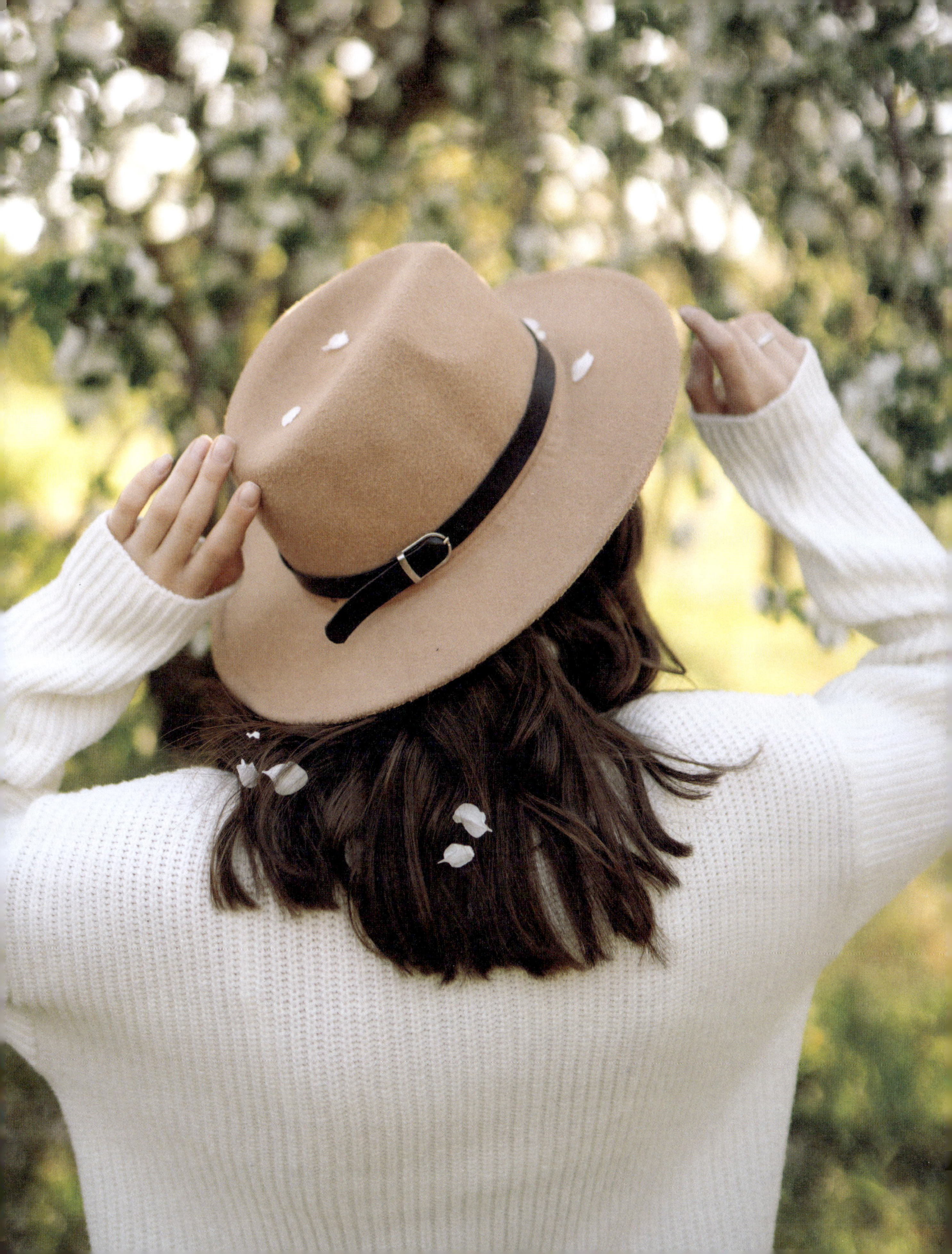

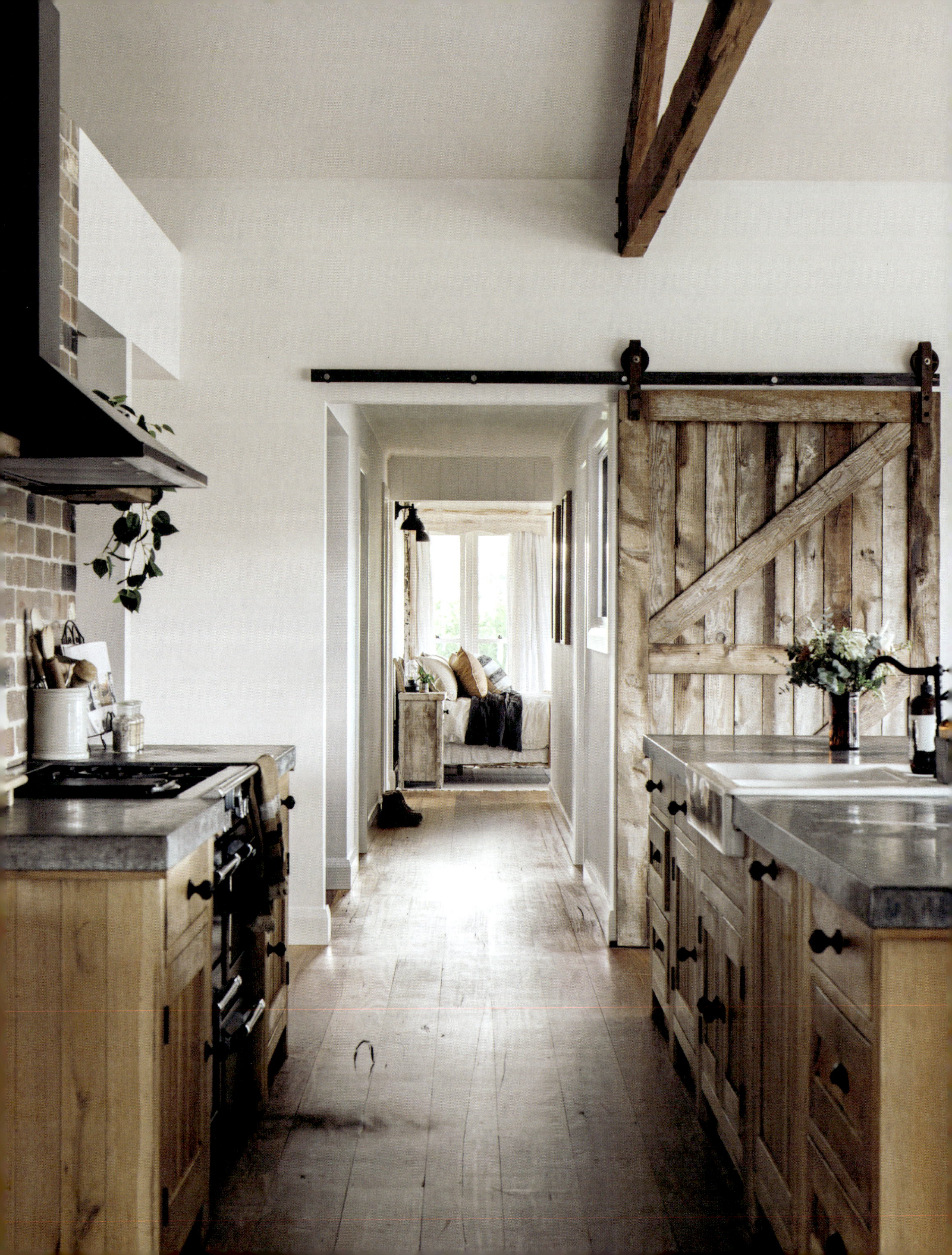

The mood is soft and welcoming. The vibe is unpretentious comfort. The values are honesty and integrity. The energy is soulful, and the promise is timeless.

Modern Australian country style embodies all of this, seemingly without effort. These core values are blended with a simple (and sometimes minimalist) aesthetic to create a version of country style that feels fresh and contemporary too.

Country style is an emblematic form of Australian interior design, traditionally warm, homely and nostalgic in feel.

This tone is set through the use of traditional materials, such as stone, wood and metal. Reclaimed timber and metal (such as brushed nickel, pewter and brass) often feature prominently in the structure and finishings of the country home.

Natural textures and materials like leather, jute, hemp and linen are integral to fabrications and furnishings, providing a softer finish to compliment the wood, metal or stone foundations and fittings. Oversize rugs add style and resilience to tough timber floors that historically absorb heavy feet.

The spectacular Australian landscape offers rich opportunities for a colour scheme to set the mood – a neutral base of warm whites and greys can be accented by the muted blue, green, terracotta and ochre tones found in nature, to create a seamless blend between inside and out.

Modern country design represents a subtle shift from the traditional. Floral, fussy and over-cluttered makes way for clean lines and contemporary styling, with items on display chosen with precision. The consistent use of materials and colour tones delivers a warm and inviting spirit – even though you may be nowhere near a farm.

TOP FIVE

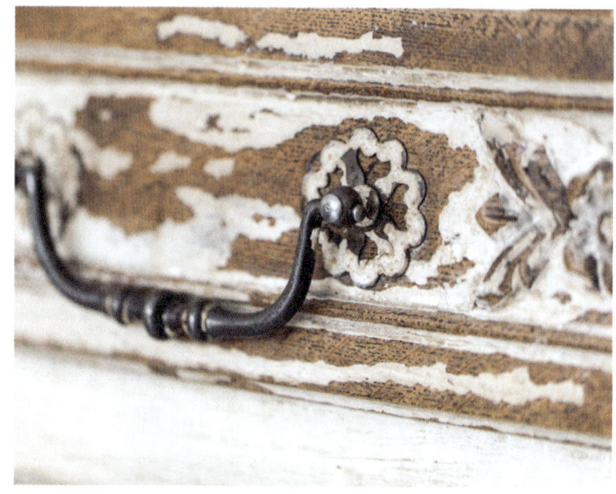

1.

Cool, clean and refined — rustic elements are balanced with crisp styling

2.

Honest materials – timber, stone and metal

3.

Hints at time-honoured craftsmanship

4.

An element of the unexpected

5.

Wooden dining table at the heart of the home

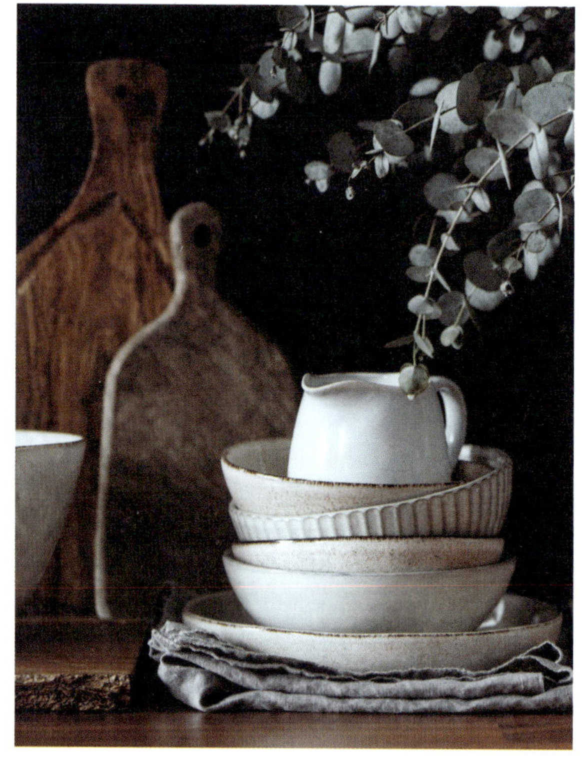

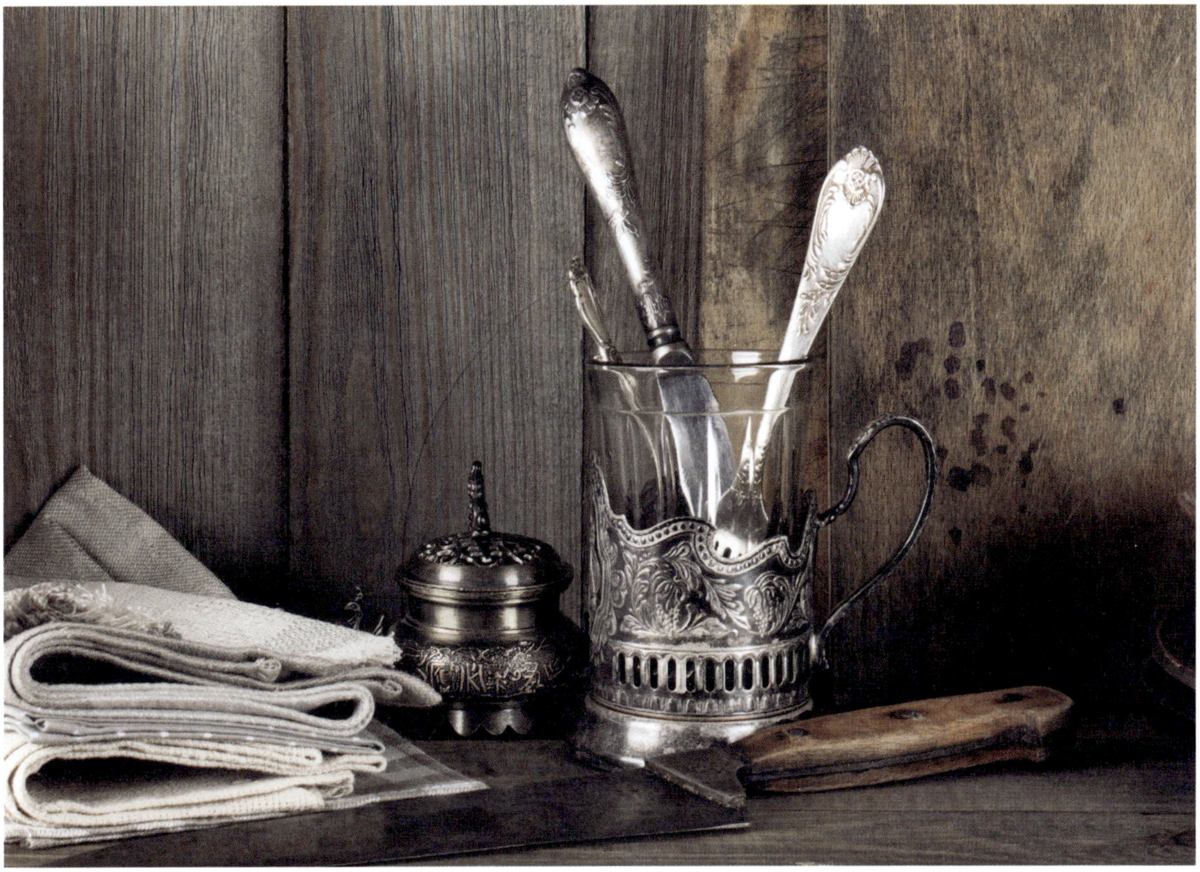

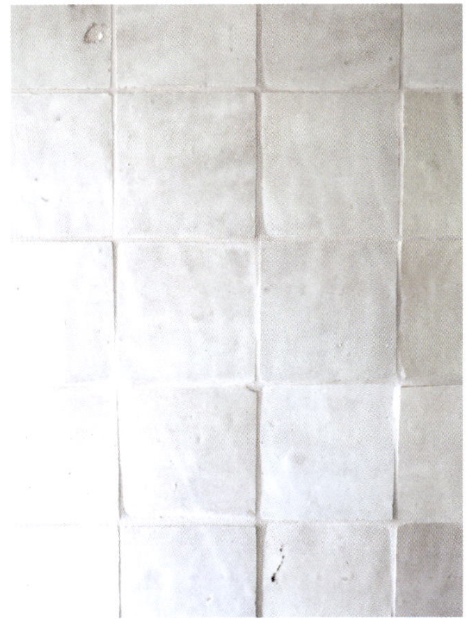

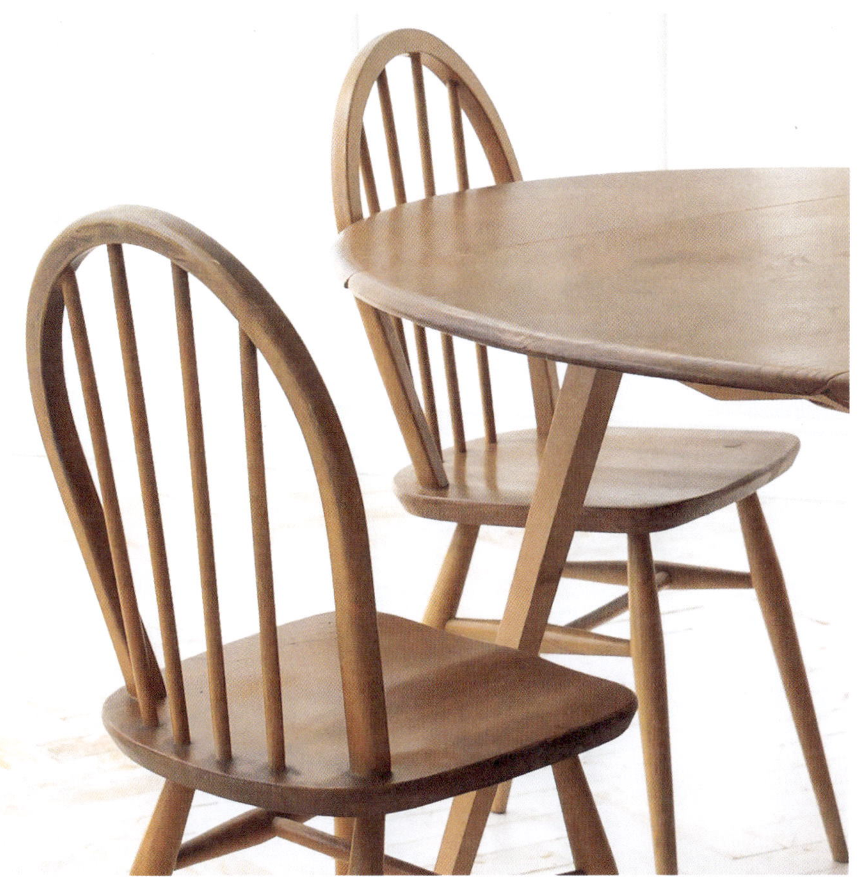

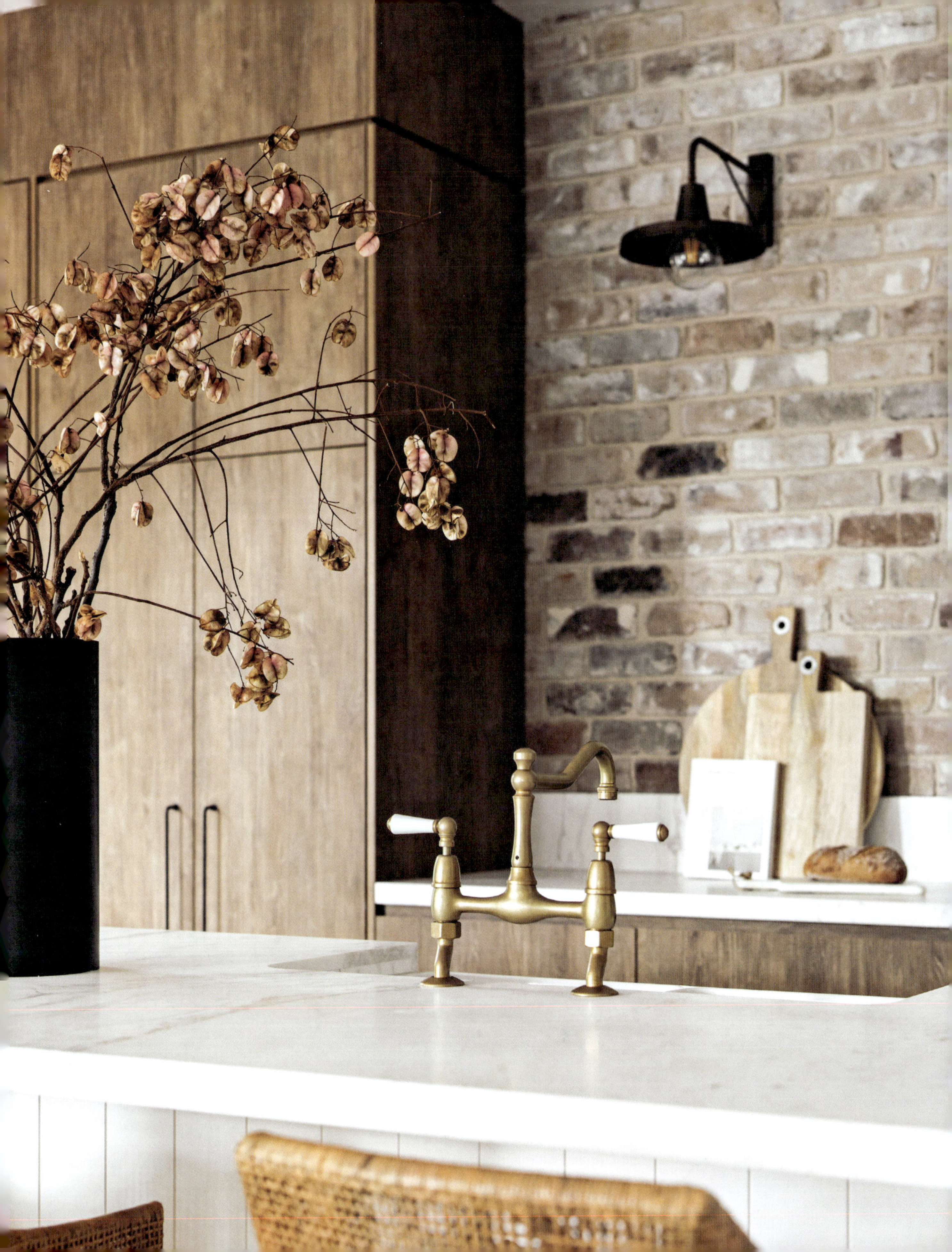

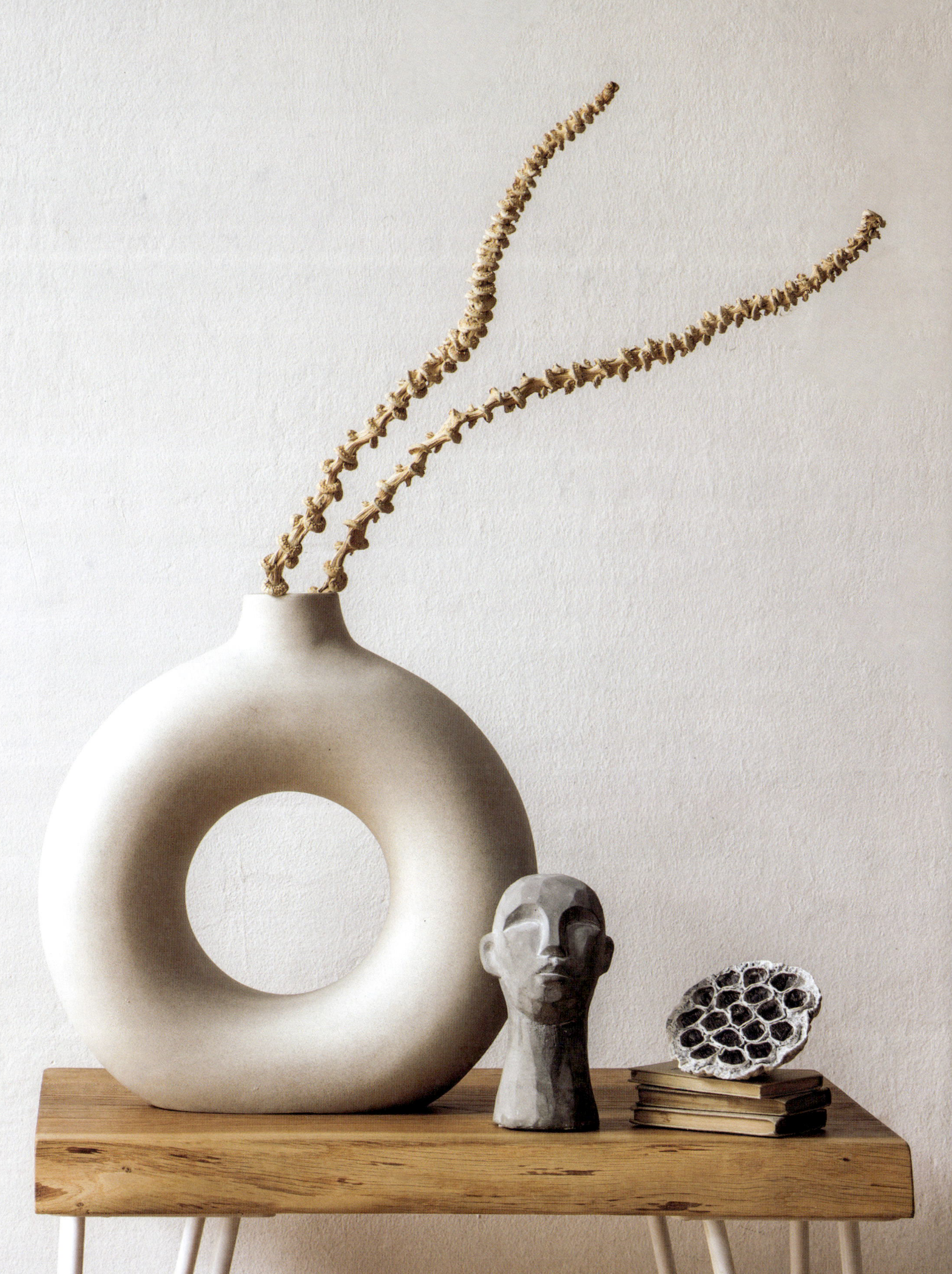

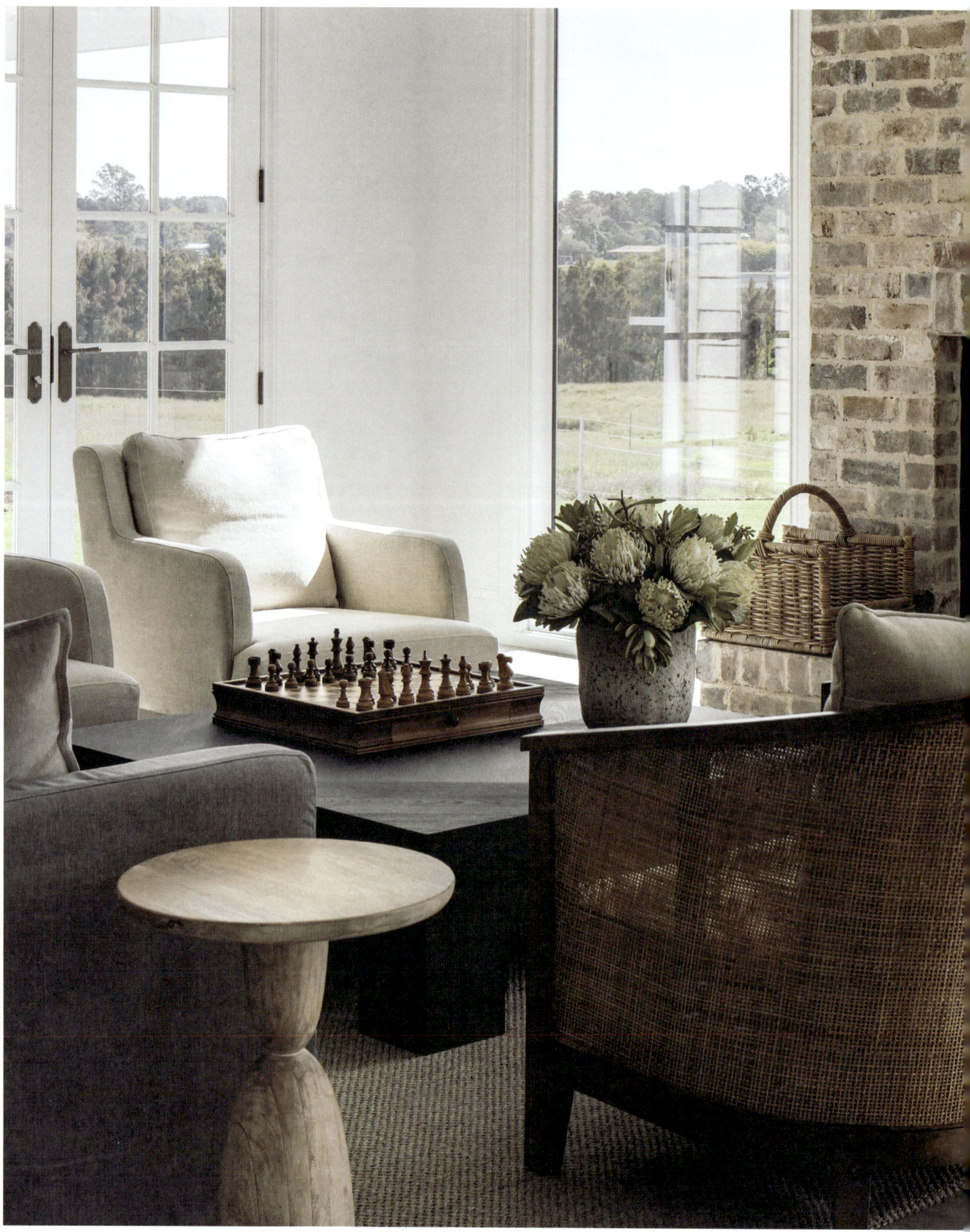

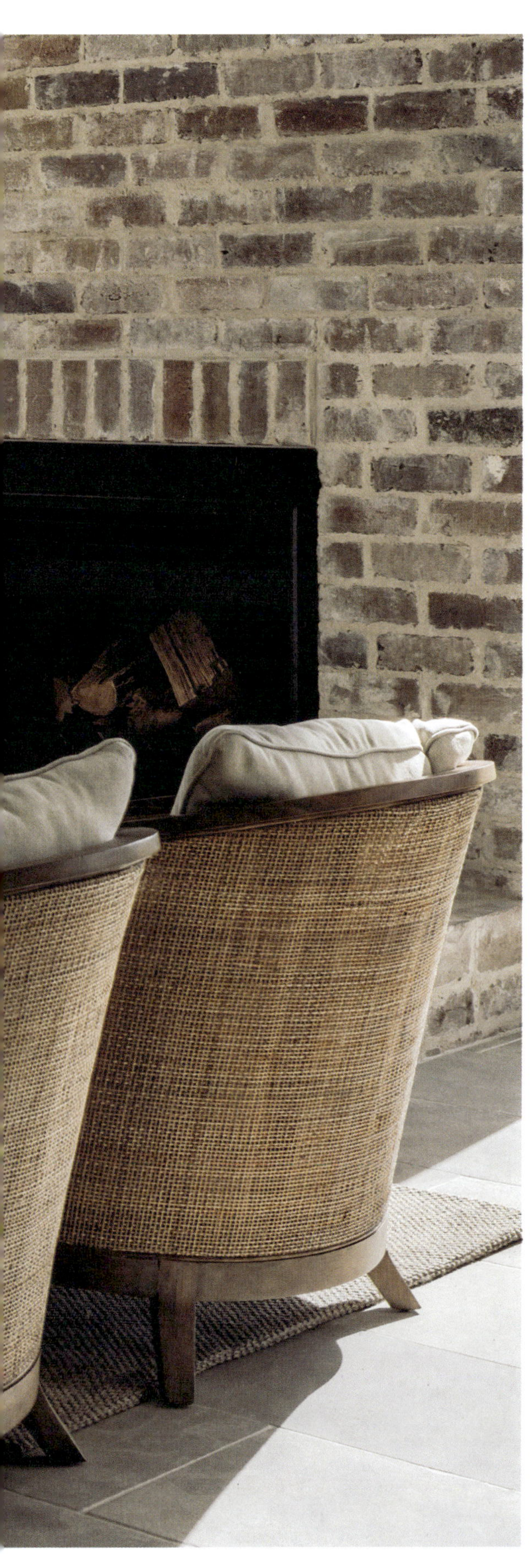

Historically a fireplace in a farmhouse has been a functional necessity. Today, it's both a comfort and a design choice. If you are lucky enough to have one, consider brick or stone surrounds to cement the country look, and don't overlook the styling opportunity provided by wood storage.

Horses are beloved creatures of Australian country life. While it might not be practical to own one, to help set the mood consider equestrian-inspired artwork or decor details in the home.

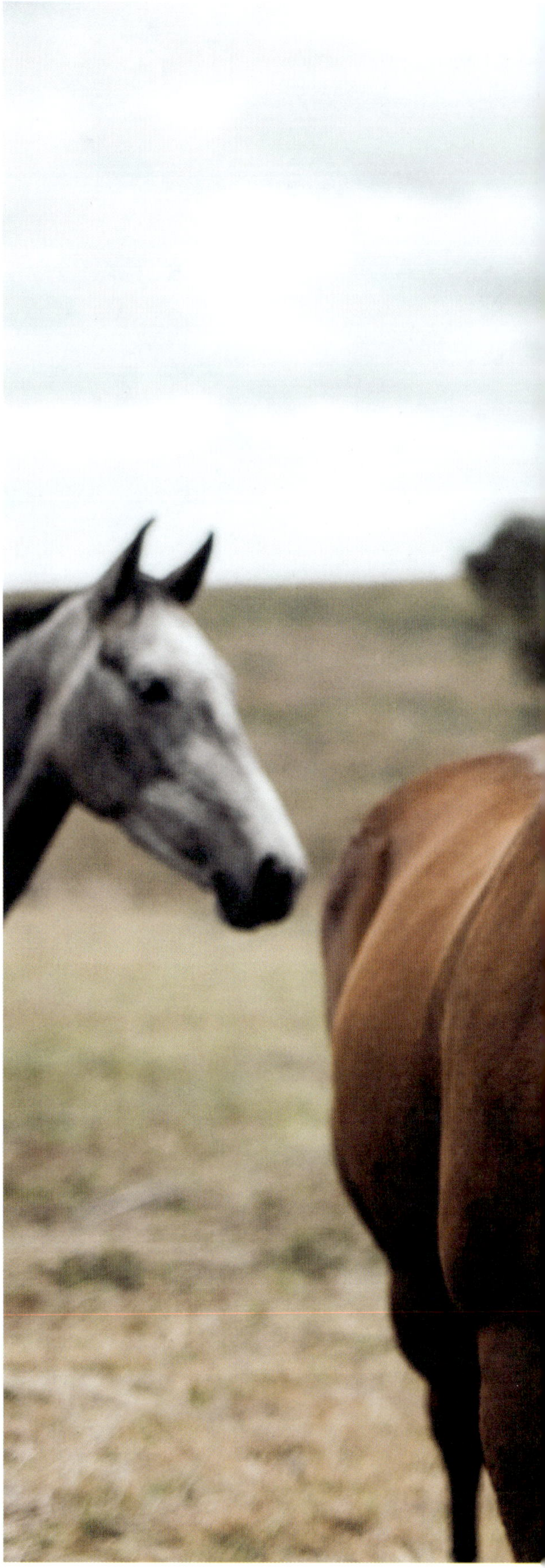

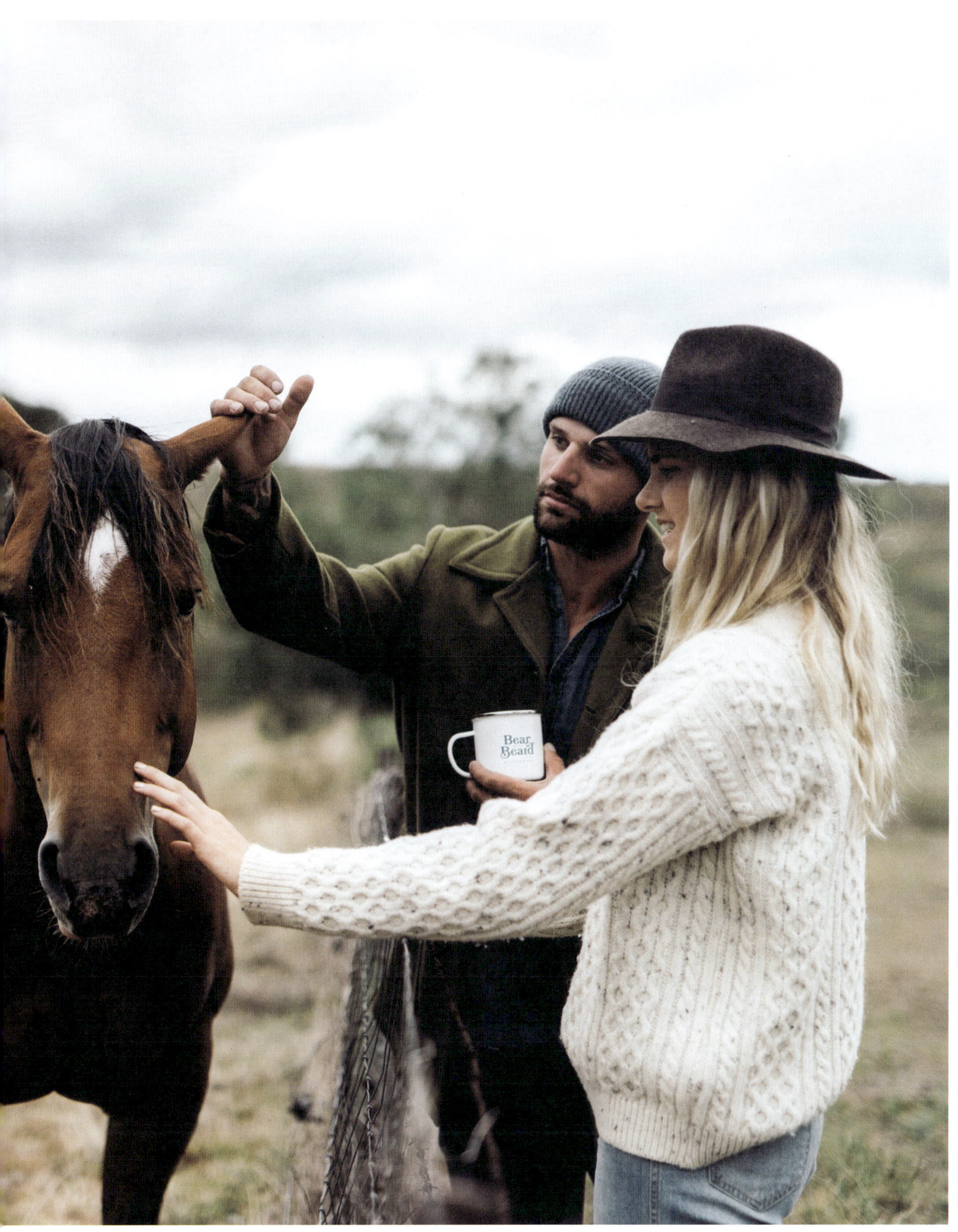
Bear
Beard

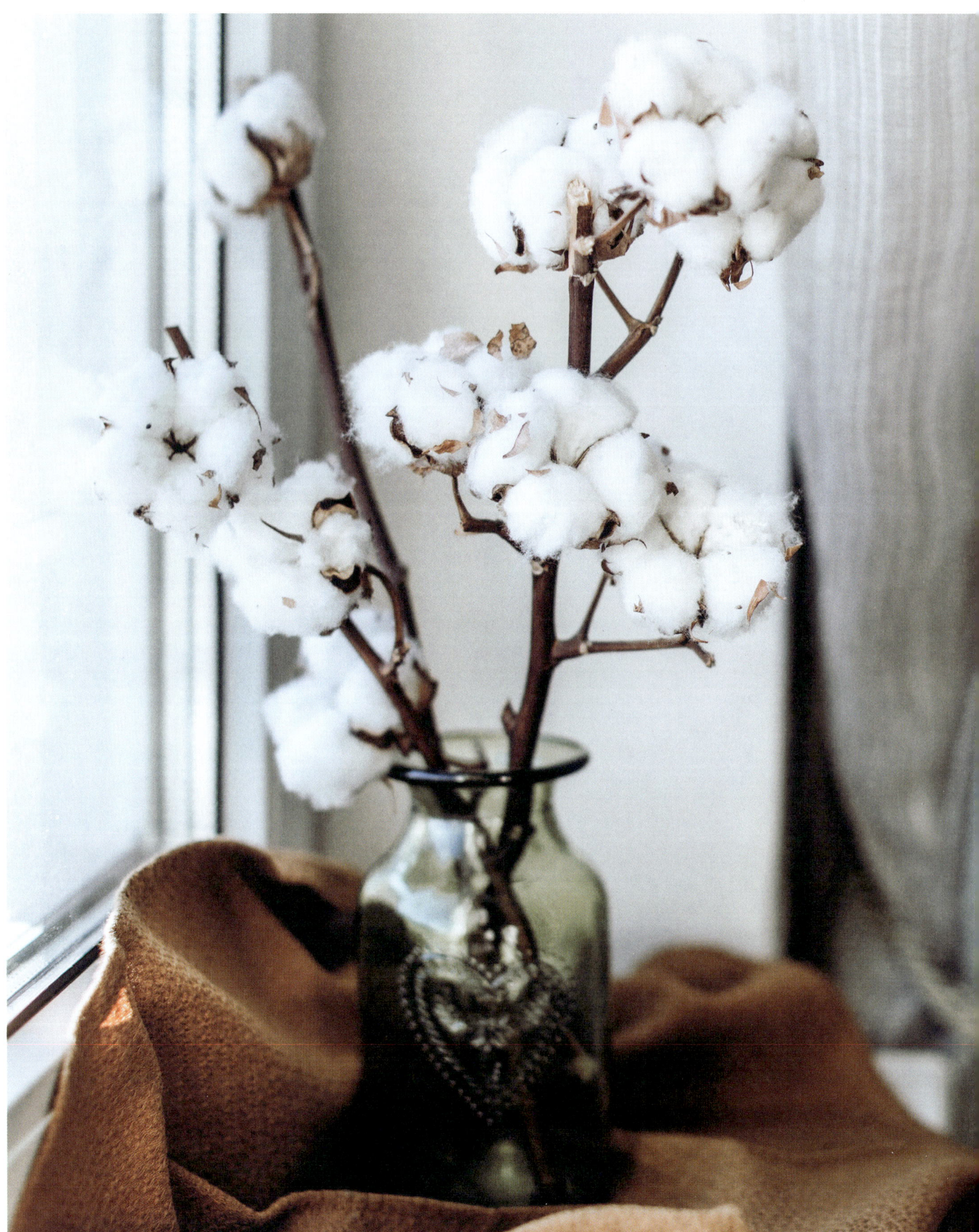

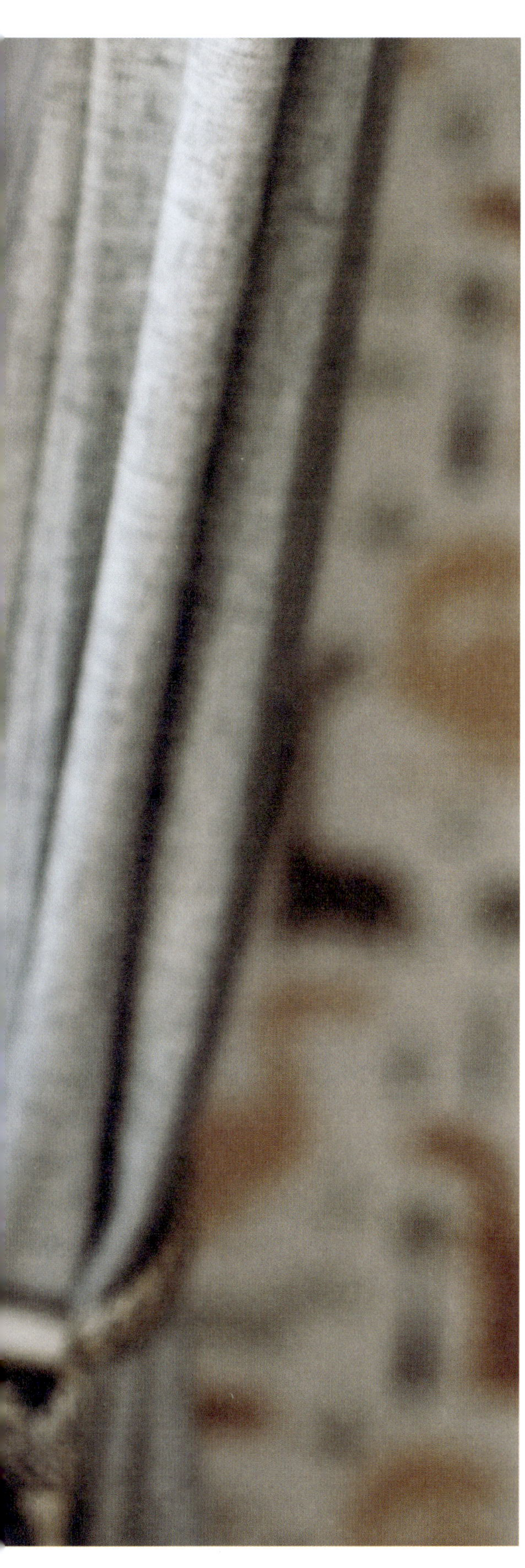

In the language of flowers, cotton is thought to symbolise good fortune and wellbeing. You can welcome these positive vibes into your home with bunches of dried cotton flowers, that also add romance and nostalgia to the country styled home.

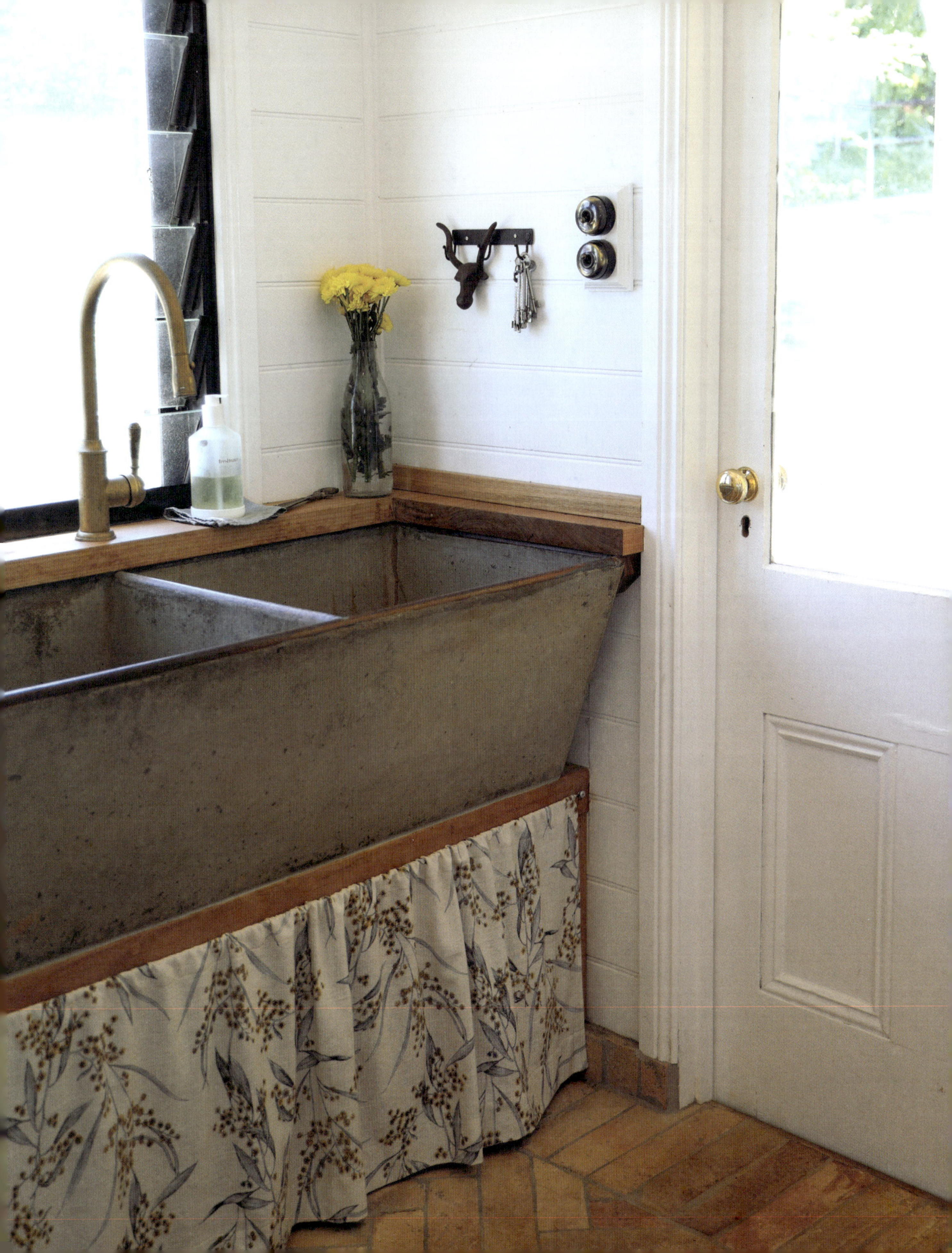

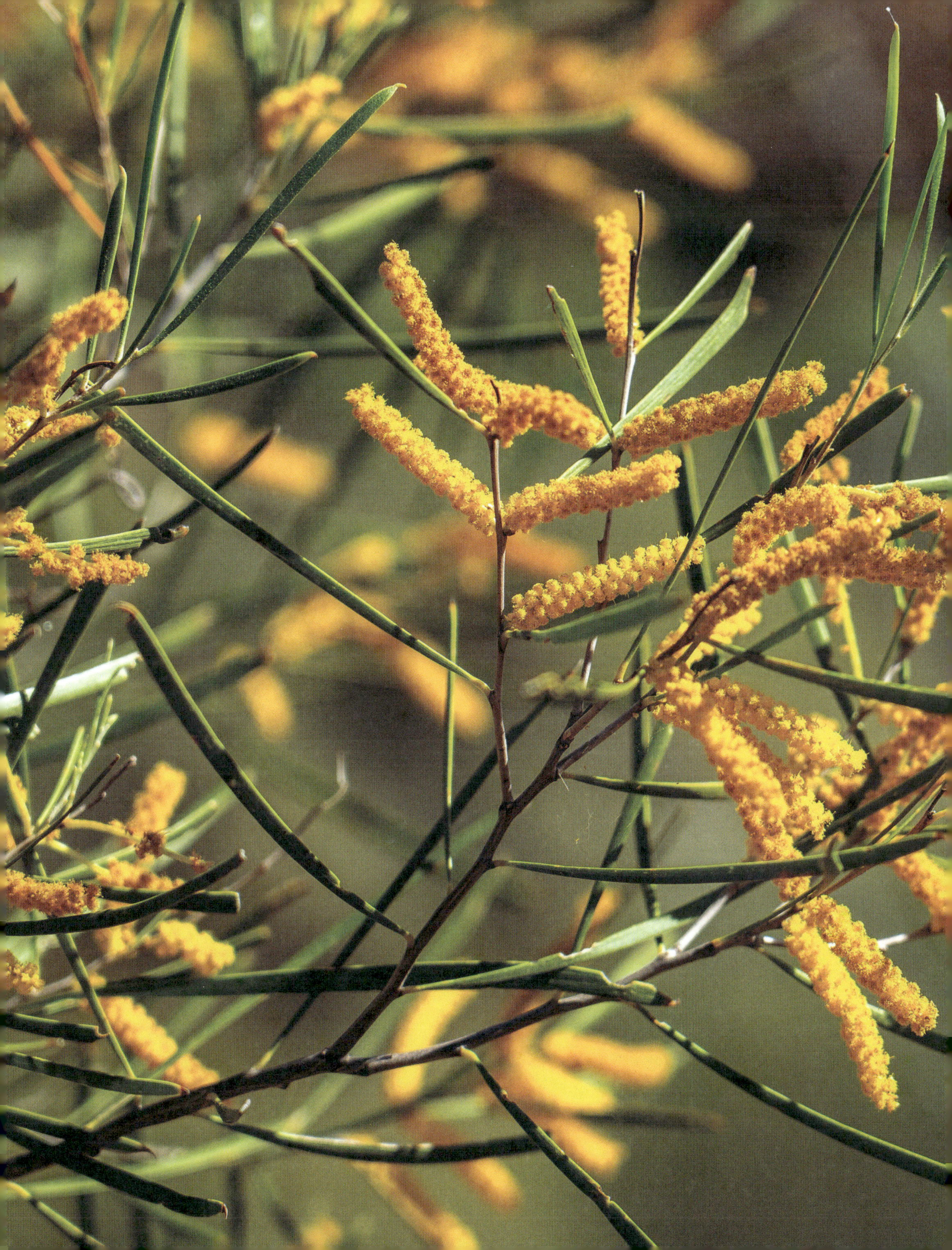

Kitchen items on show create a mood of cosy familiarity, and are suggestive of a busy, productive family life. A selection of dried pulses and beans in jars provides a nod to natural food and the respect for real food which is central to country life.

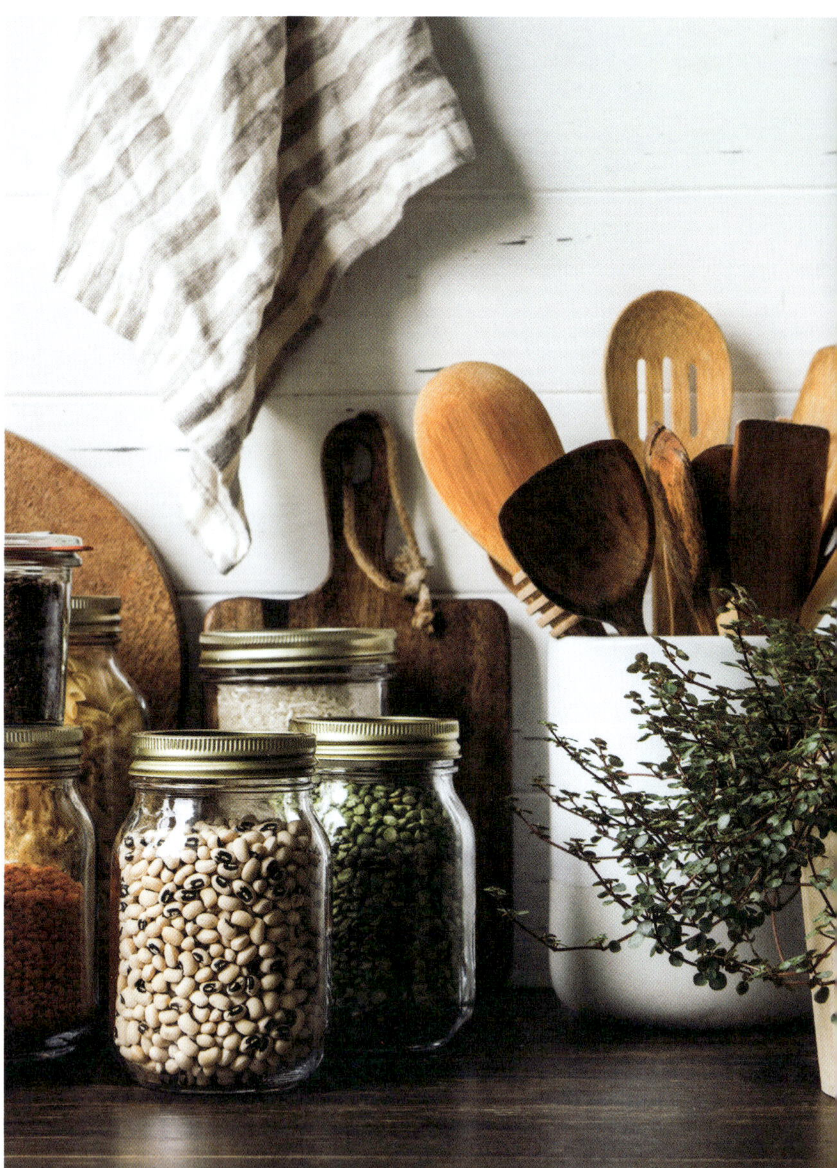

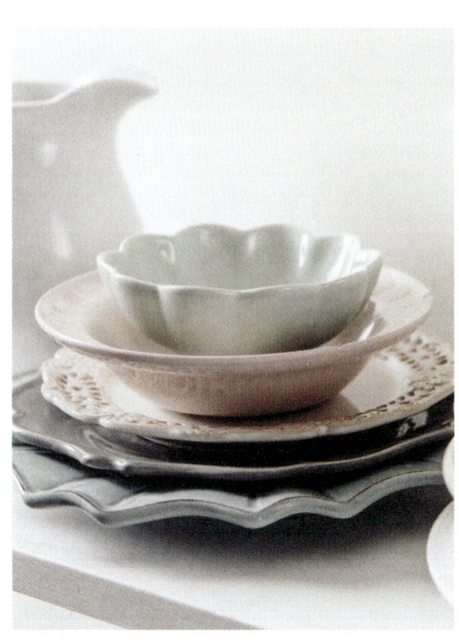

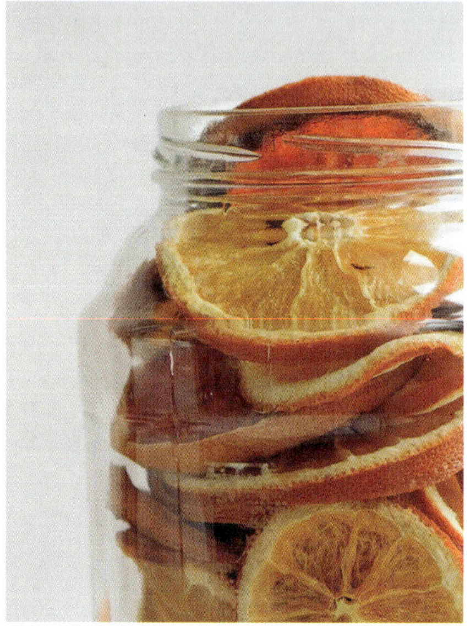

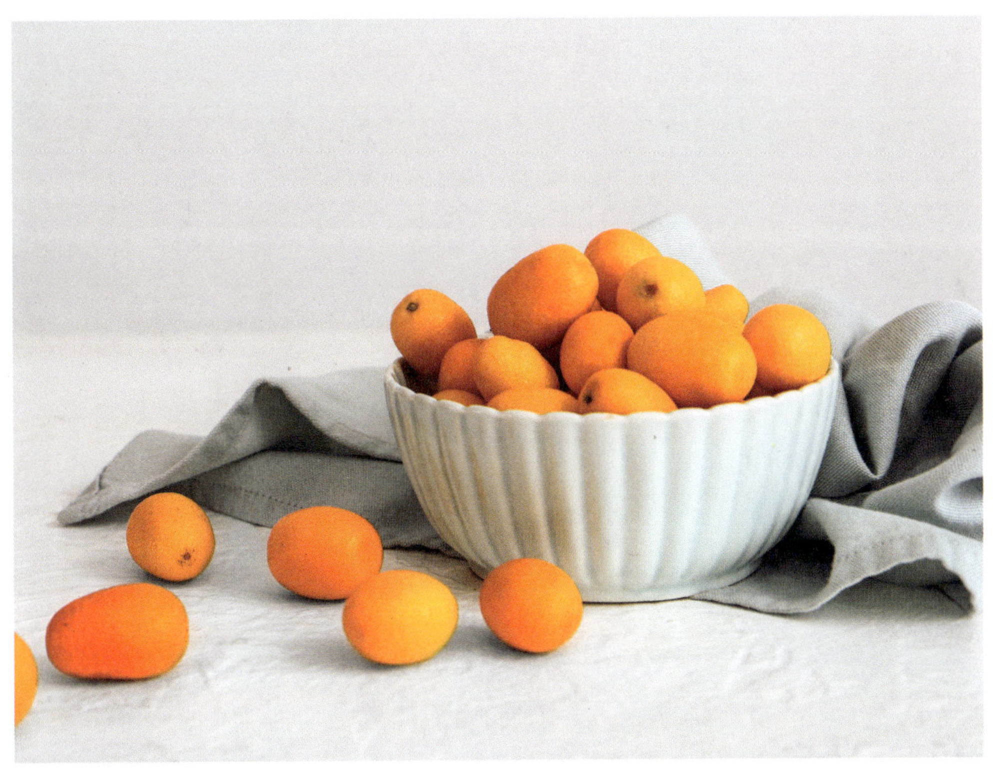

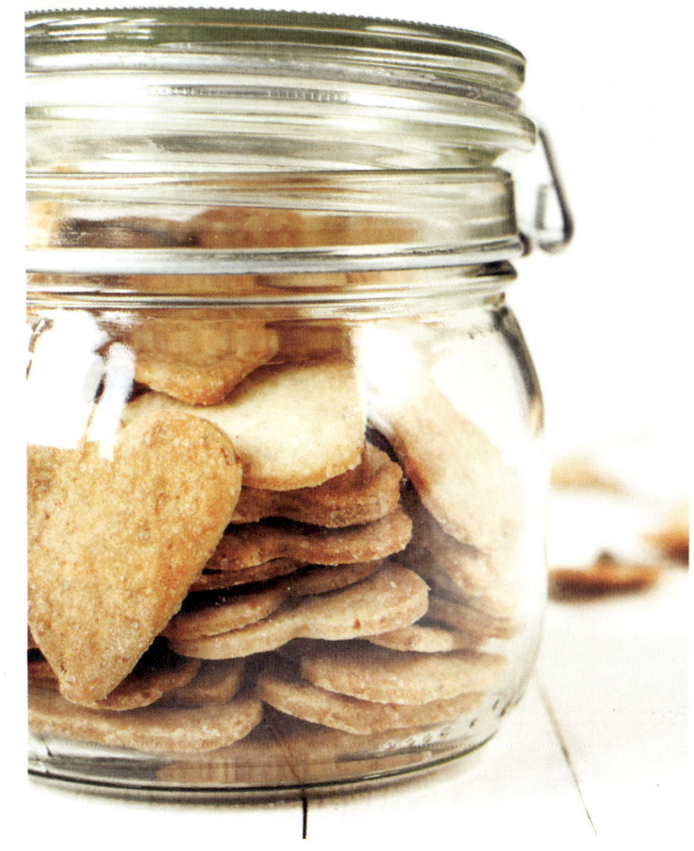

Central to modern country style is the notion of a happy, convivial life shared between family and friends. Home-baked cookies, vintage tea sets, full fruit bowls or other indicators of hospitality help convey this invitation to residents and visitors alike.

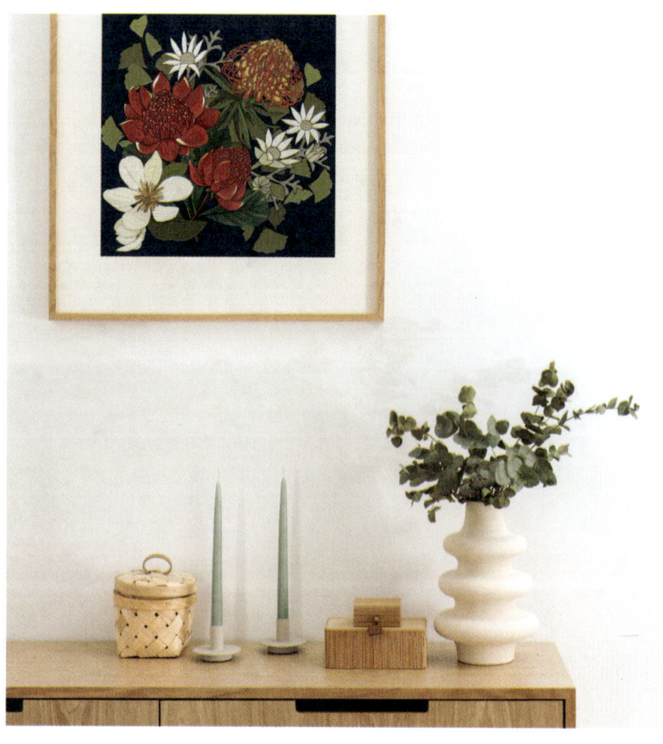

Modern country bedrooms ooze comfort and simplicity. The colours and design choices are natural and muted, not contrasting or too lively. The overall mood is one of calm tranquillity, perfect for restful sleep.

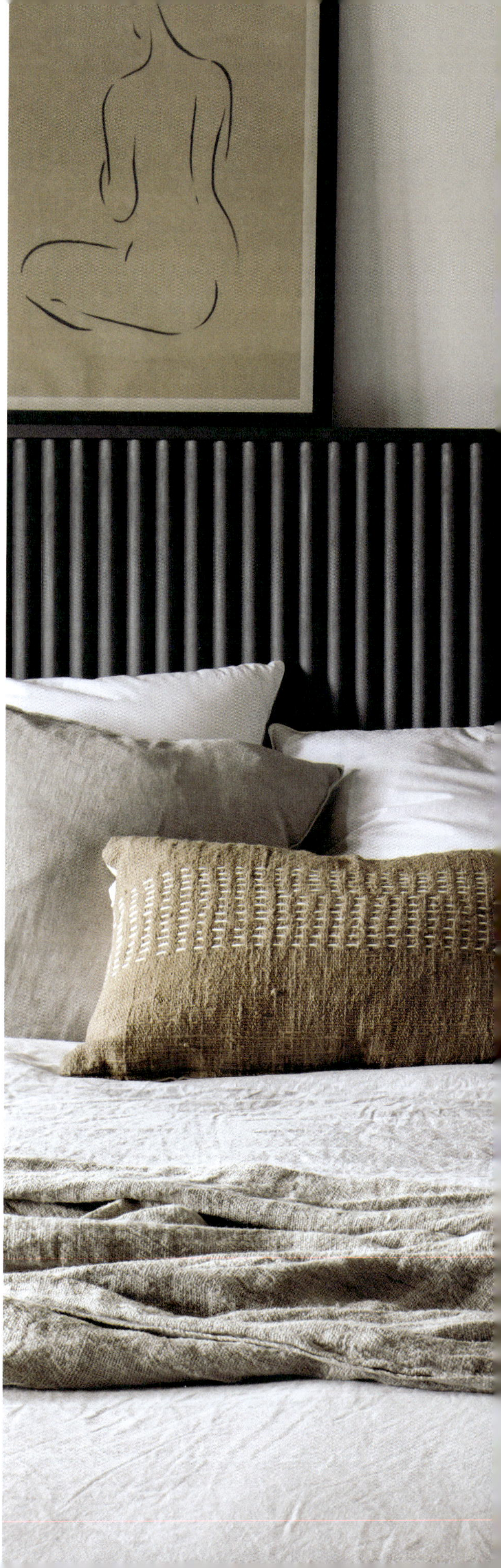

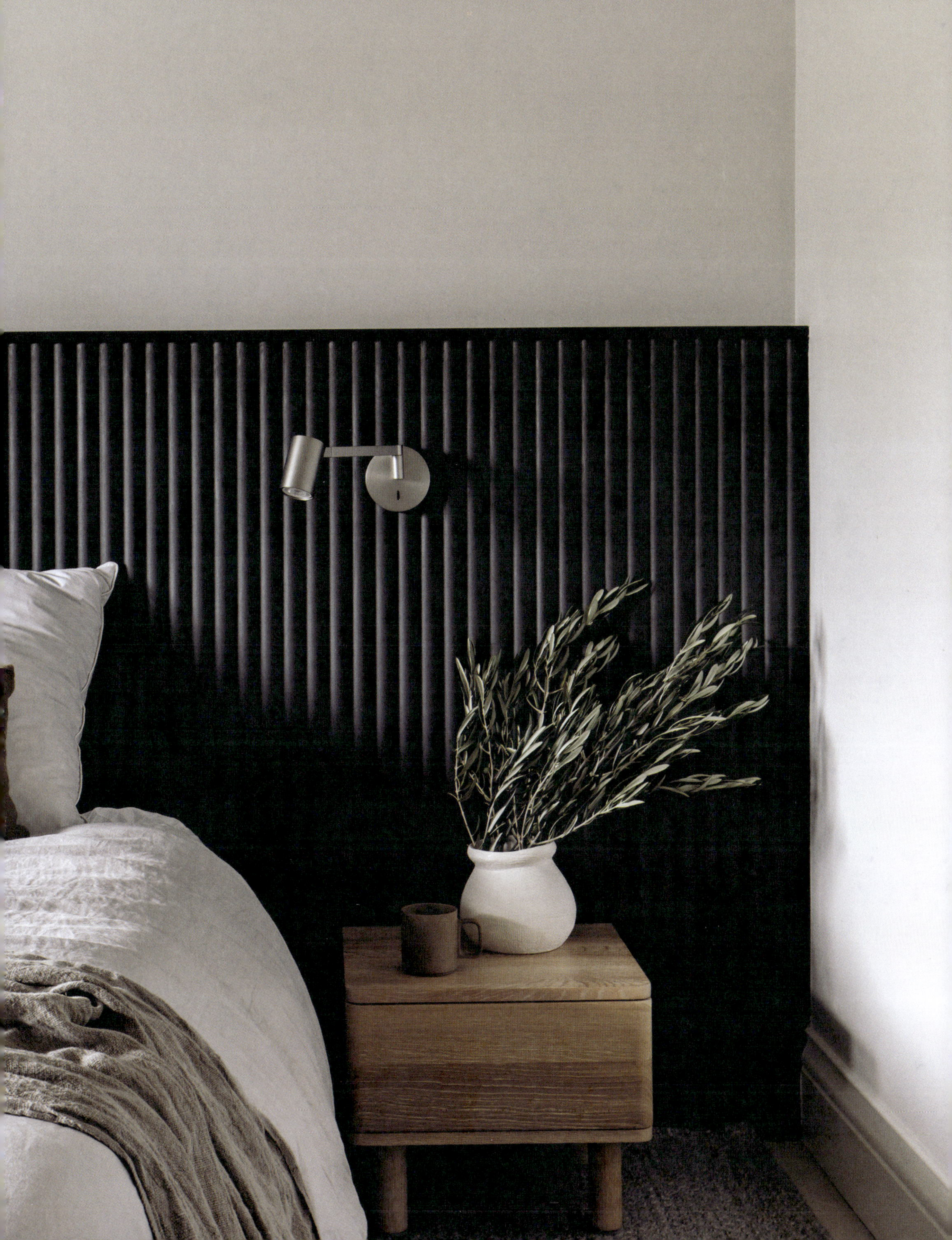

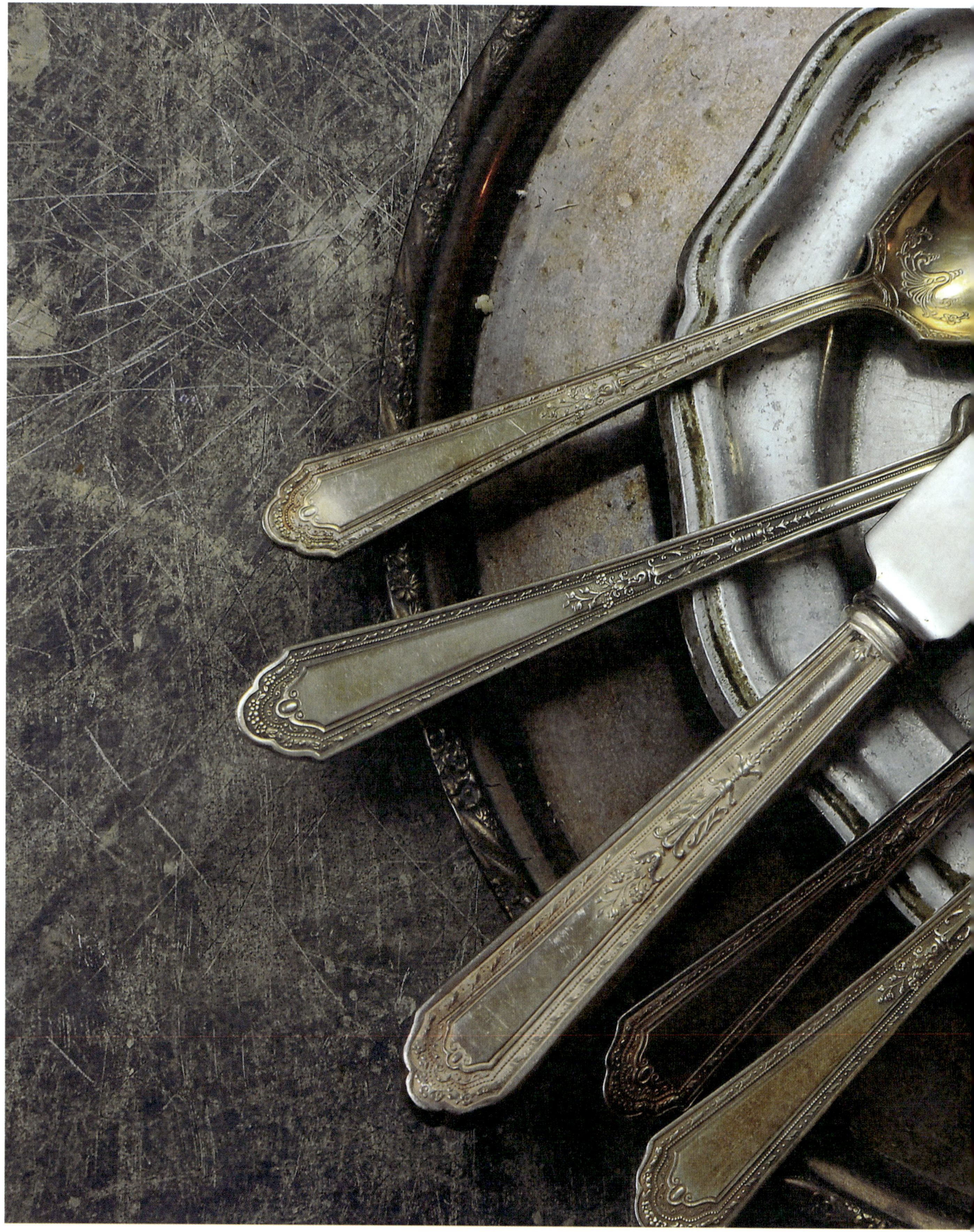

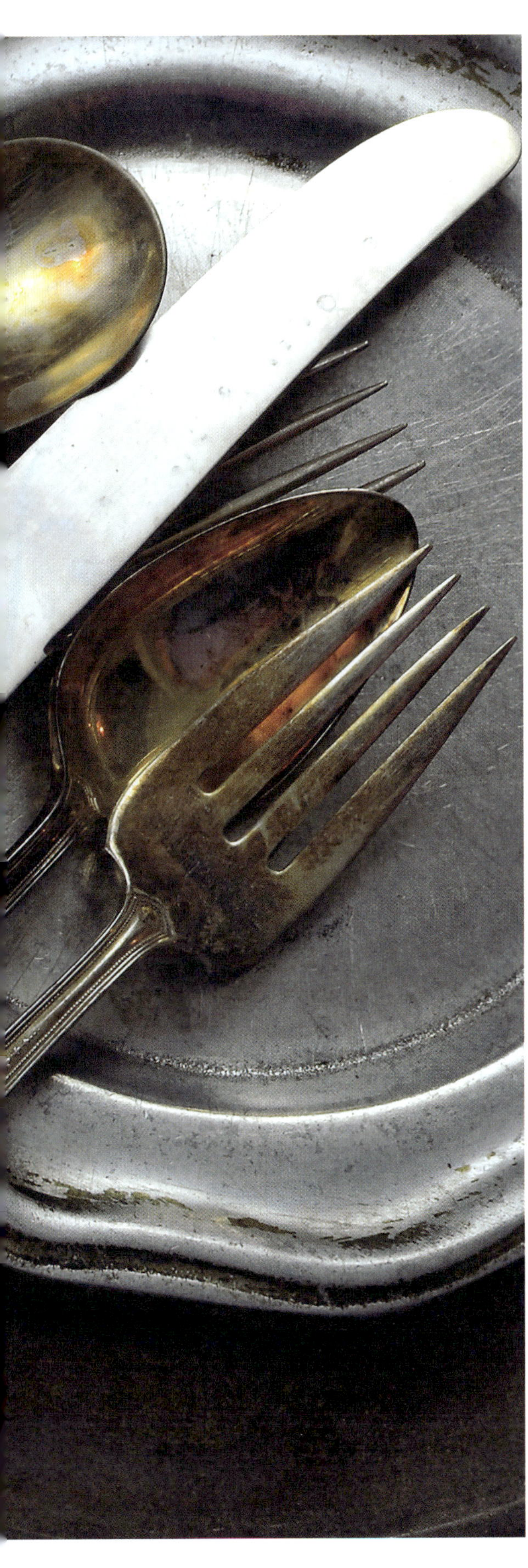

Vintage pieces are essential elements of the modern country look. These tarnished pieces of silverware set the mood perfectly, evoking a sense of familiarity and inviting connection with the past.

The Quick List

Sheer curtains to let the natural light flow

Handmade pottery mugs exuding the cosy vibe

Vintage items adding authenticity and character

Layered natural textures to create warmth and harmony

Fluffy rugs, extra cushions: it's all about comfort

Beautiful books on display – they invite the feeling of a mental pause

Storied treasures – personal items that surprise and intrigue

Curved vases or asymmetrical mirrors to create a soft mood

Objects with imperfections to add a timeless feel

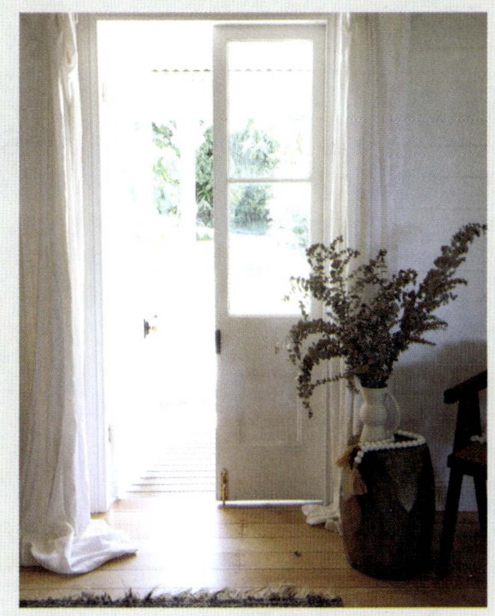
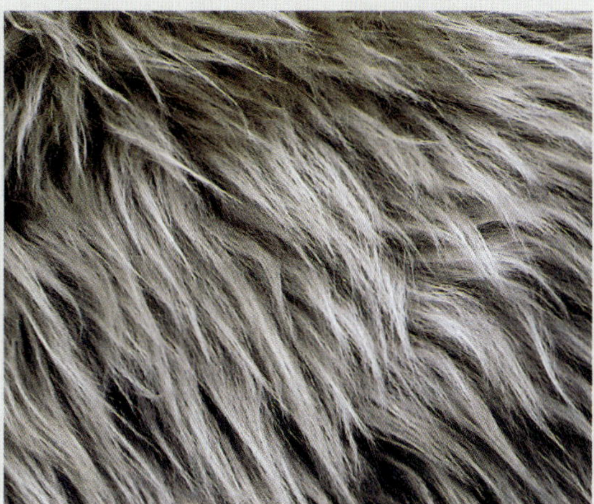
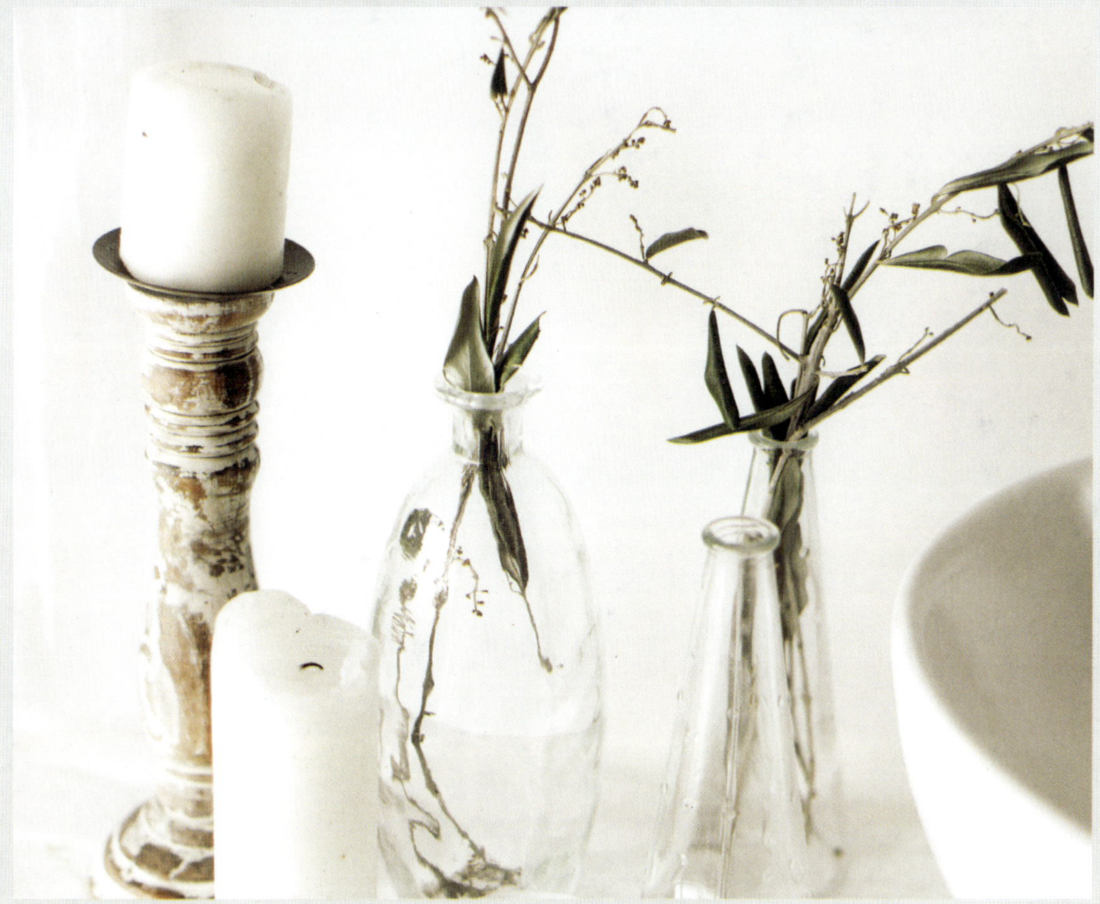

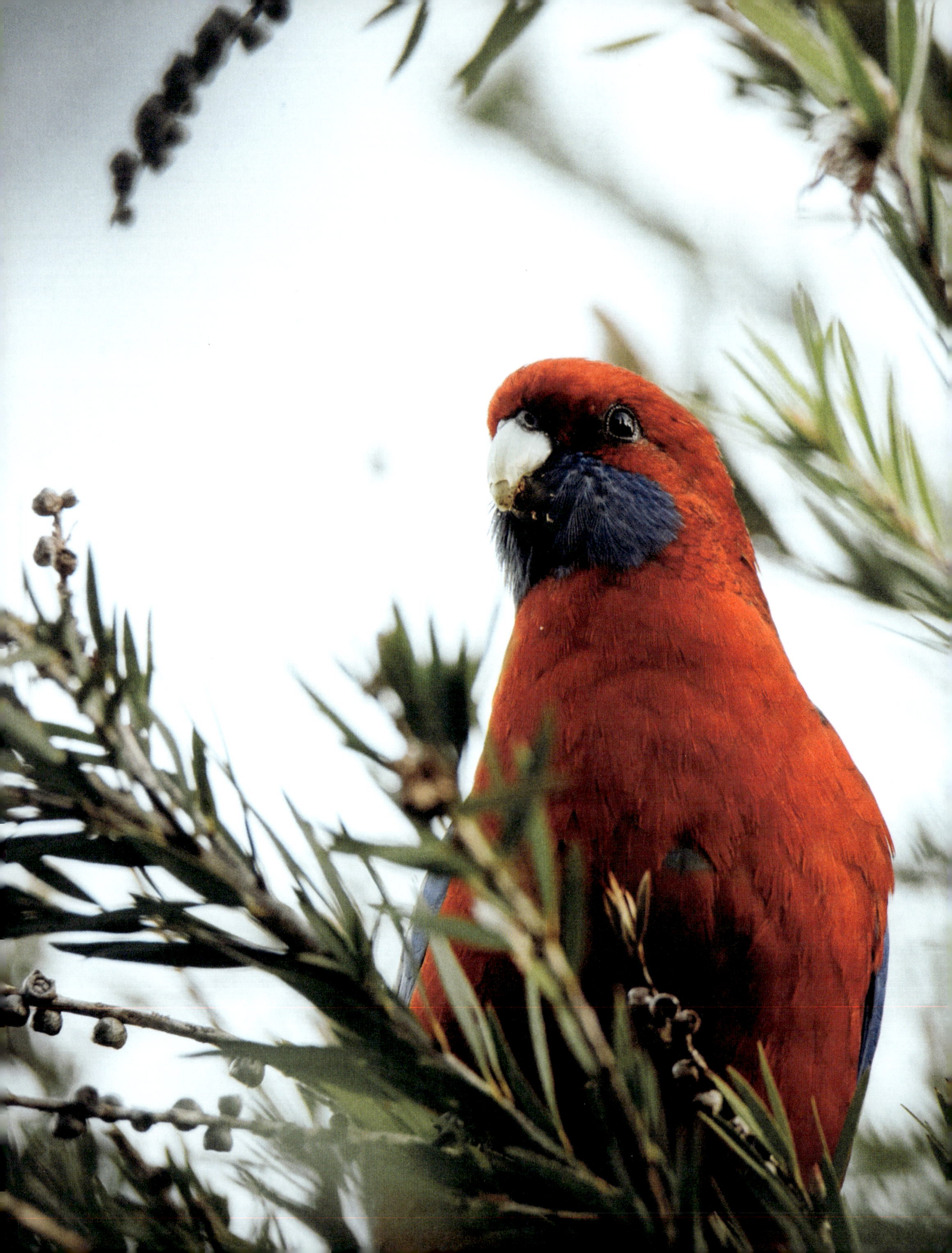

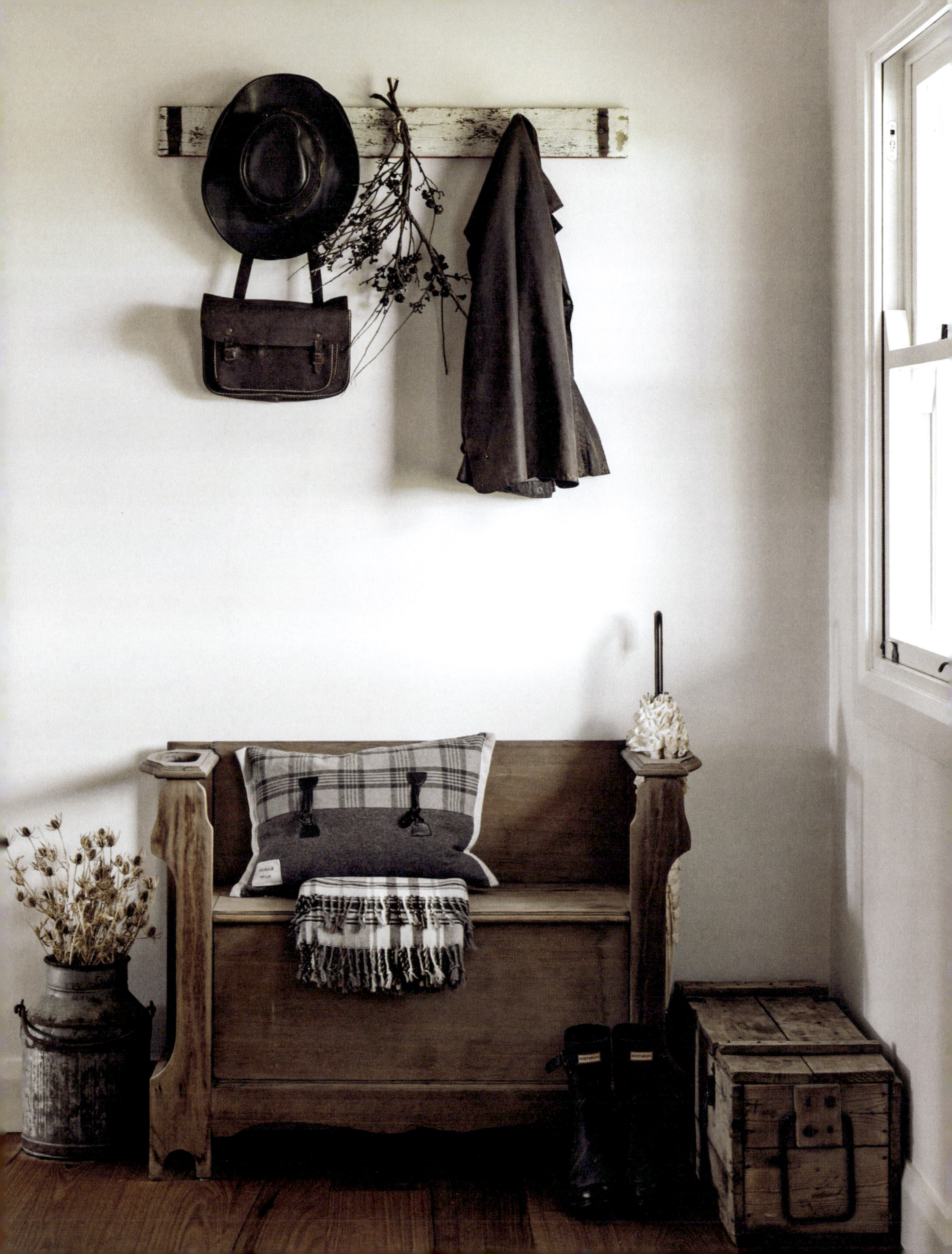

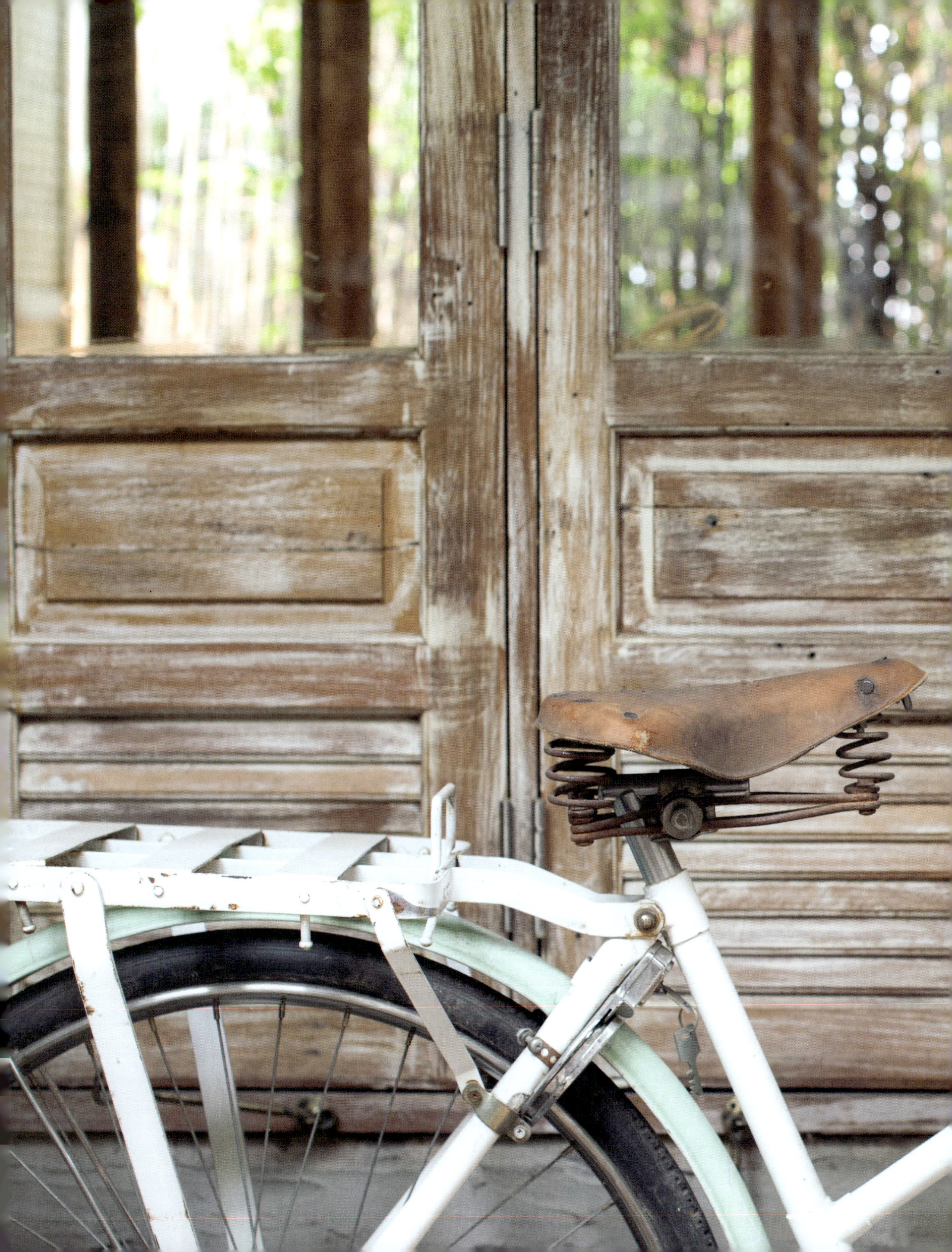

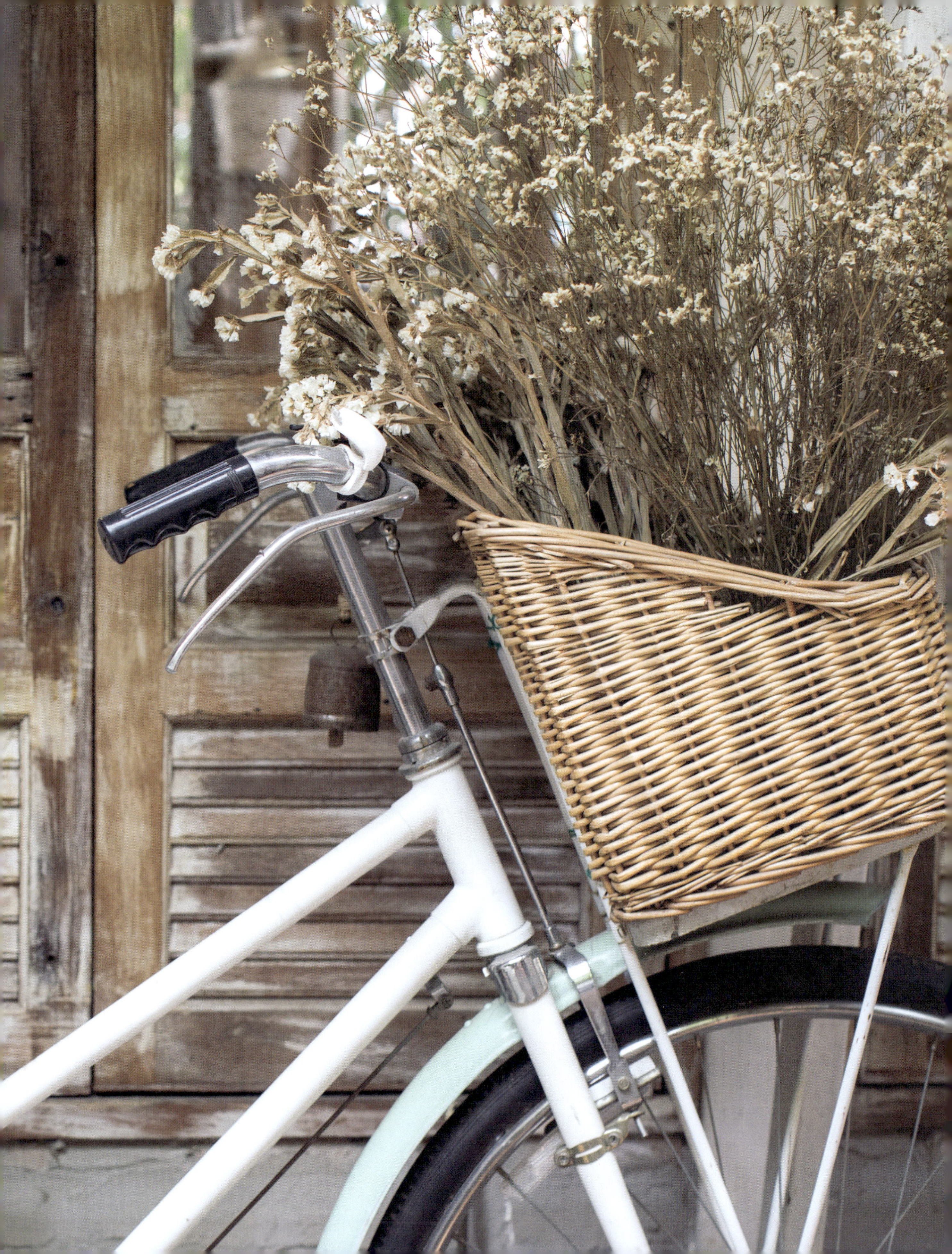

chapter two

colour & texture

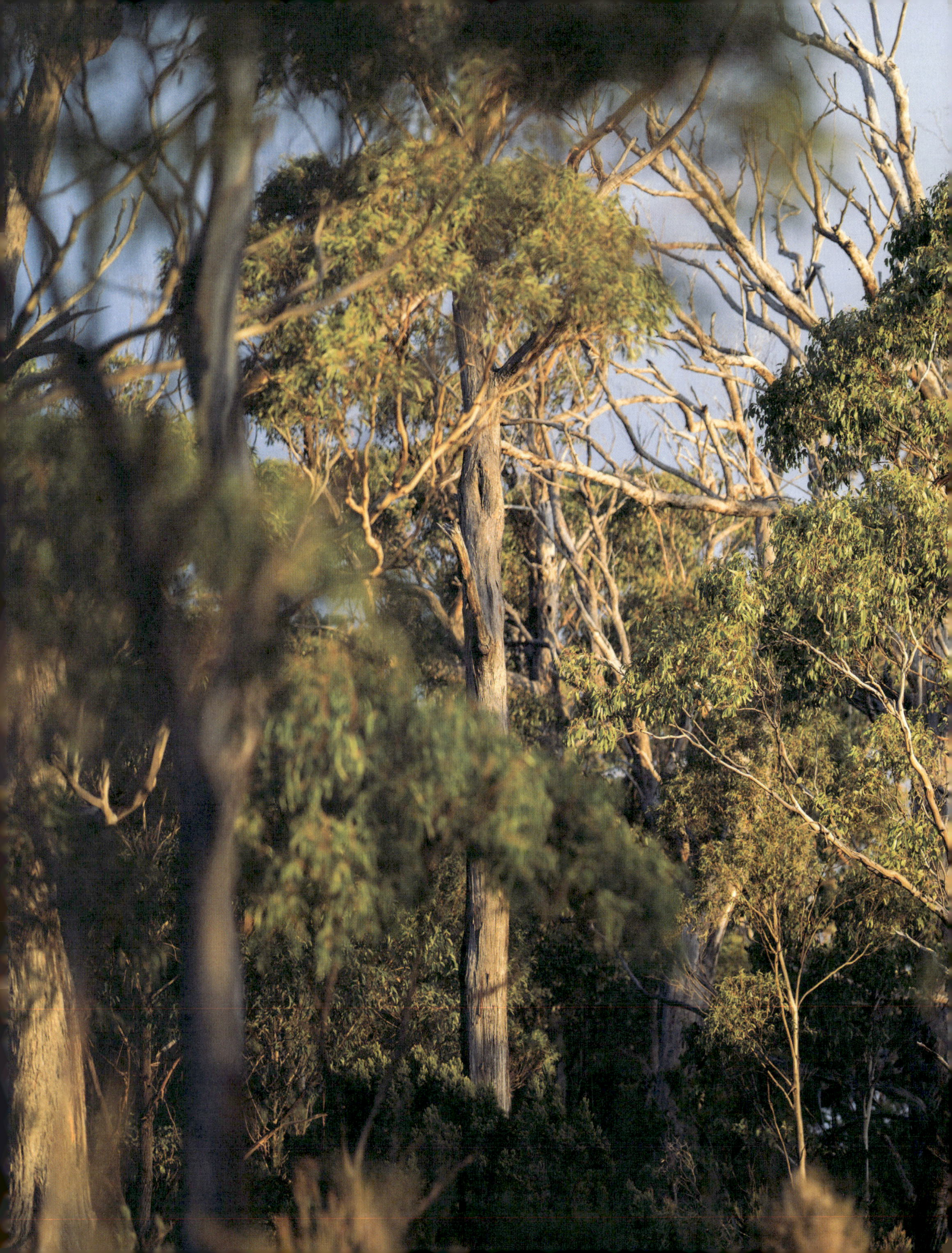

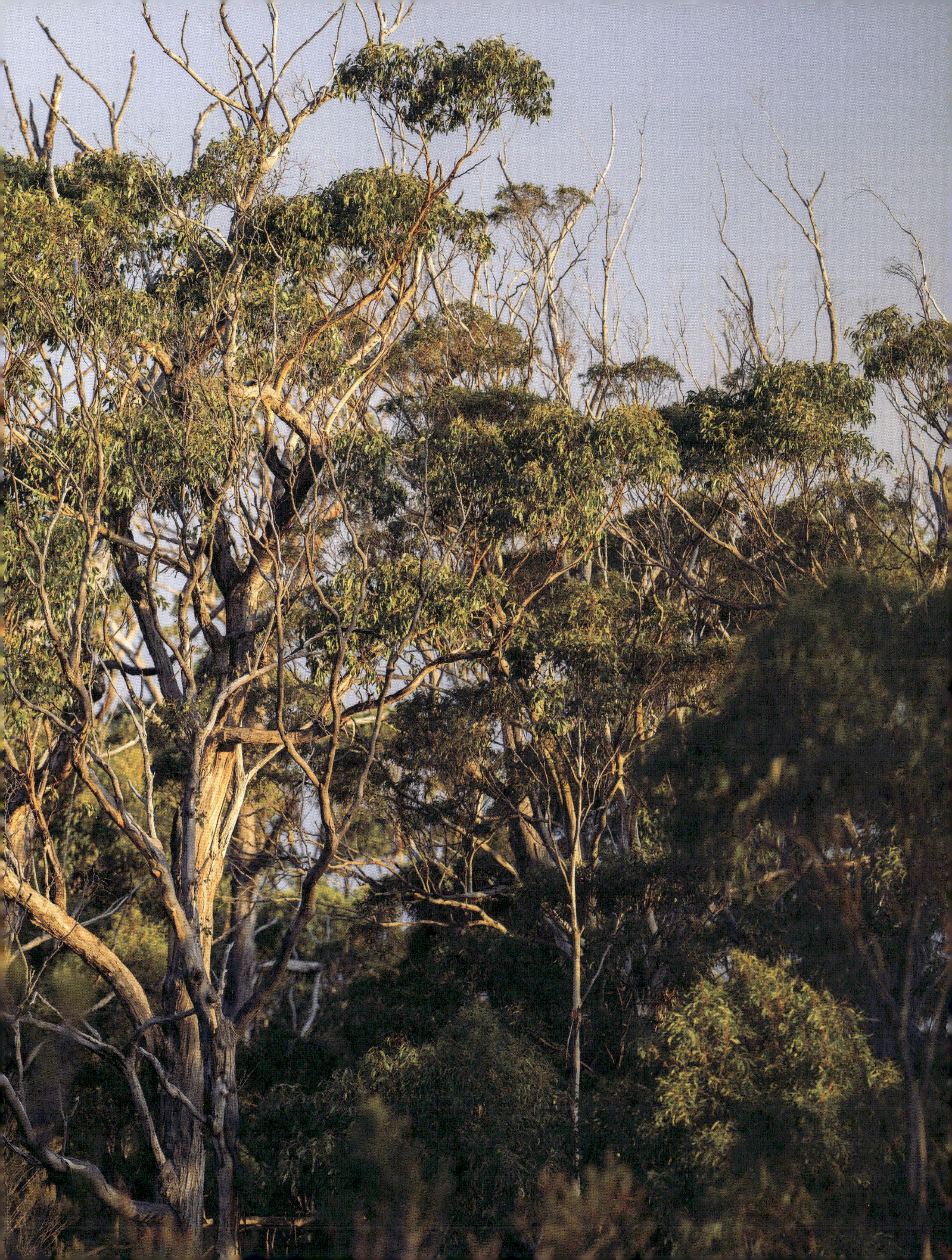

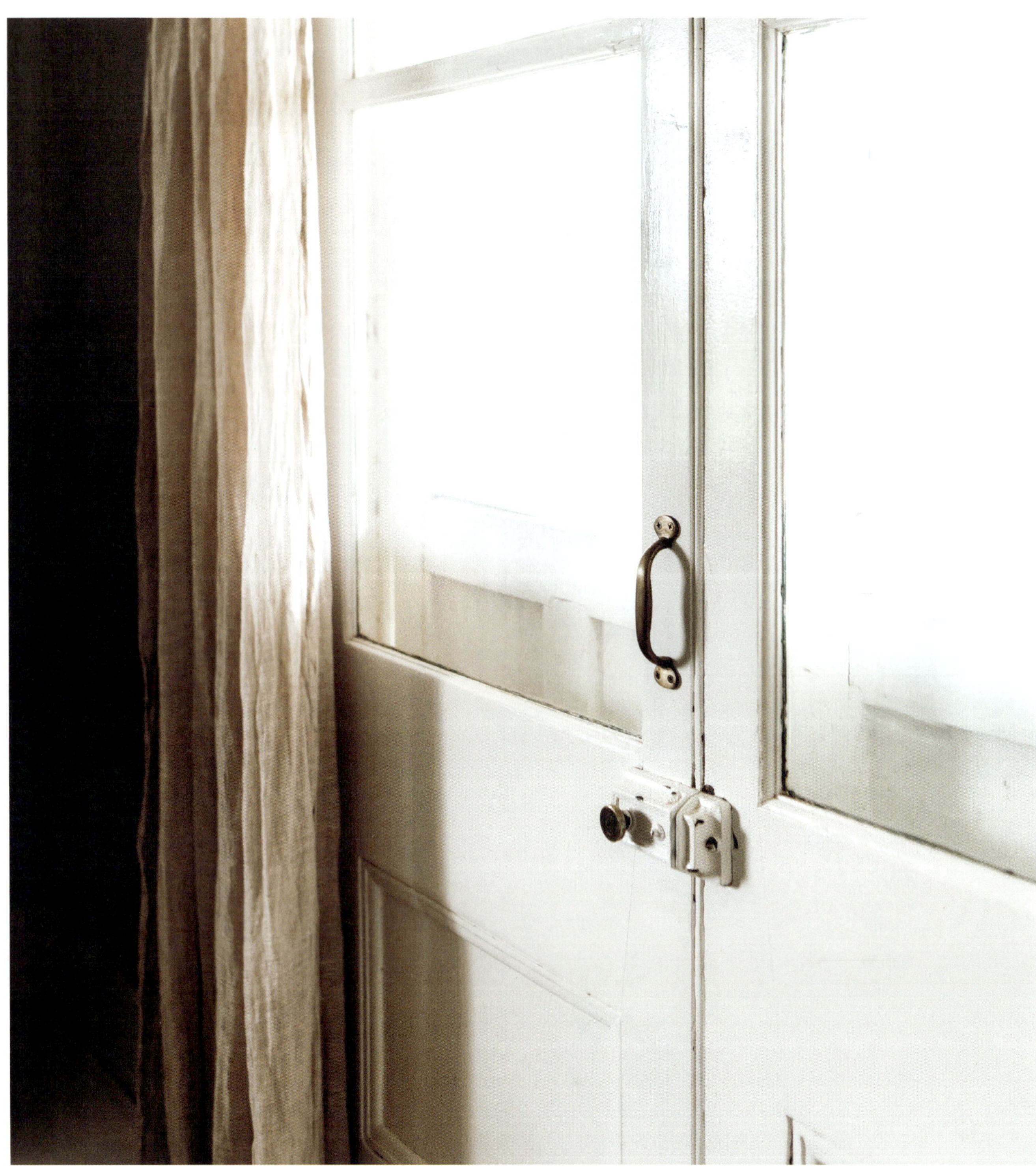

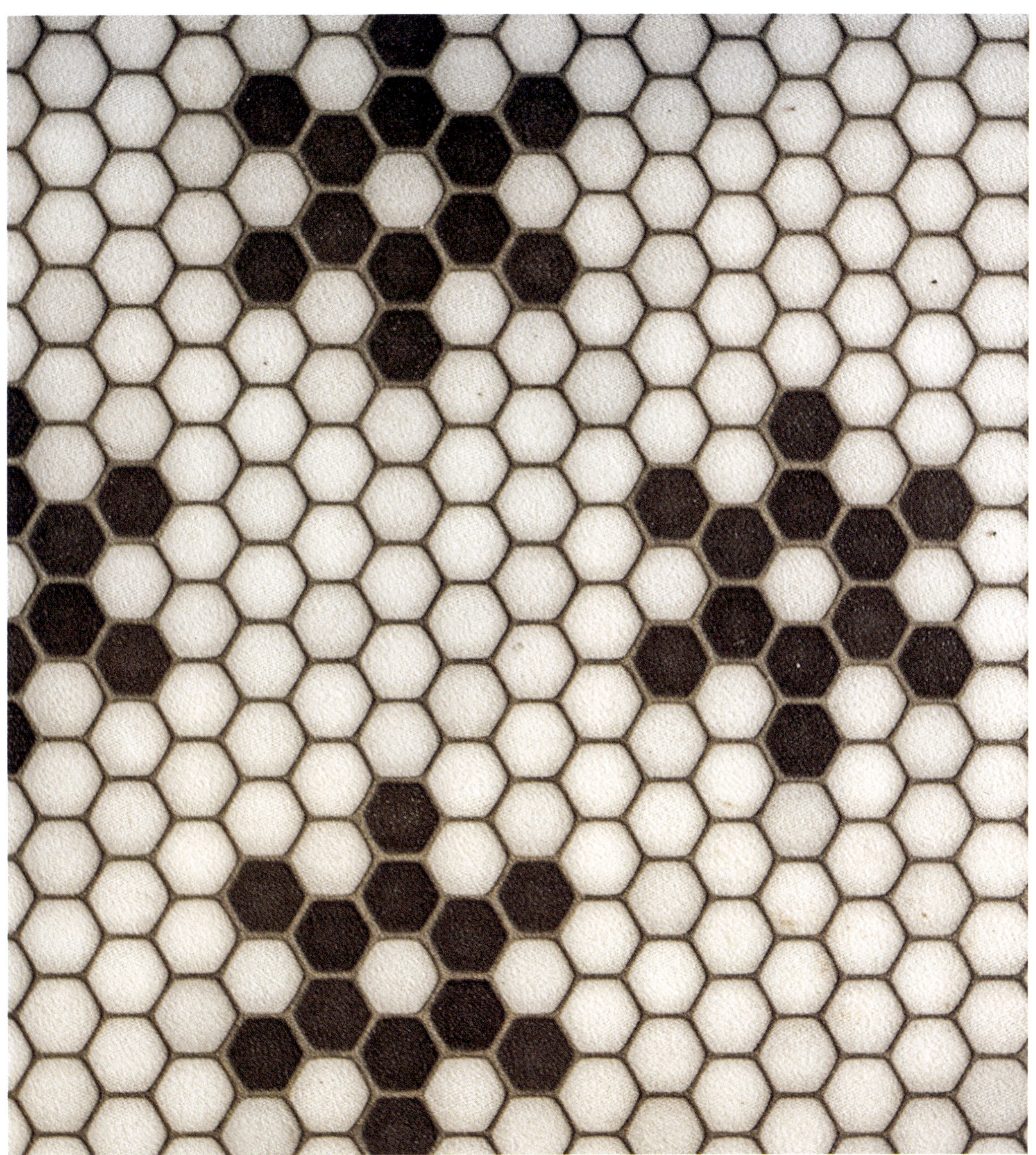

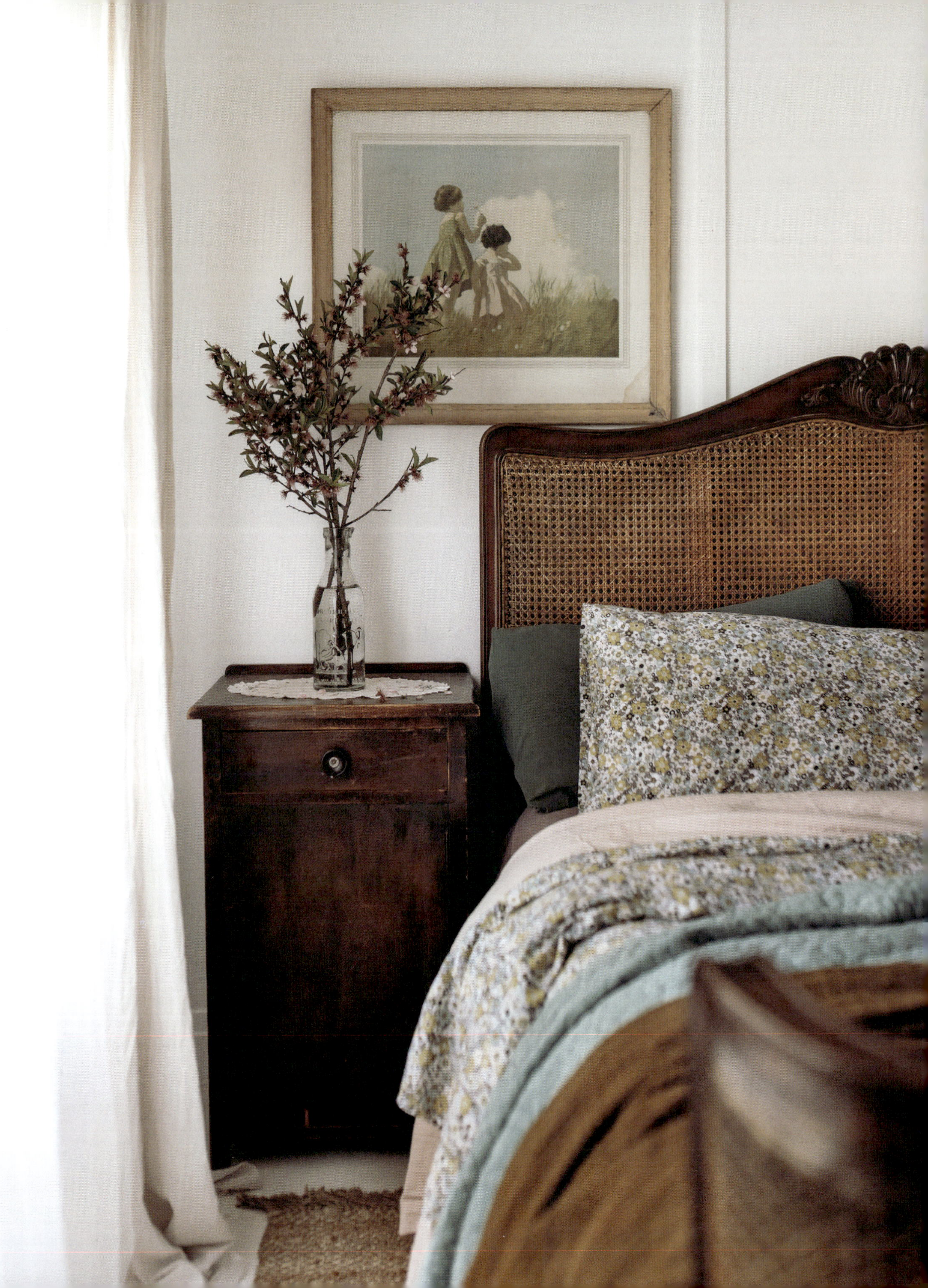

Anything that feels earthy, natural or organic is a perfect fit for the modern Australian country style.

When it comes to textiles, that means soft materials like pure linen, wool or cotton – beds and sofas adorned with throws and cushions in these materials are luxuriously desirable and right on trend.

For fixtures and fittings, and furniture, think wood and metal – preferably reclaimed timbers and tarnished or aged metals, evocative of farm life in days past. These add authenticity and a sense of nostalgia to create a cosy and intimate feel.

Whichever materials you choose, it's all about combining those tactile and visual elements for maximum effect. Layered and soft bedding combined with a wood and jute headboard, as pictured opposite, illustrates this unity of look and feel.

While the modern country look is clean and sophisticated by comparison to the traditional form of this style, it's still acceptable (desirable, even) to have a few rough edges here and there. Vintage items or well-loved treasures can certainly be incorporated, and their uniqueness will add charm and personality to the home, as well as hinting at a yarn that longs to be told.

Colour is key. Starting with a neutral base is always a good idea – whites and greys create a calm backdrop and allow for the introduction of pops of colour. When choosing these accent colours, look to nature for clues. Think the green shades of eucalyptus trees; oranges and yellows that evoke rusty farmyard metal, the red dirt of the outback or natural pigments like ochre; and muddy blues that bring to mind a creek at sunset, or a slate tile.

With these key elements of texture and colour in place, a modern country look is much easier to engineer with the rest of your styling touches.

TOP FIVE

1.

Organic materials – linen, cotton and wool

2.

Reclaimed timbers or limewashed wood

3.

Tarnished metals: brass, copper, nickel, pewter and wrought iron

4.

A neutral backdrop

5.

Accent colours derived from colours in nature

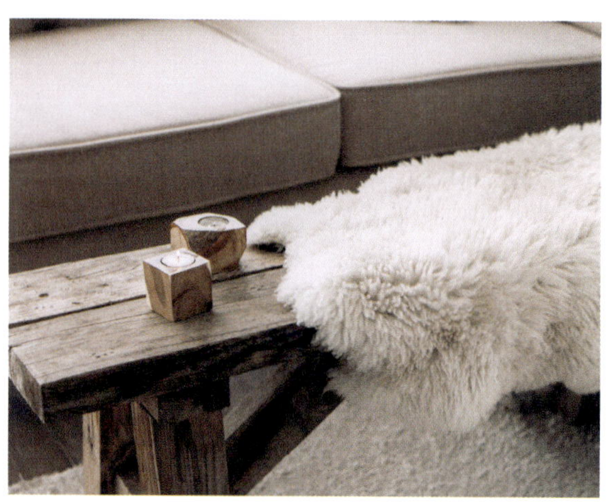

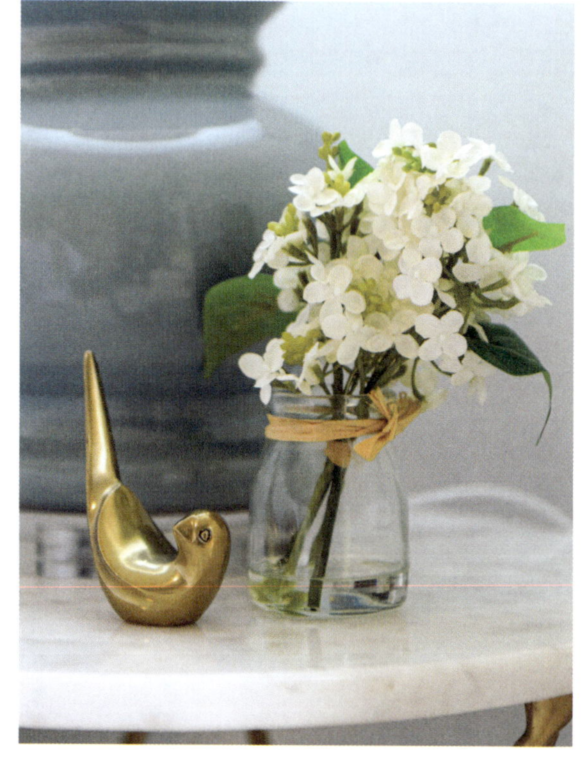

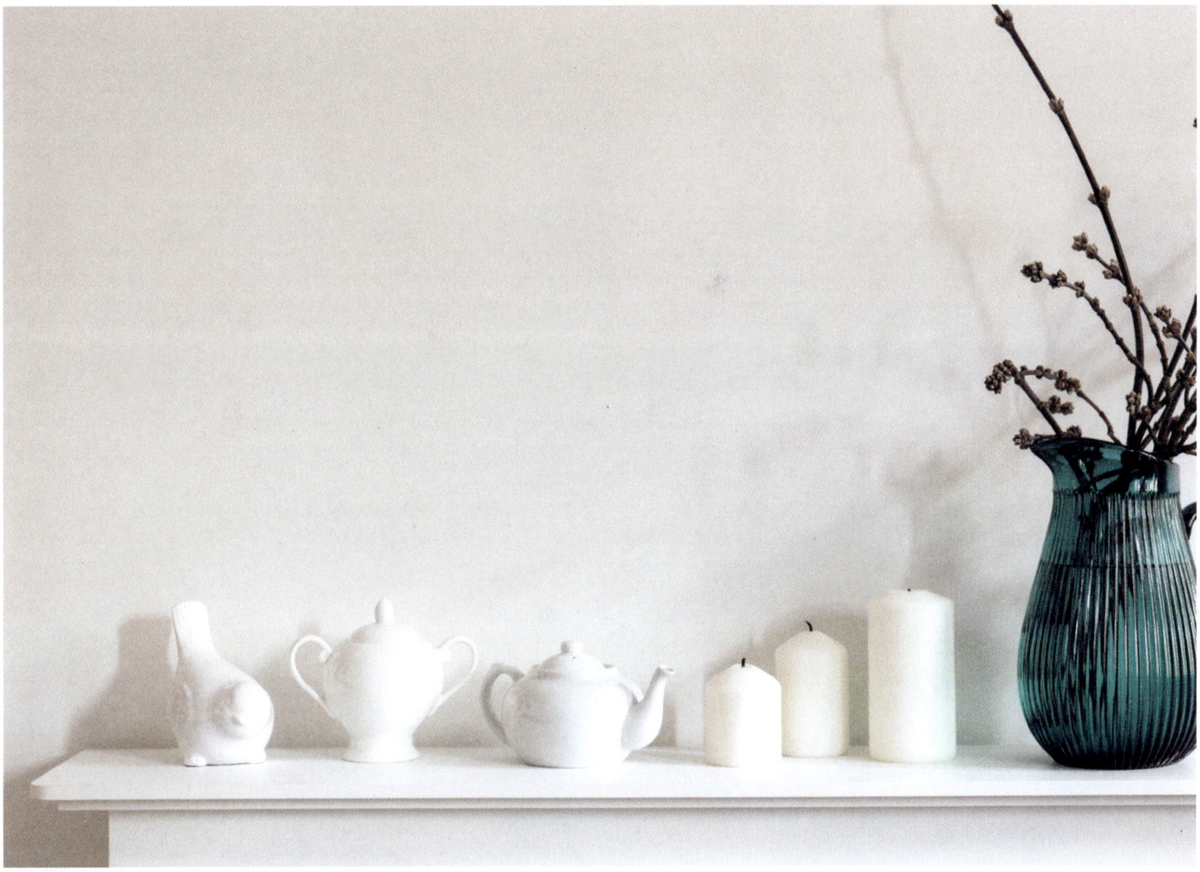

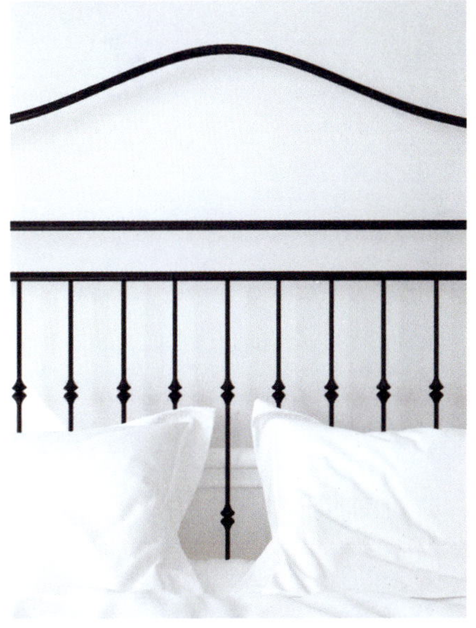

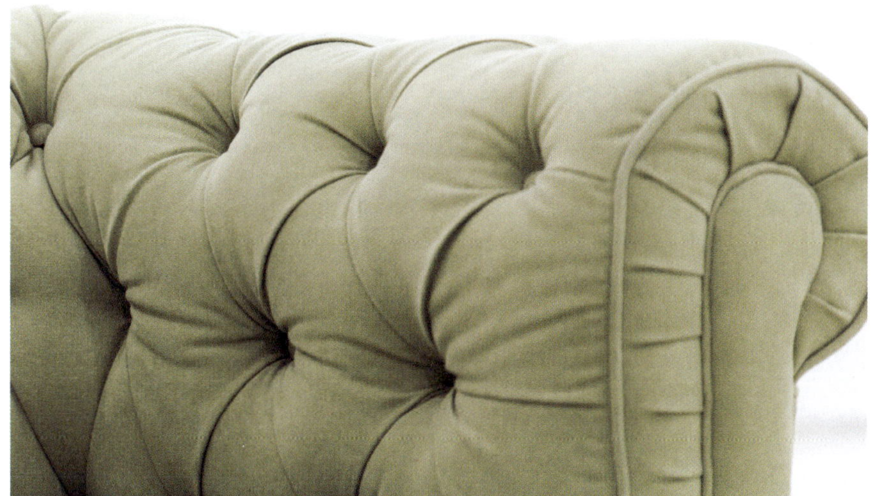

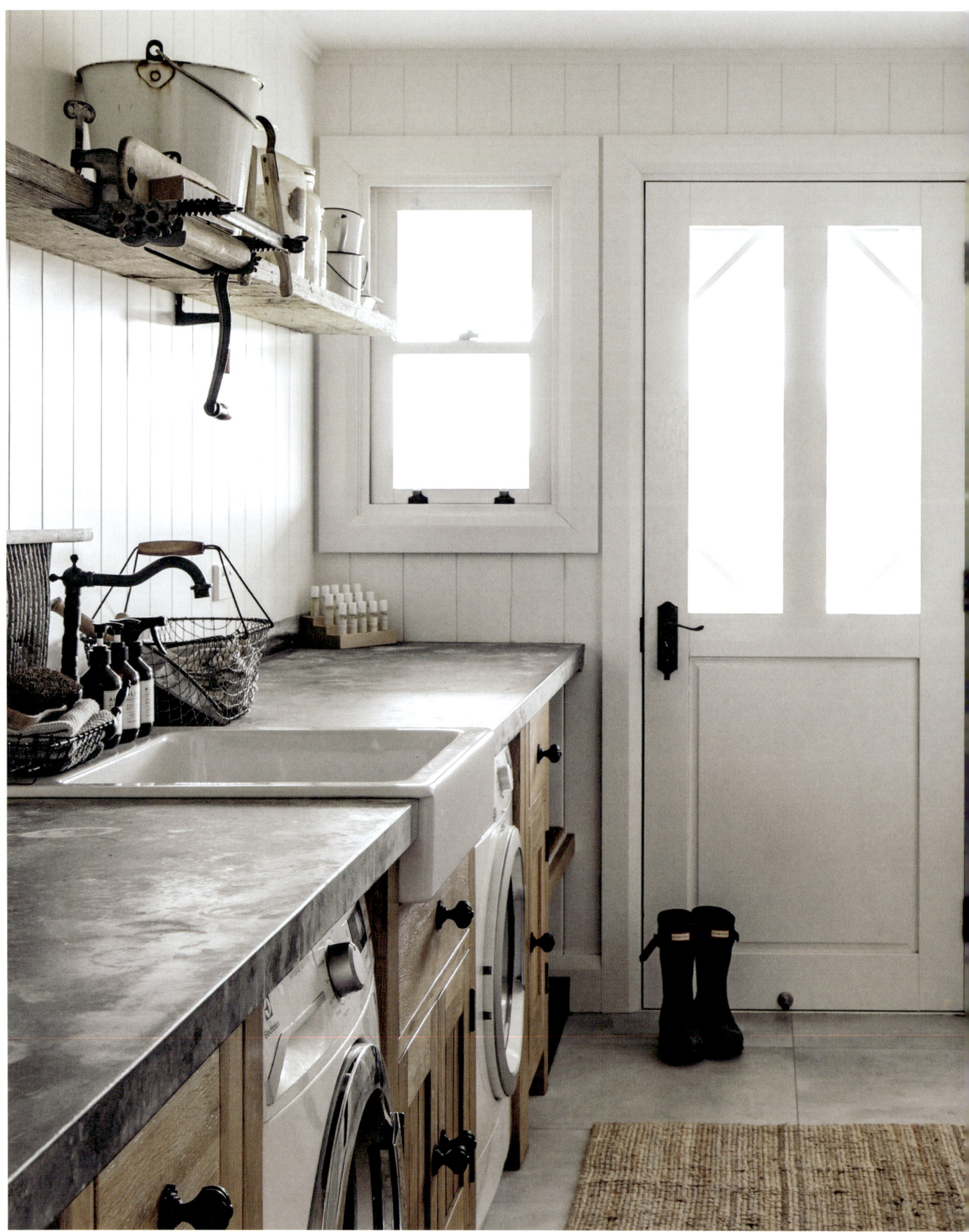

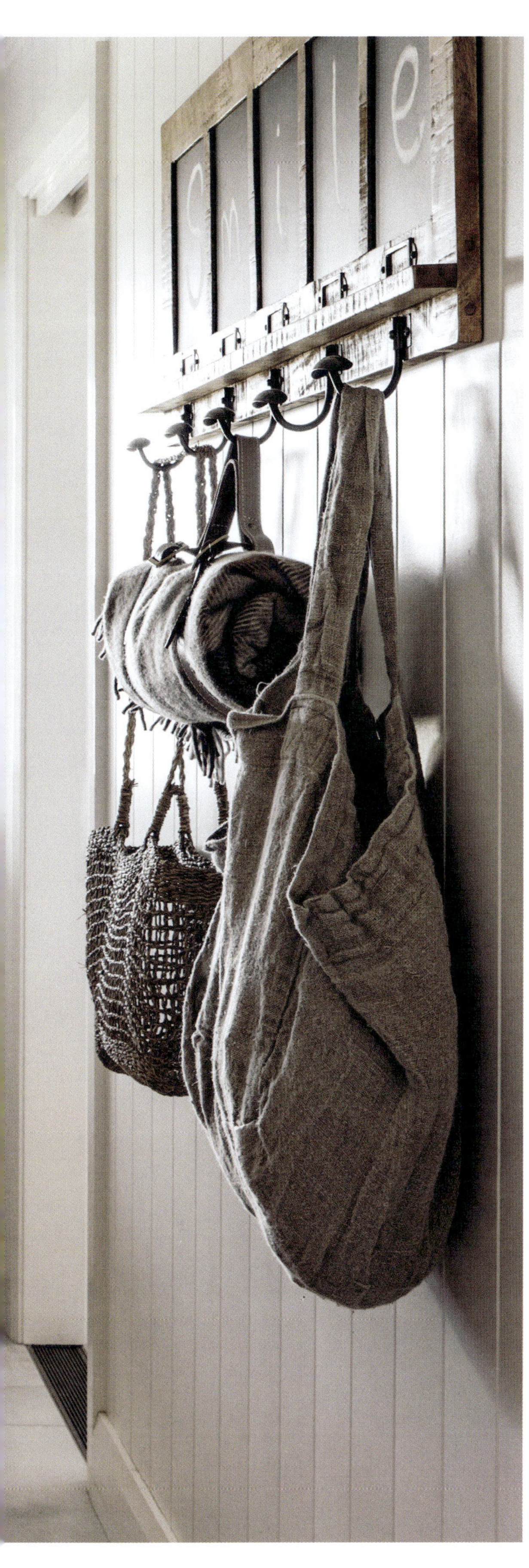

This lovely laundry combines many key elements of modern country style from the bright white backdrop to the combination of timber, stone and metal hardware, but it's the vintage enamel buckets and mangle (laundry press) mounted on the shelf that cement the look.

This fireplace vignette is perfectly styled, delivering both personality and elegance. The earthy brown hue of the wall colour is delicately complimented in the choice of artwork, the floral display and the deer statuettes. This illustrates how tones of one colour can be used to great effect.

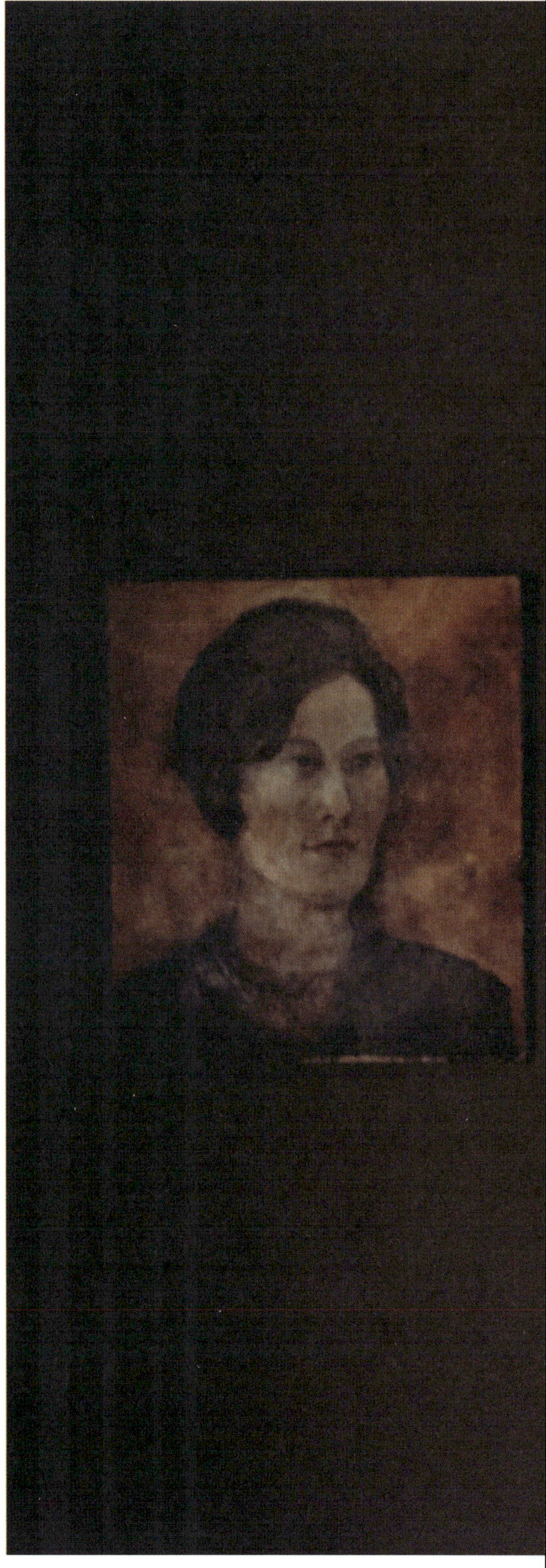

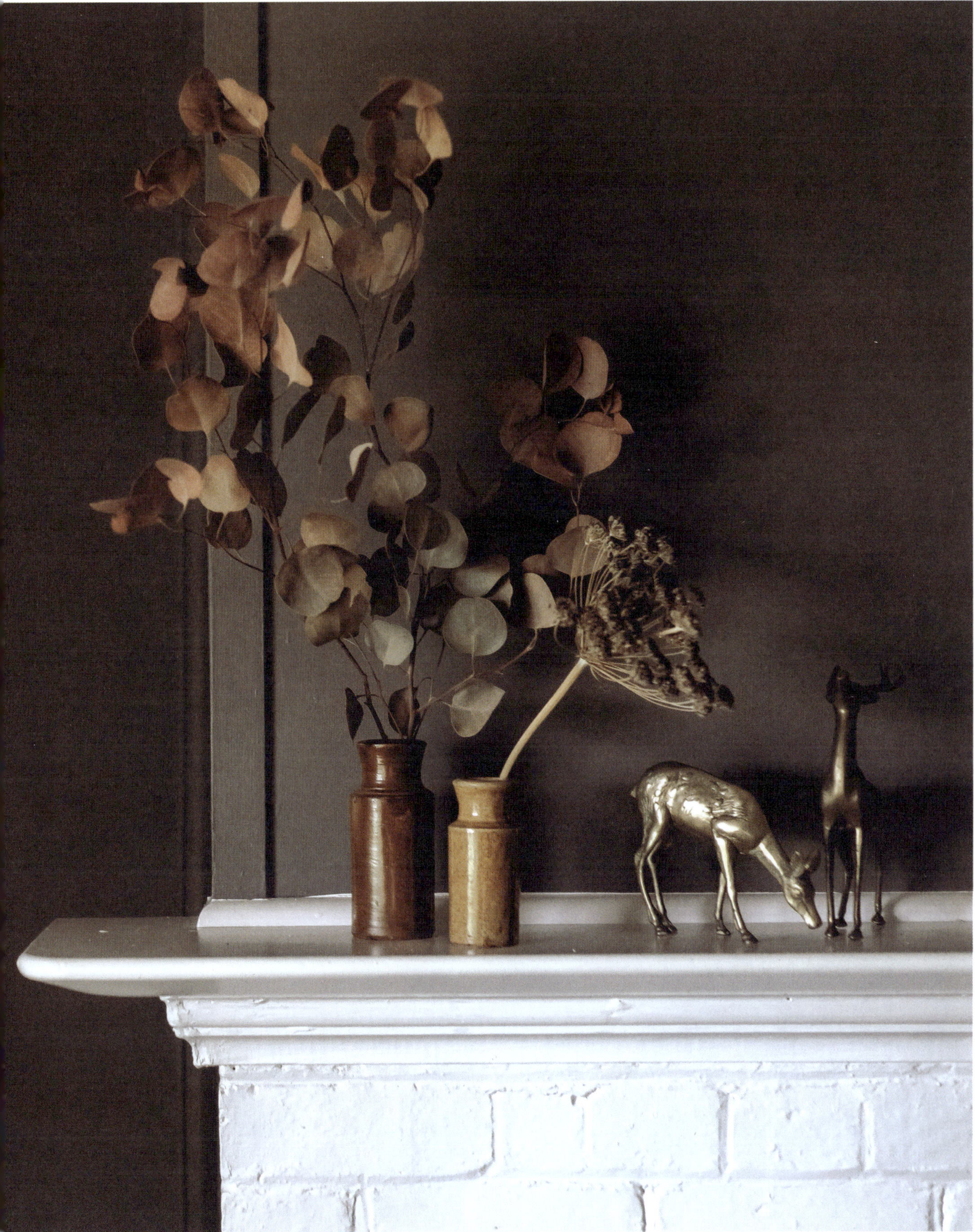

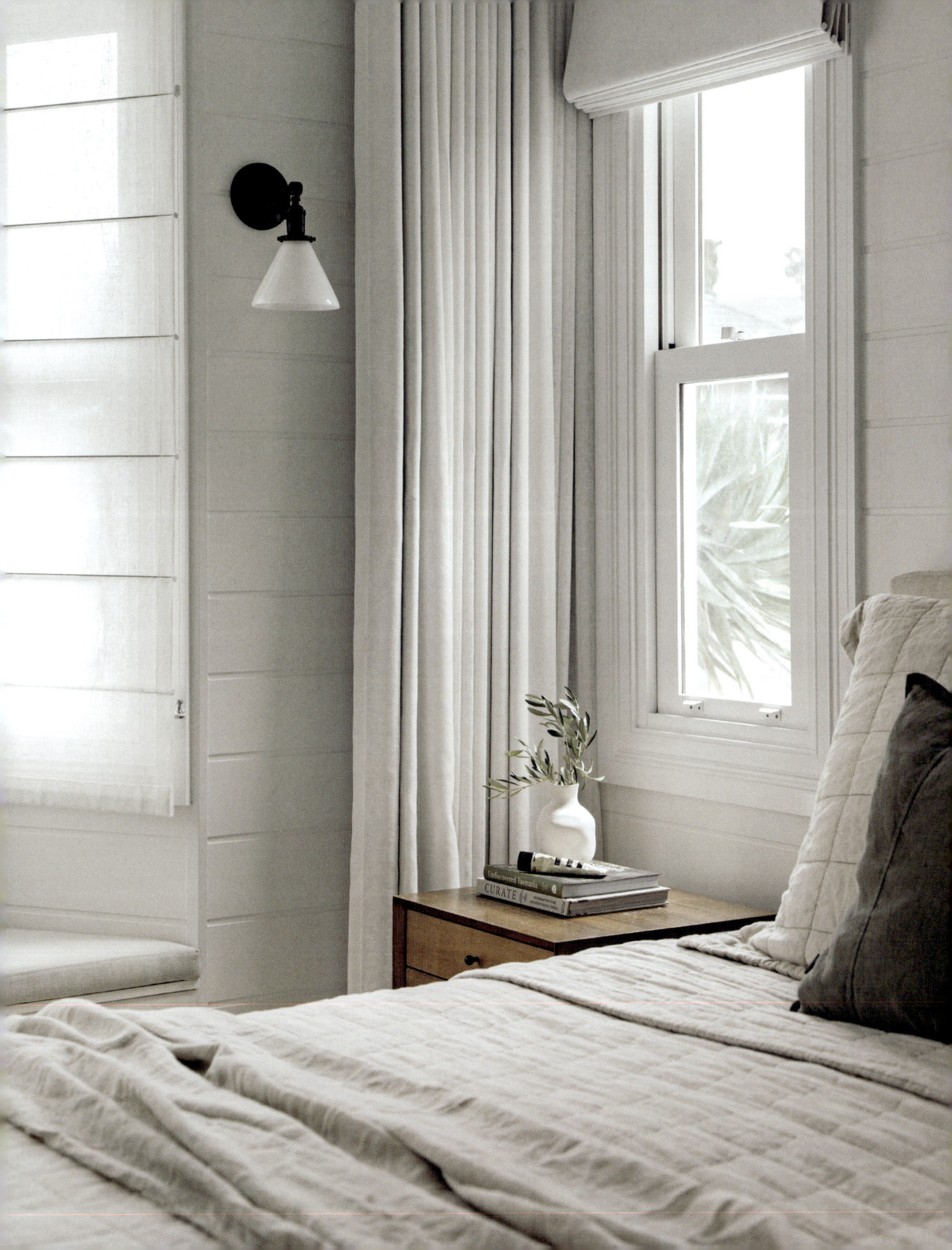
Undiscovered Tasmania
CURATE

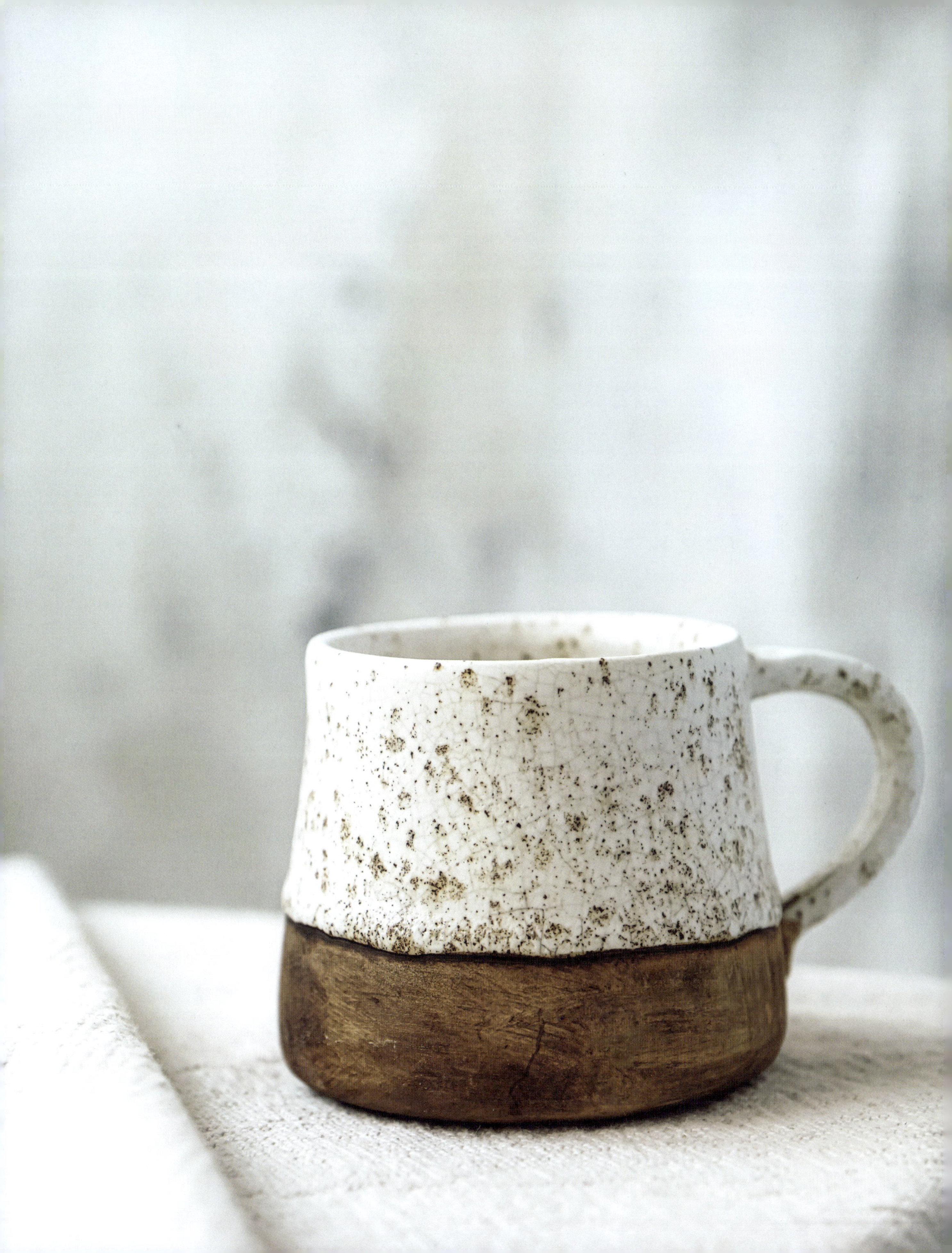

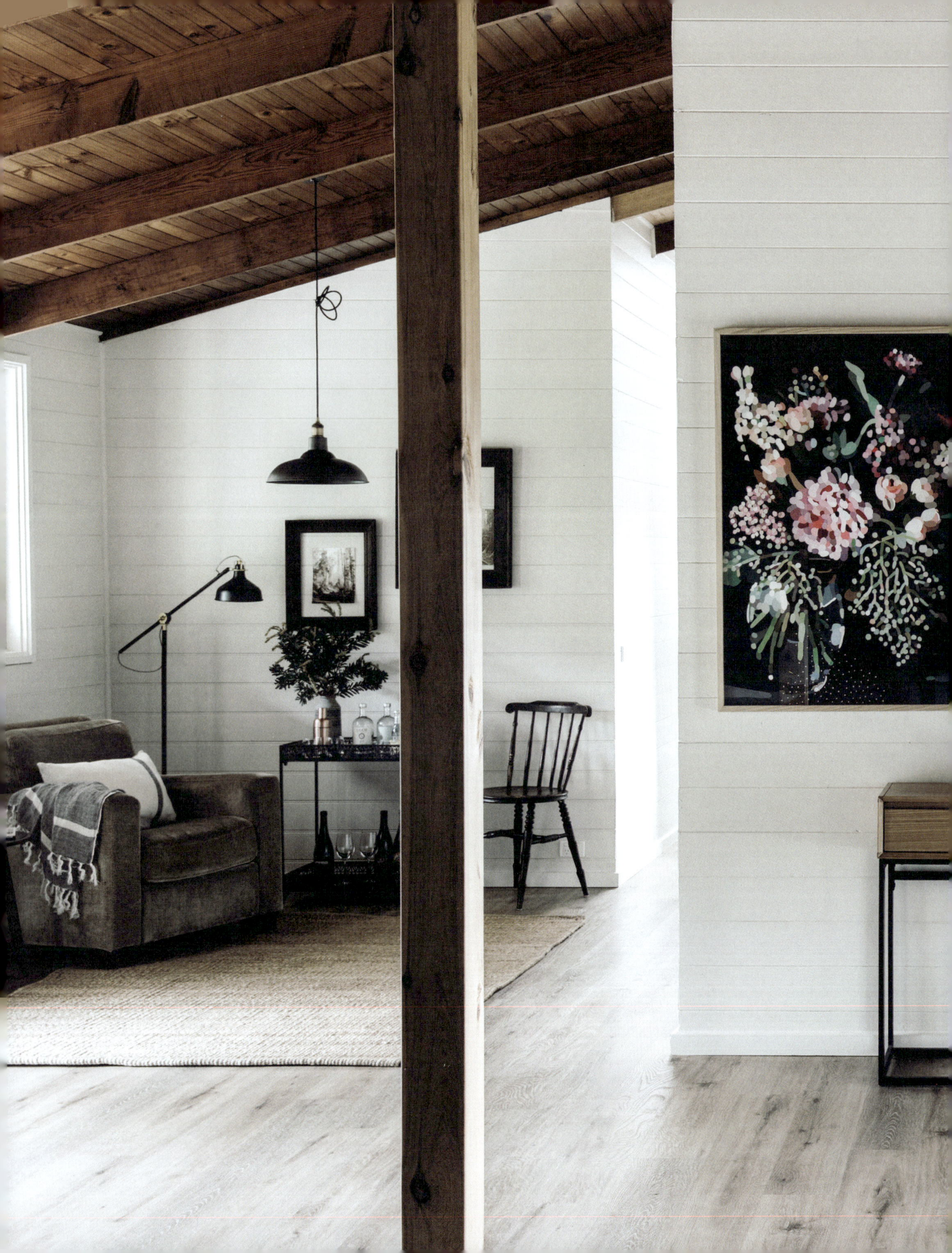

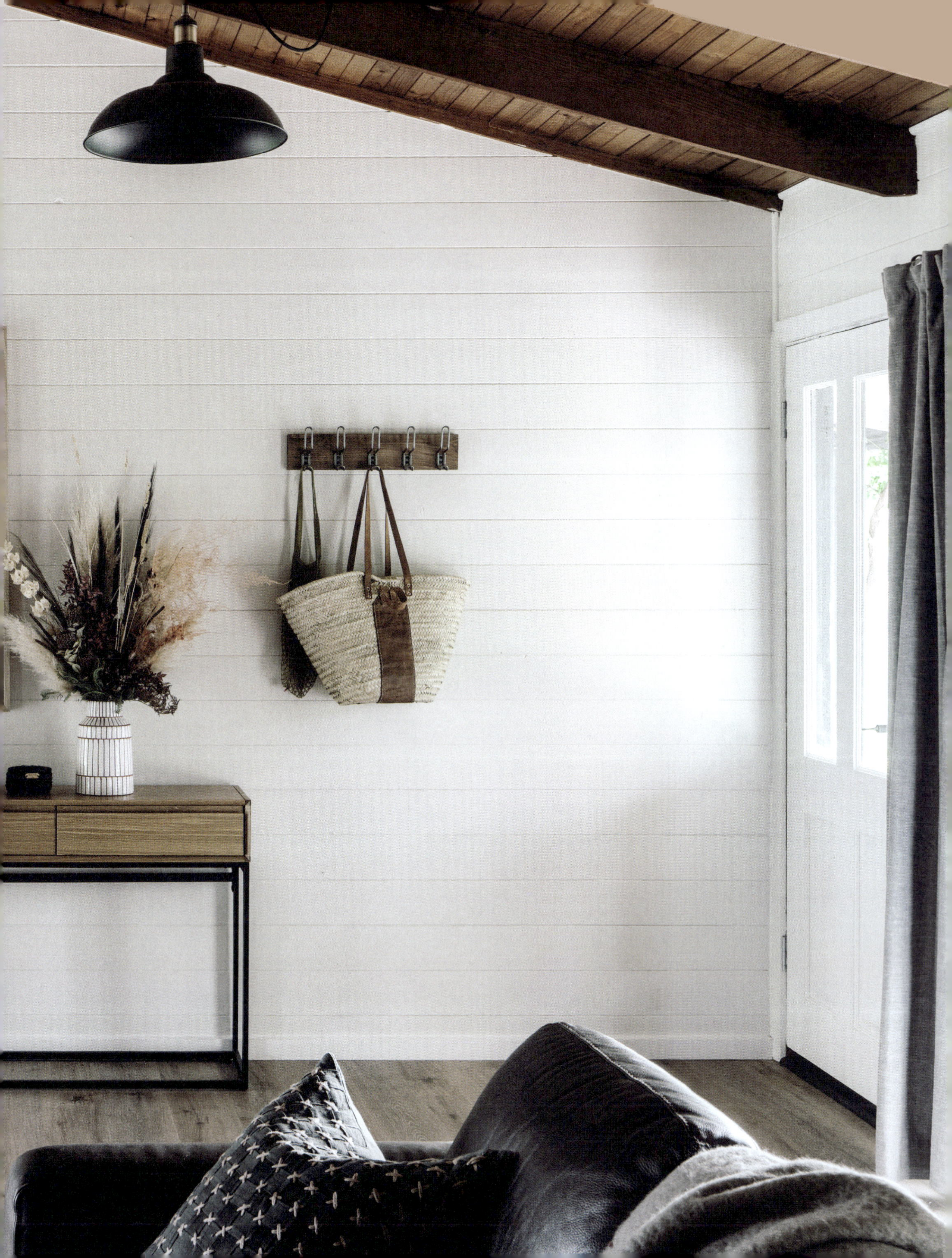

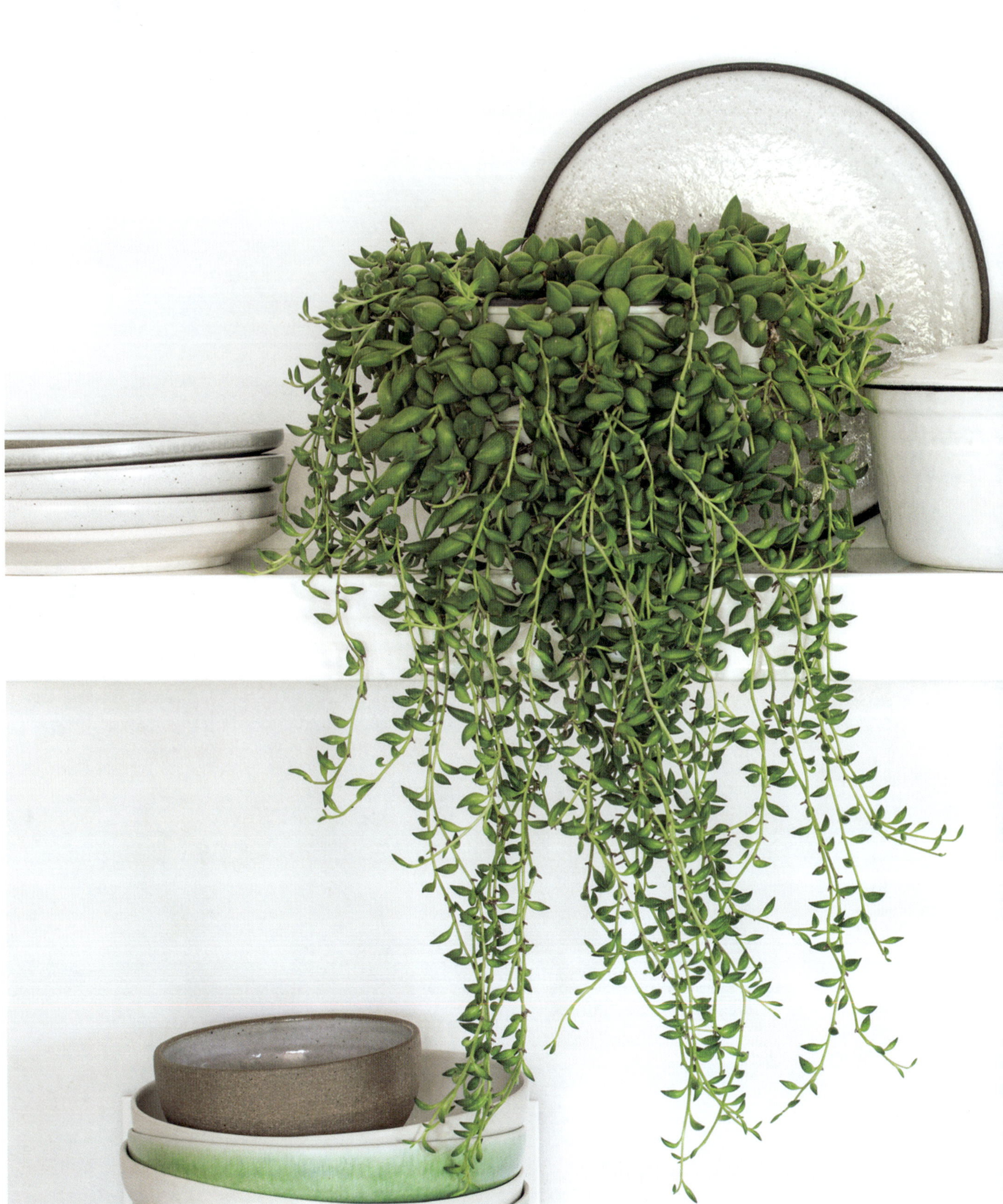

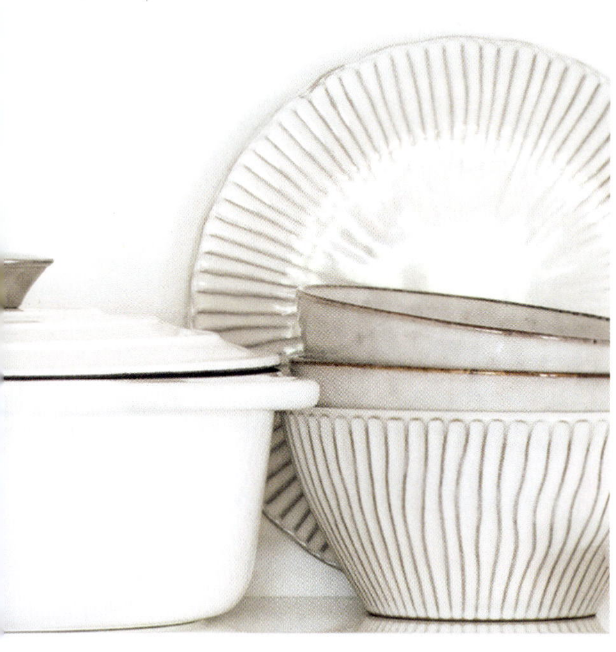

Bright white is the perfect setting for this display of crockery and greenery that leans into the contemporary edge of modern country style.

Soft blues and greys are cleverly offset by a striped pillow in tones of chocolate and rust, which is echoed in the vase on the bedside table. This subtle connecting use of colour and pattern works well in modern country styling.

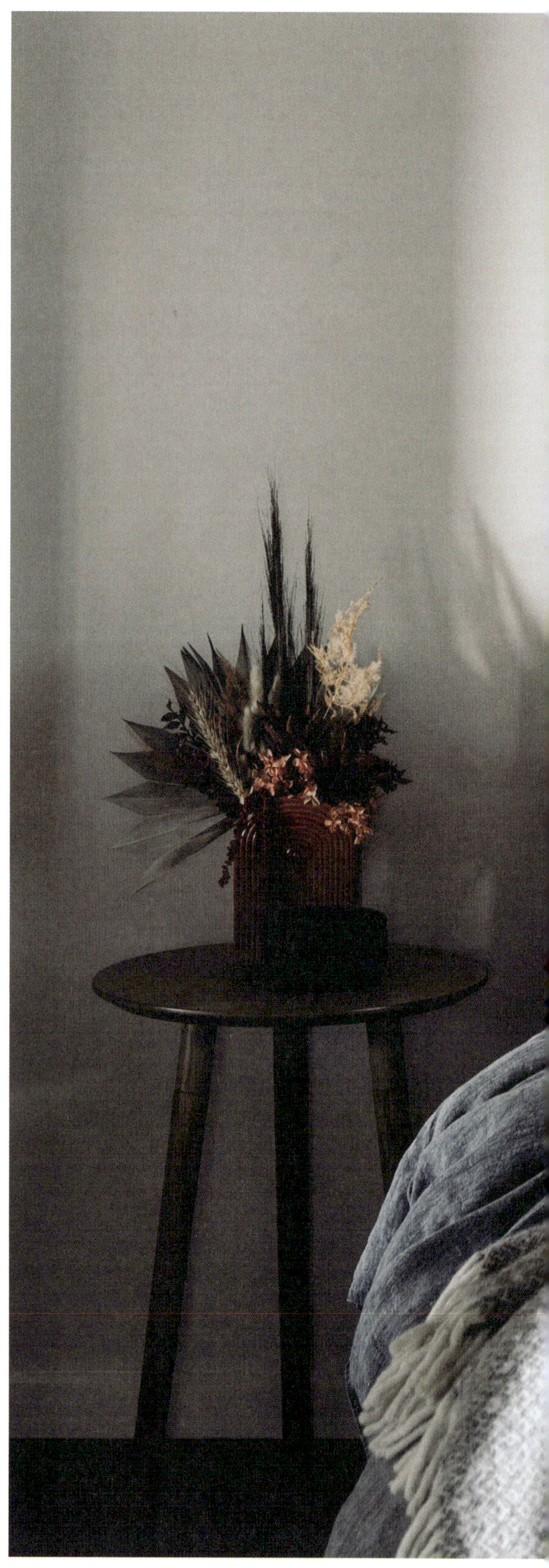

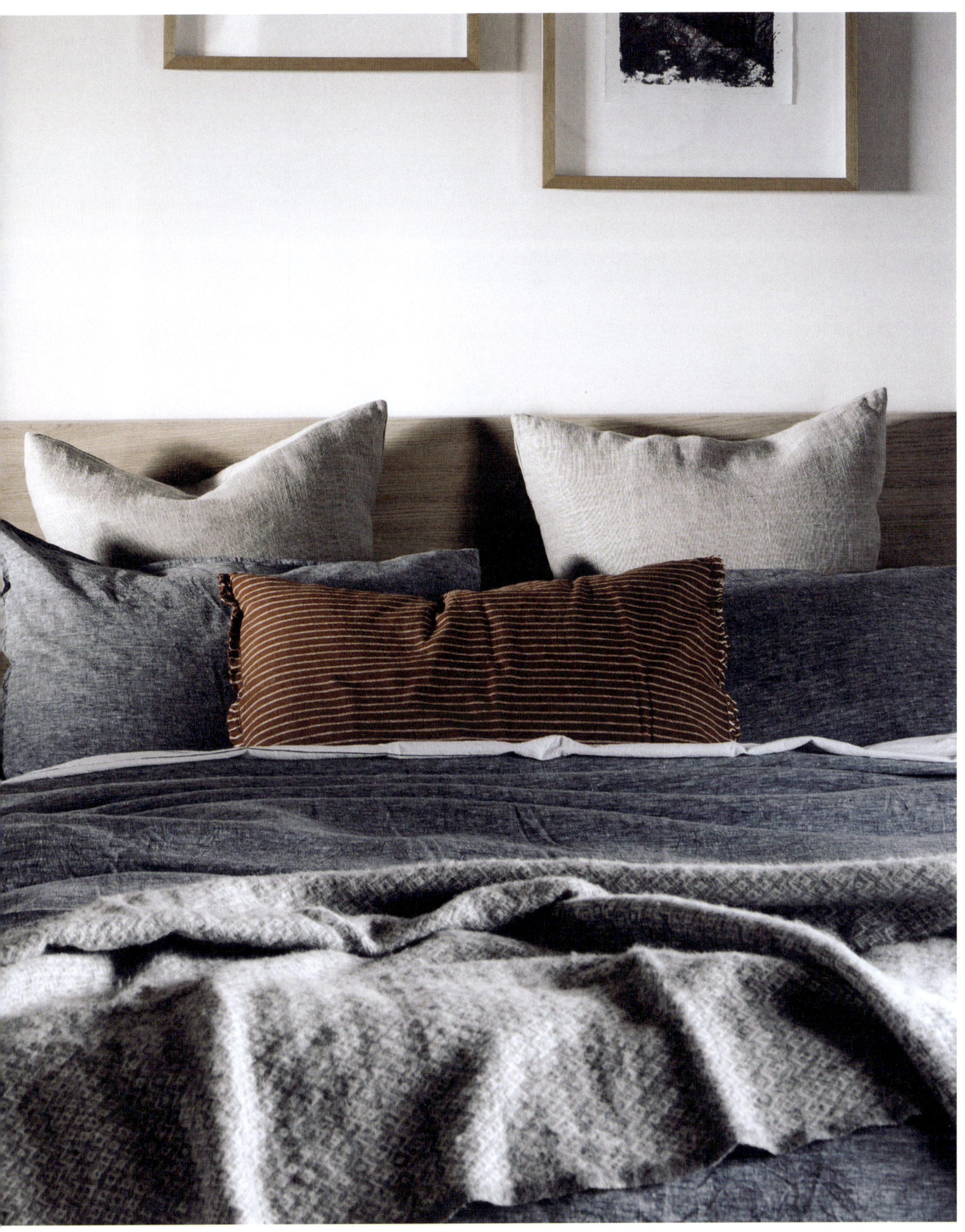

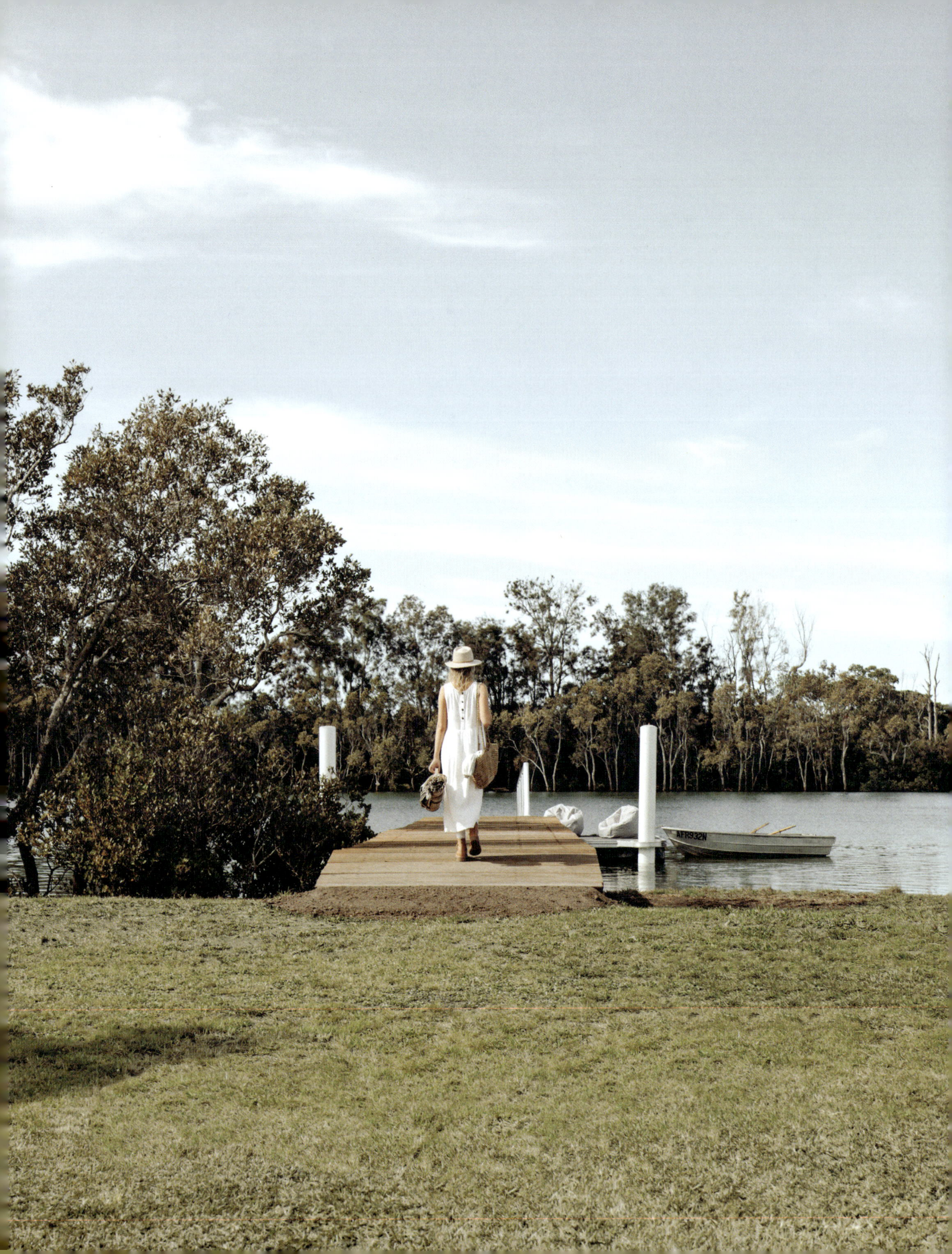
AFR932N

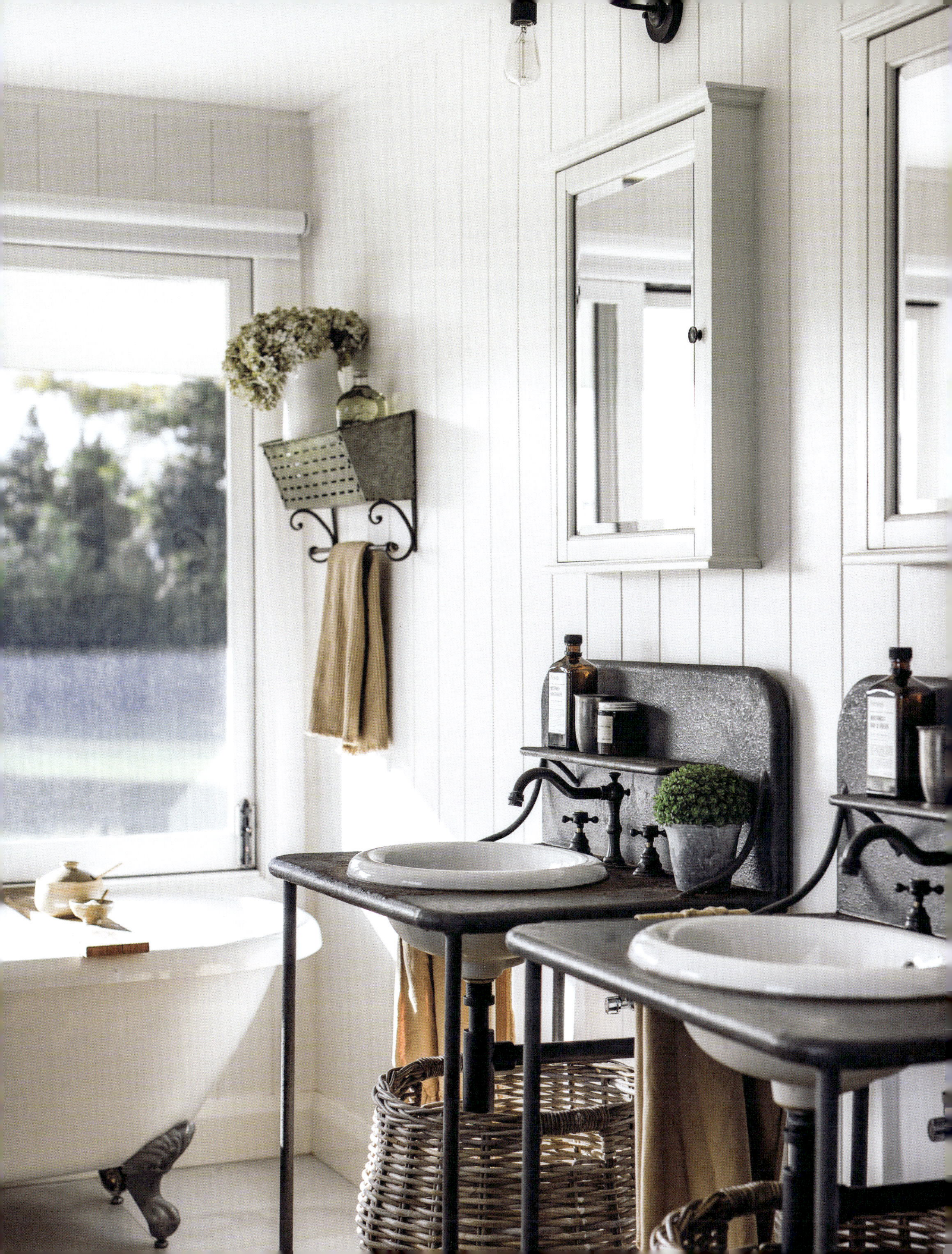

A neutral base colour makes the home seem bright and spacious. When layering with whites, it's important to consider the base tone, which will be enhanced as you add more items. A blueish white will look all the more so as you add other tones. There is no right choice of white, though, just what works for your home.

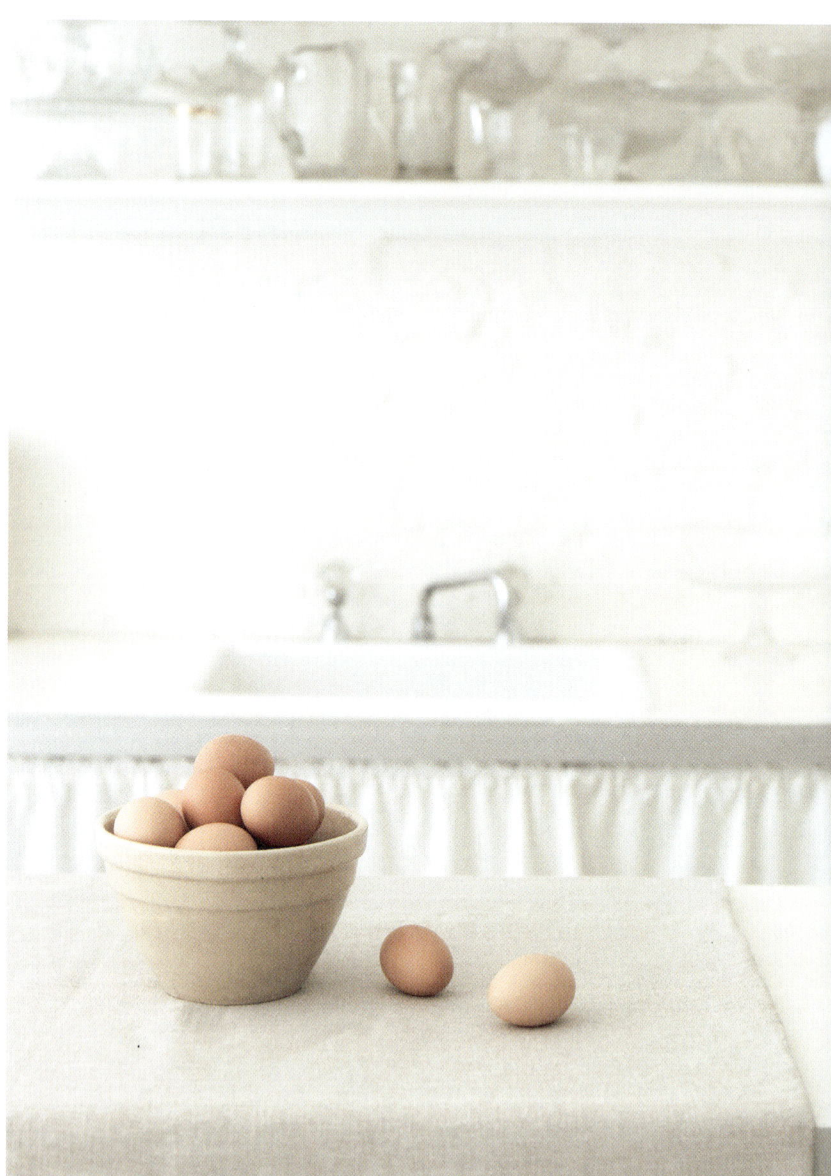

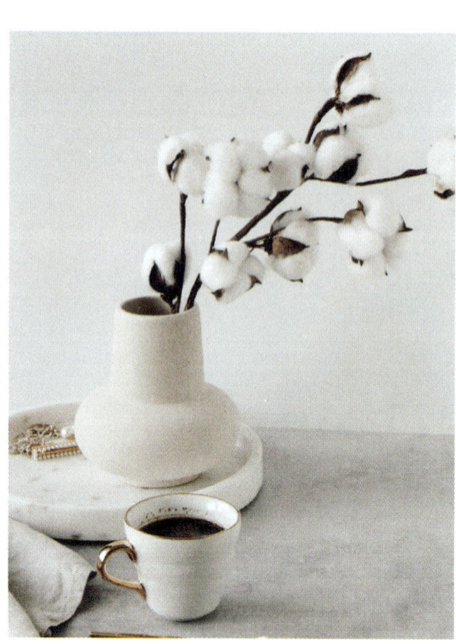

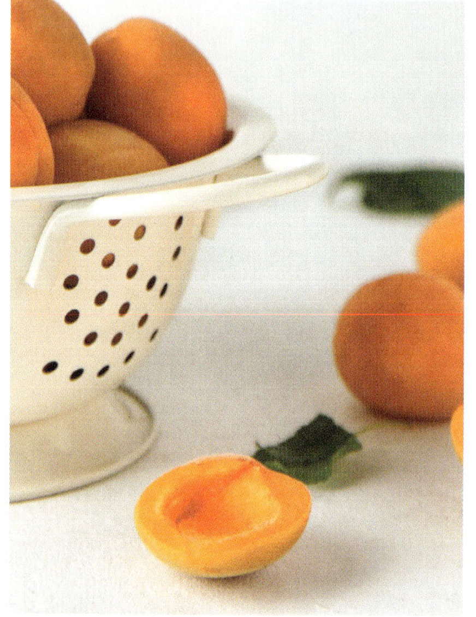

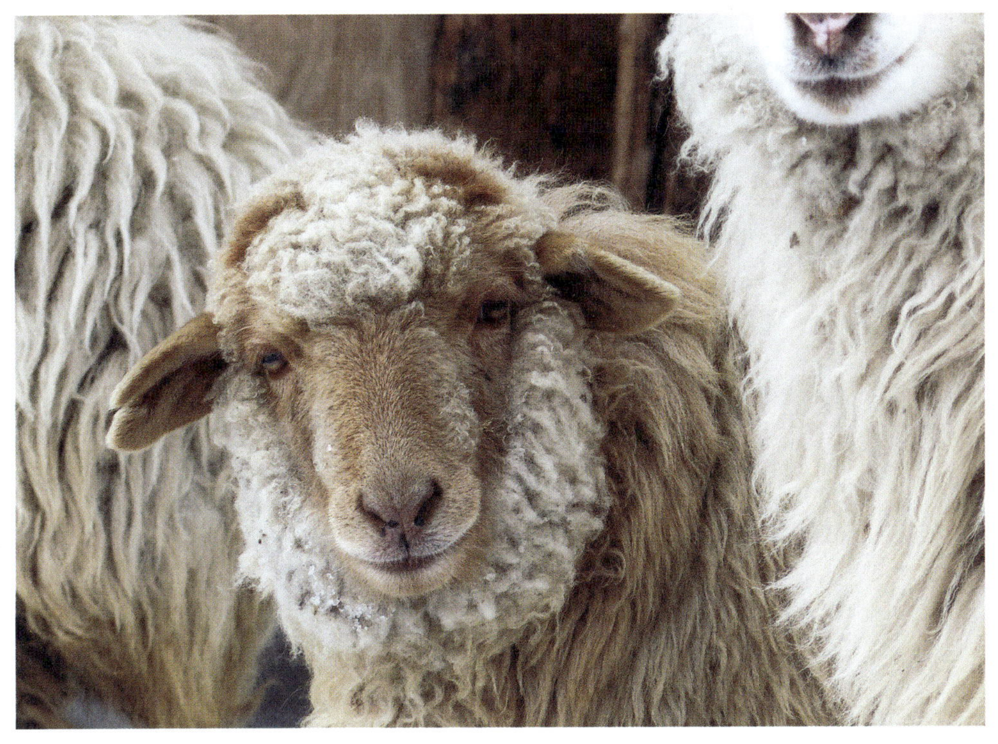

Matt finishes and soft chalky limewashes are additional paint effects that complement the style, or can be added in decor elements like the vase pictured far left.You can add pops of cream and white with fresh blooms, or eggs, too.

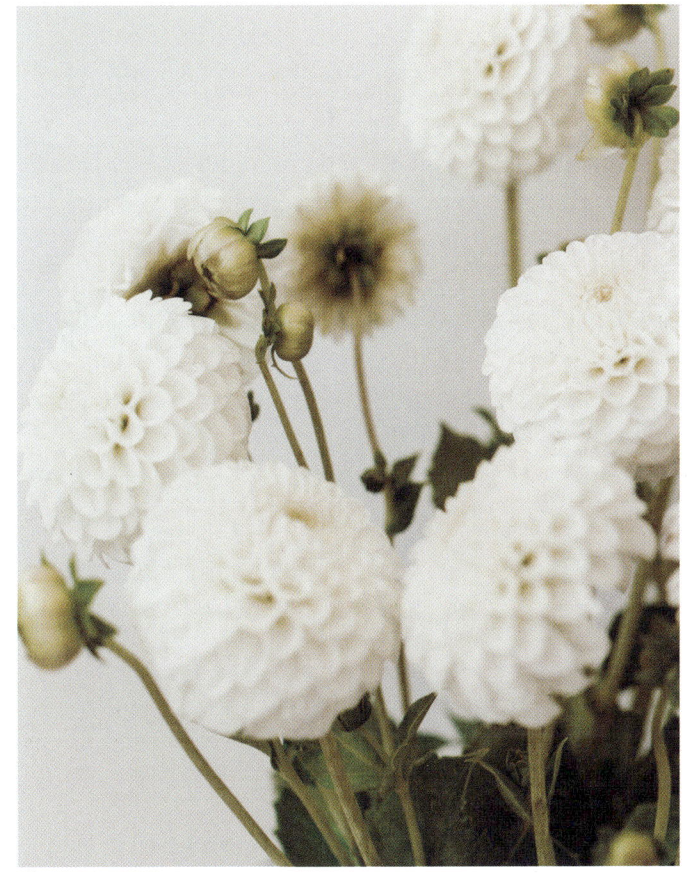

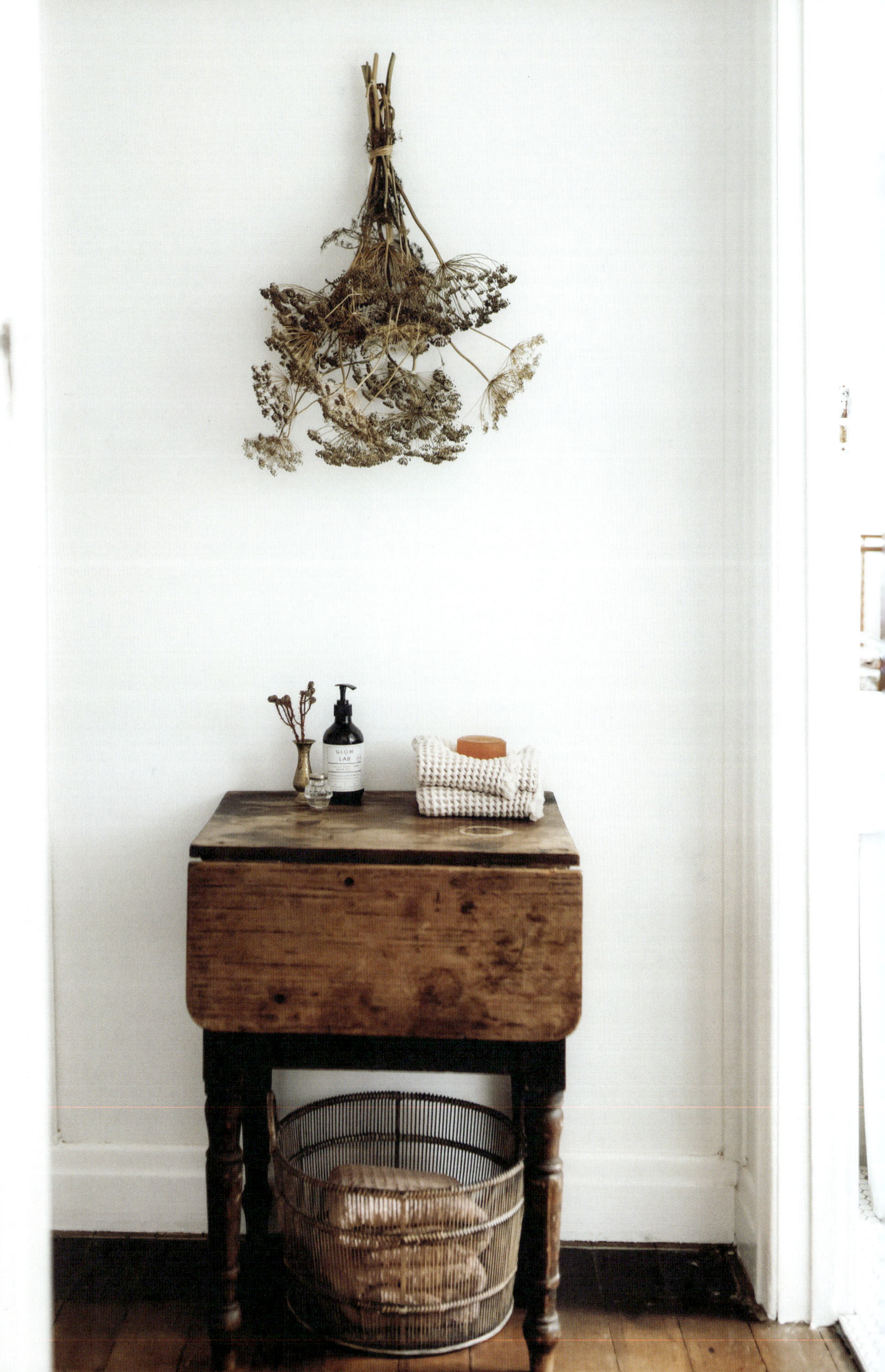
GLOW
LAB

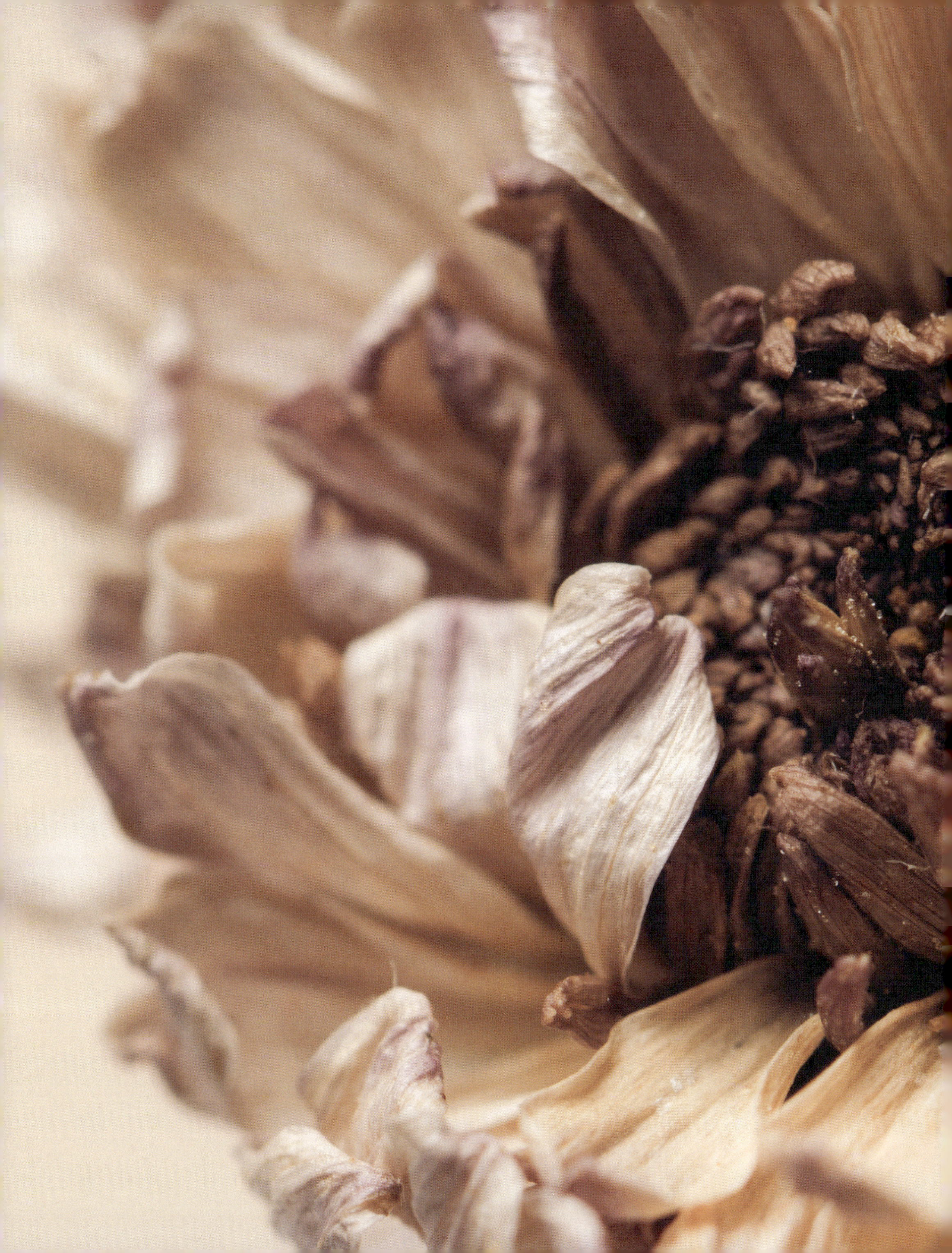

The Quick List

Bunches of dried leaves, such as eucalyptus, to evoke Australia

Vintage mirrors, which develop a beautiful patina over time

Wooden desks and tables with signs of wear and tear

Combined and layered textures, rather than added colour

Lemons or limes – they make great display items

Shades of white or soft greys providing a neutral base

Vignettes or displays in tones of one colour

Brass or other metal statuettes

Displays of vintage bottles

Subtly teased-out connections in patterns

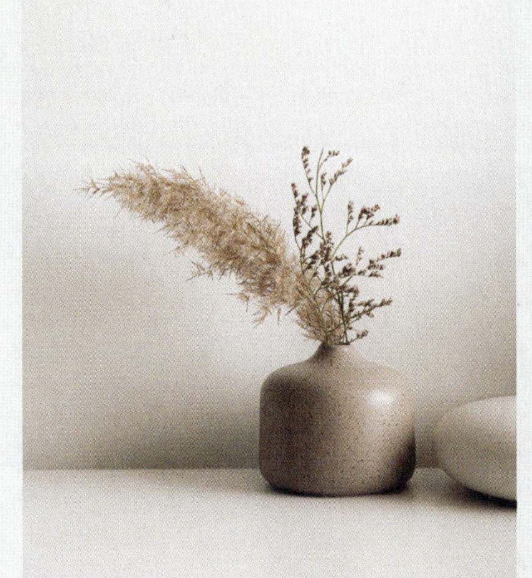
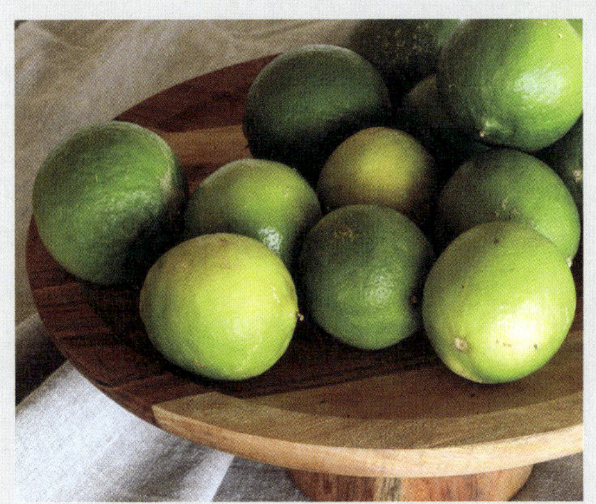

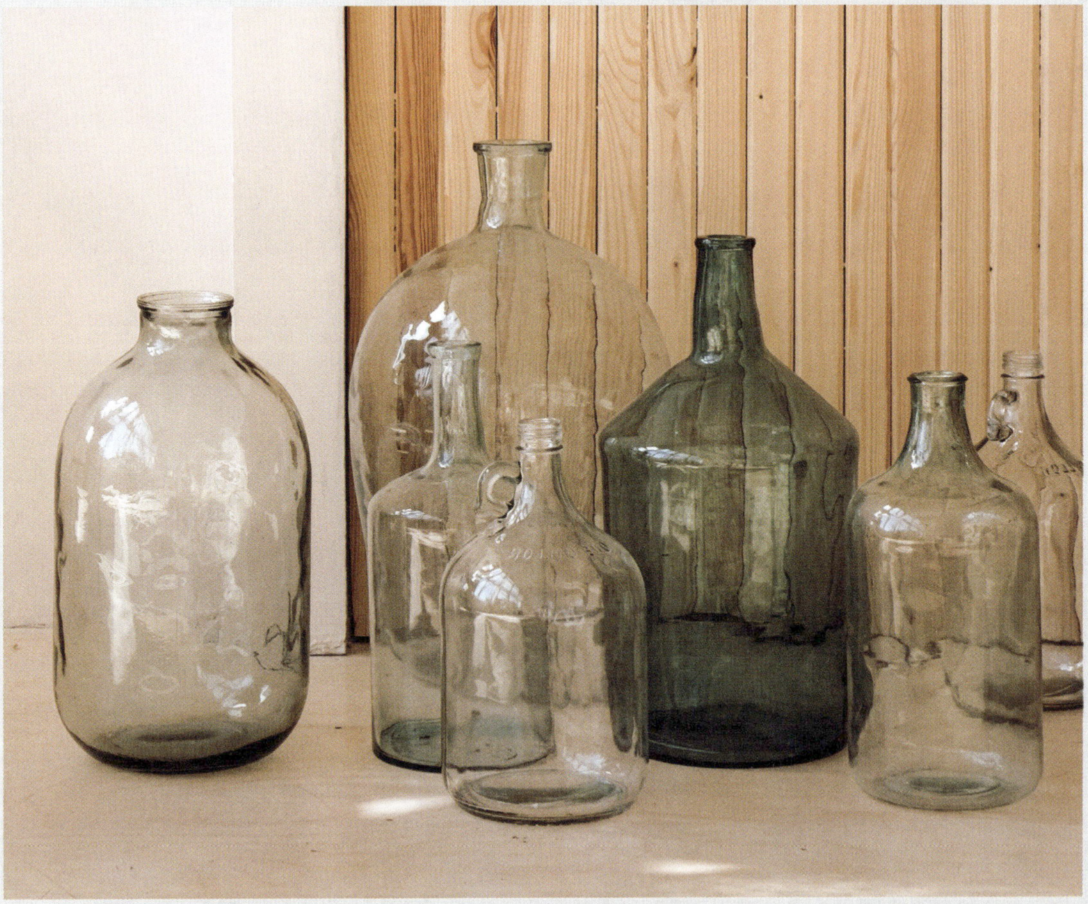

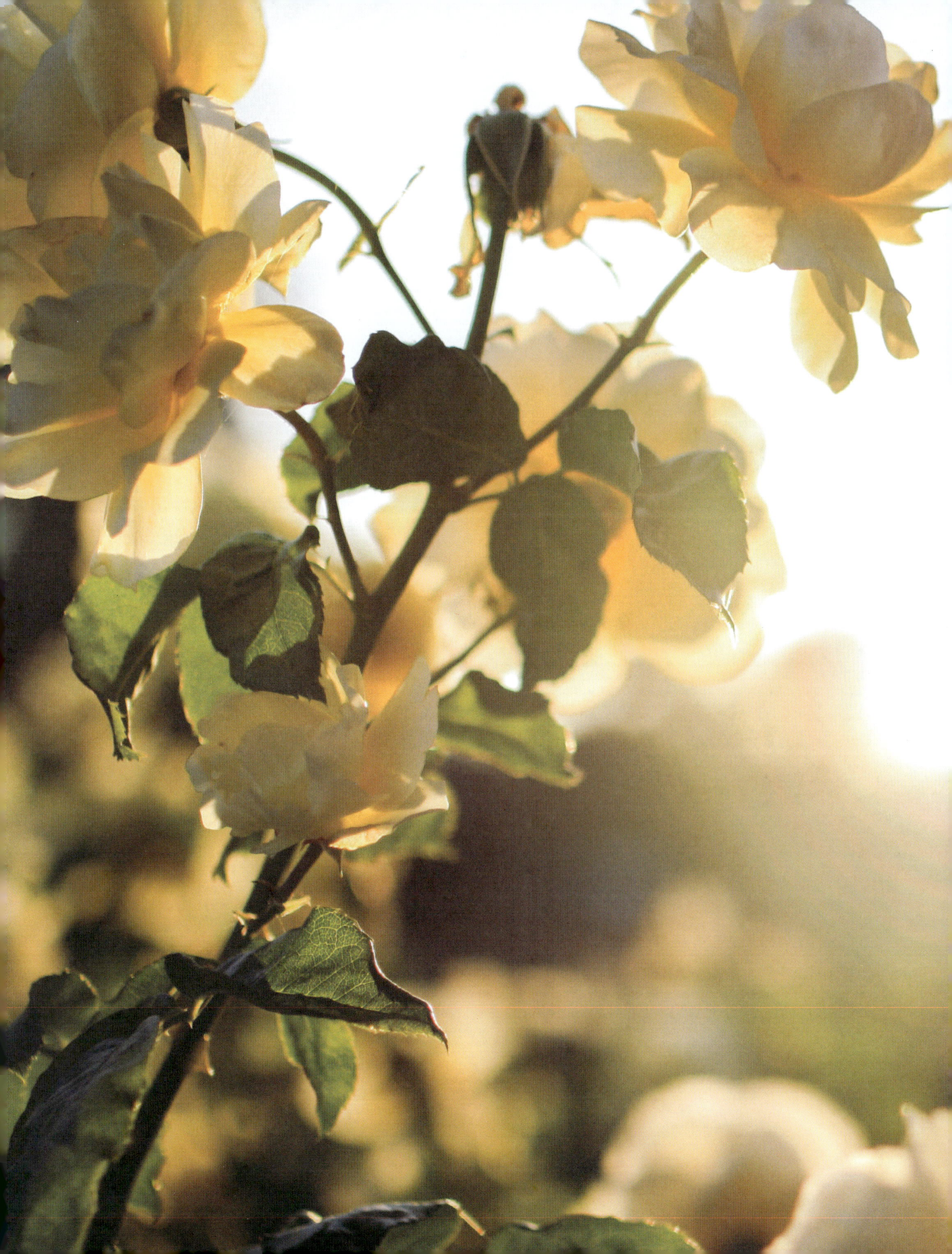

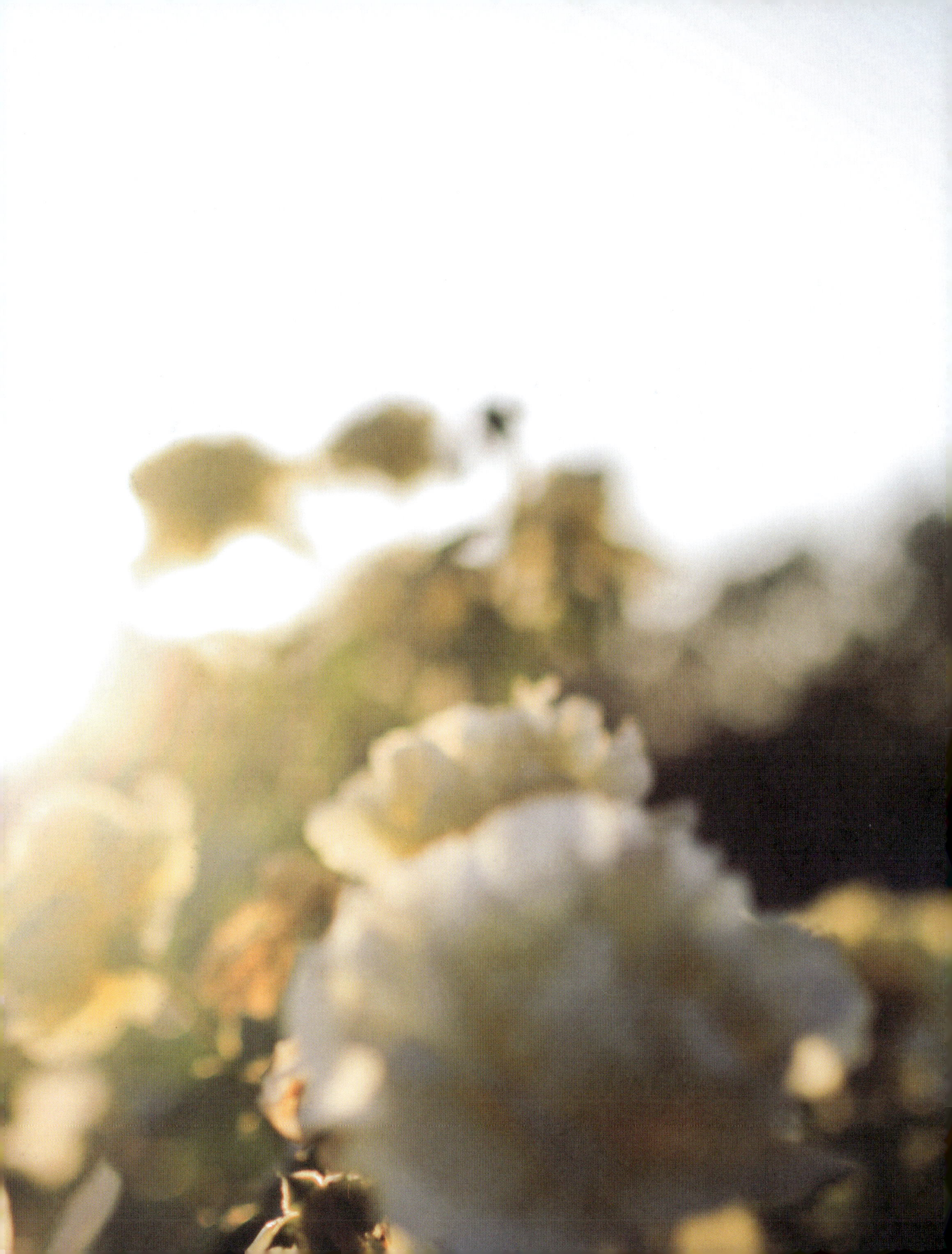

chapter three

living

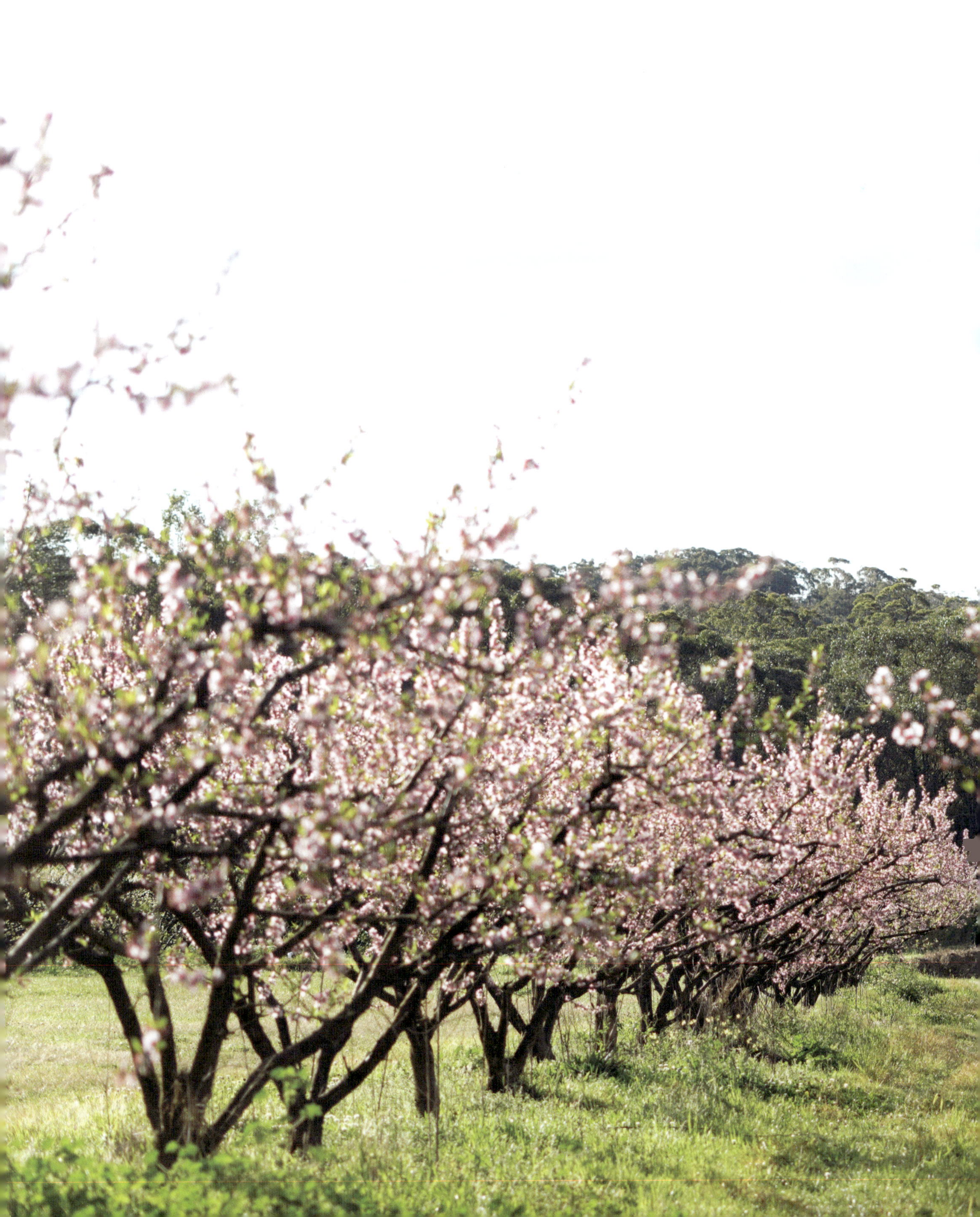

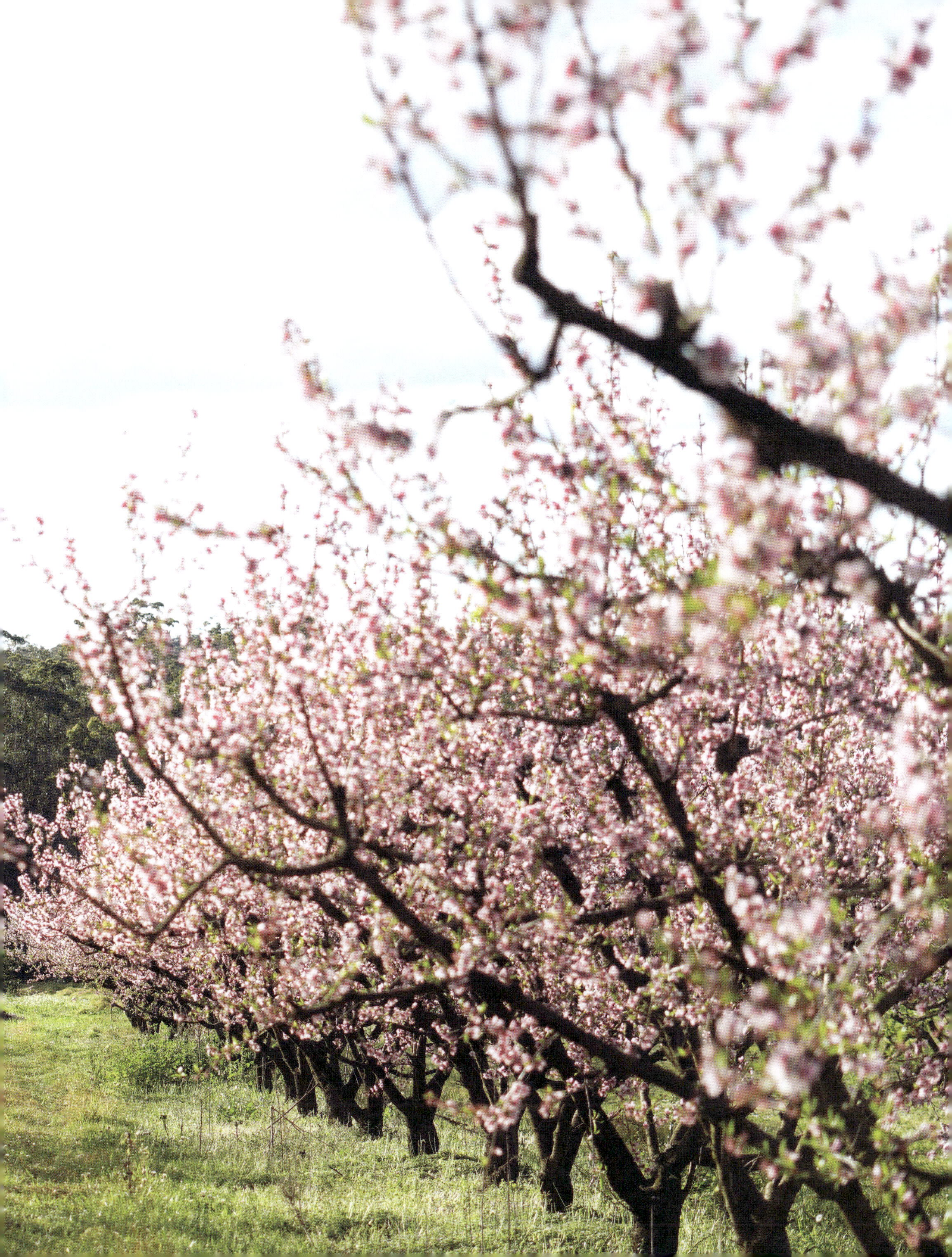

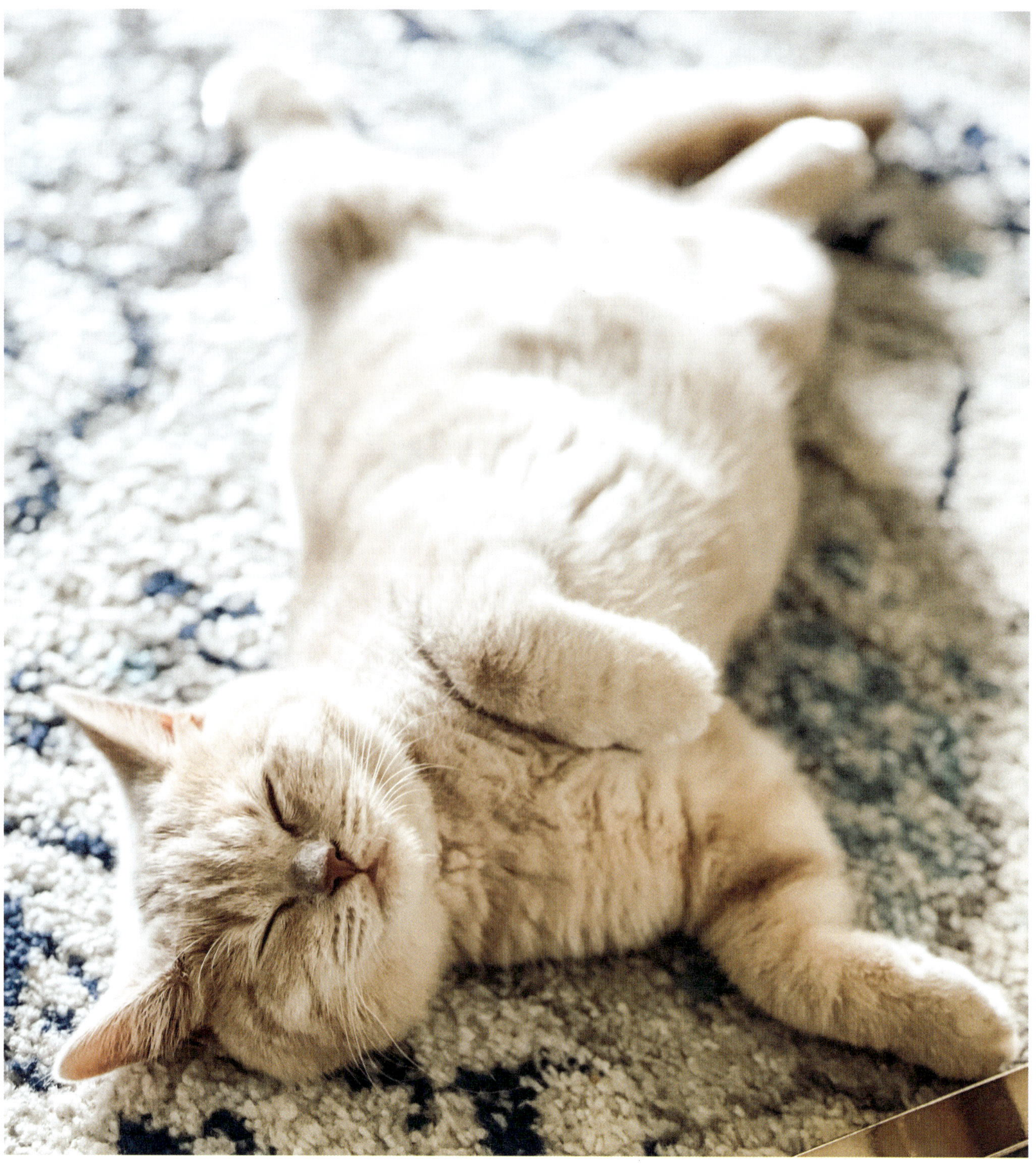

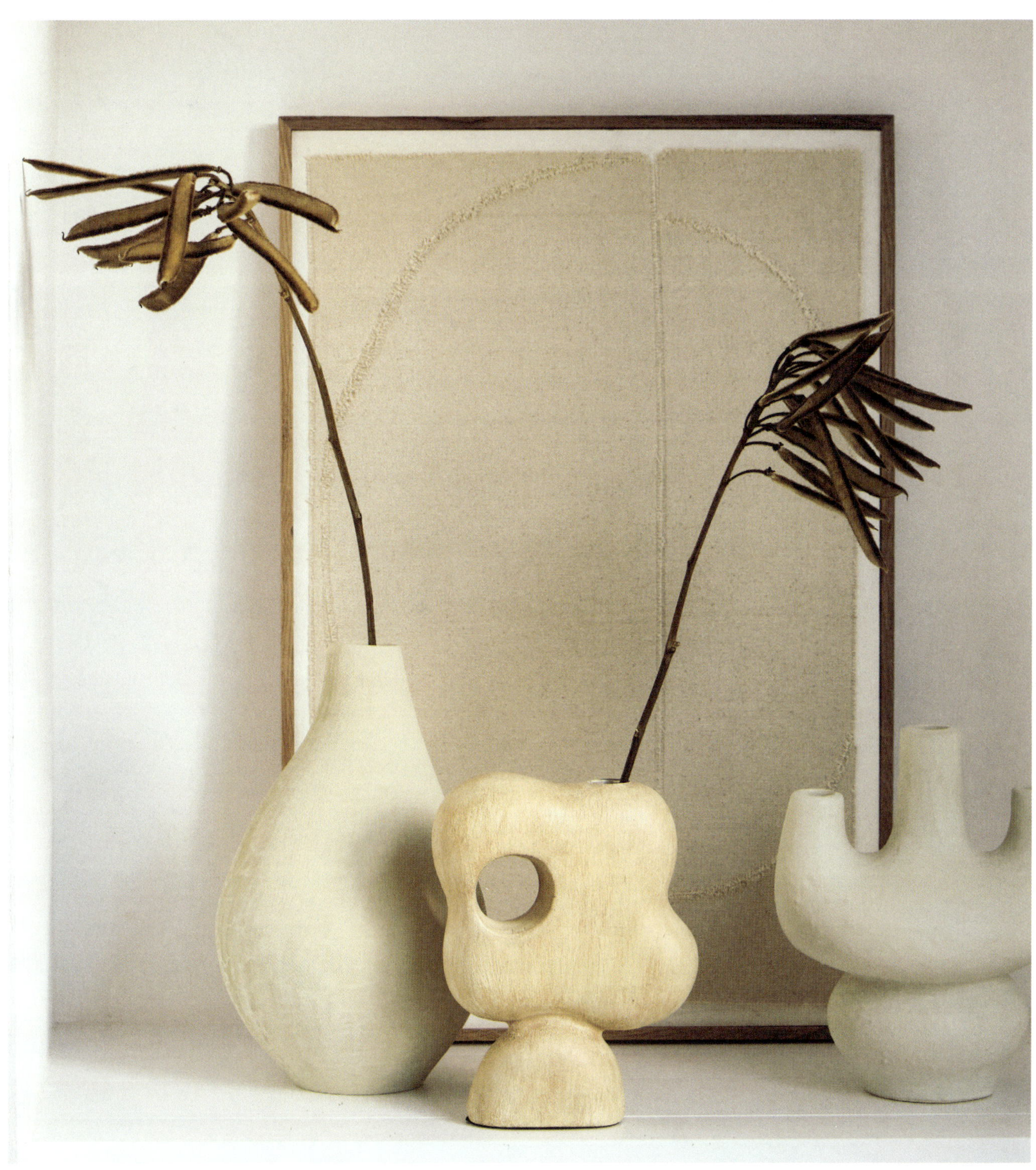

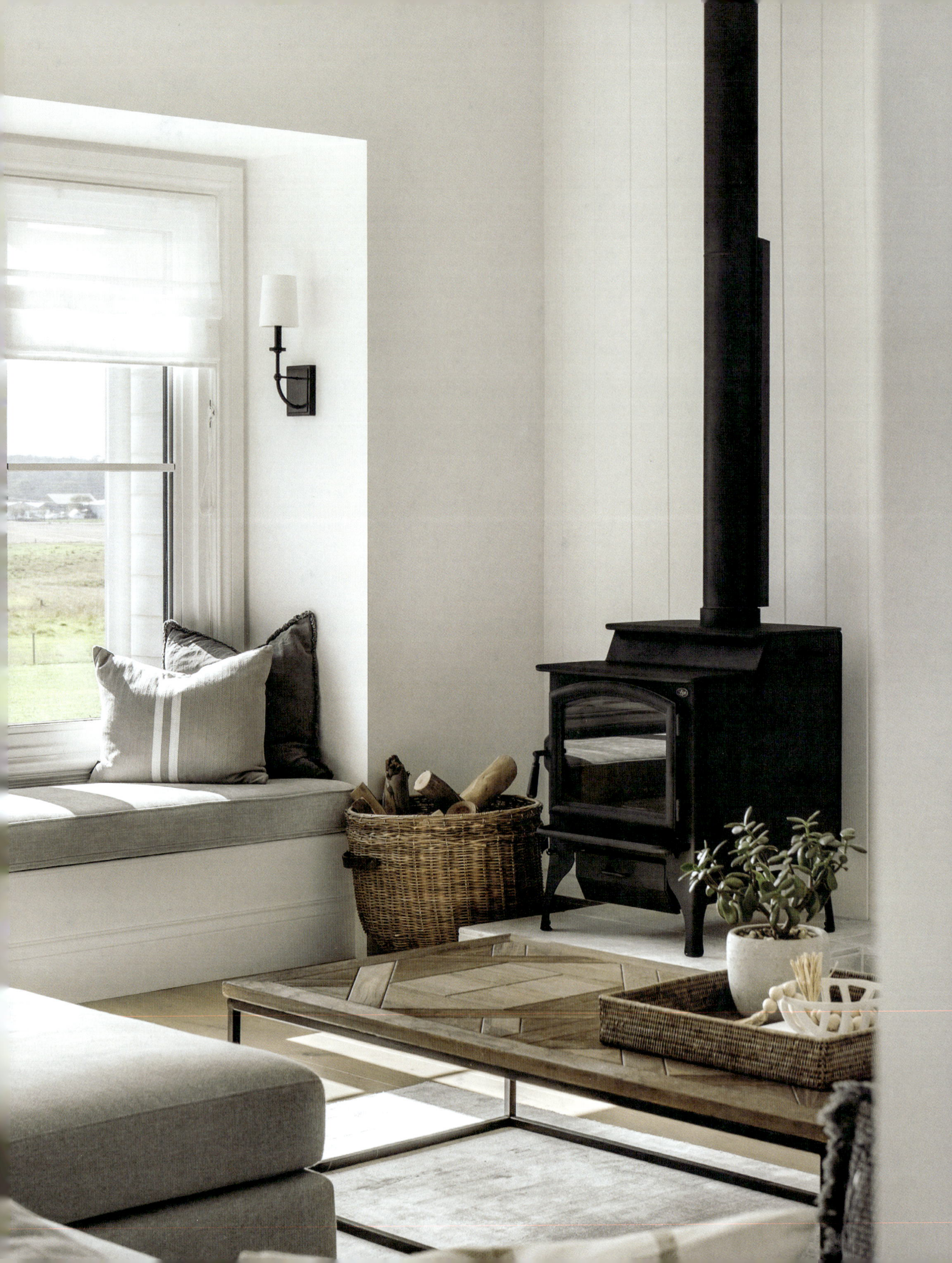

Modern country living spaces are an interplay of practicality, comfort and detail.

The practical is rarely the glamorous side of styling, but paying attention to it will pay dividends, ensuring the home is functional, streamlined and organised.

Modern country homes, especially those actually in the country, tend to see a bit of wear and tear (and they usually have a dog or two on the loose), so considering furniture and upholstery that will stand up in the face of that is important. Think blankets, throws, slips and cushion covers that are easy to replace and clean.

Alongside the need for a robustness of furnishings, the importance of lighting in country style should not be overlooked. Mood lighting can create a cosy ambience on dark and cooler evenings. A fireplace is both a luxury and a surefire way to deliver the modern country look. It's practical too, providing warmth in wintertime and a focal point for the room all year-round.

Mudrooms, boot rooms and drying rooms are all a necessary part of managing the elements in outback country life, and these practical elements have made their way into the broader look and feel of the style. Even in smaller spaces, a mudroom can make for a practical and stylish inclusion.

With practicalities in place, and comfort embedded in your furniture and furnishing choices, it comes down to the styling details that will help articulate your particular country home style. Think baskets and hats on display, greenery and bunches of flowers, stacks of carefully chosen books on the coffee table and handmade ceramics or knitted throws on display. If you love it, it's going to work.

TOP FIVE

1.

Practical furnishings that absorb daily wear and tear

2.

Books and treasured items on display

3.

Layers and textures

4.

A fireplace – the perfect style statement

5.

Mood lighting for ambience

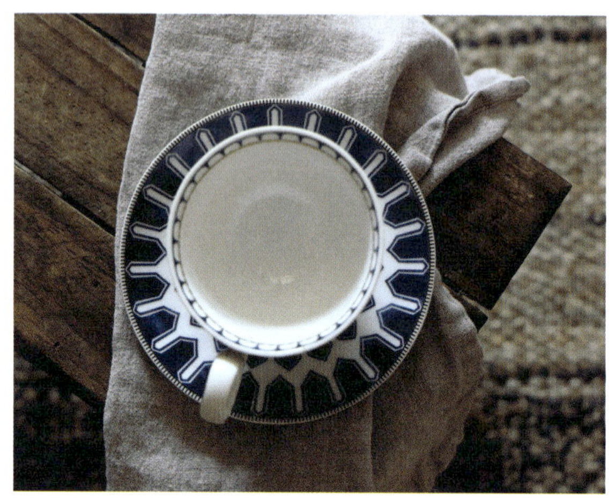

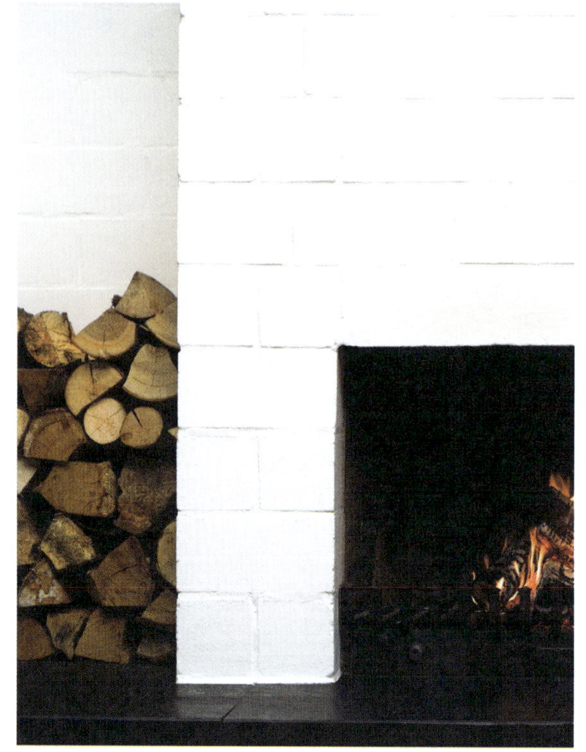

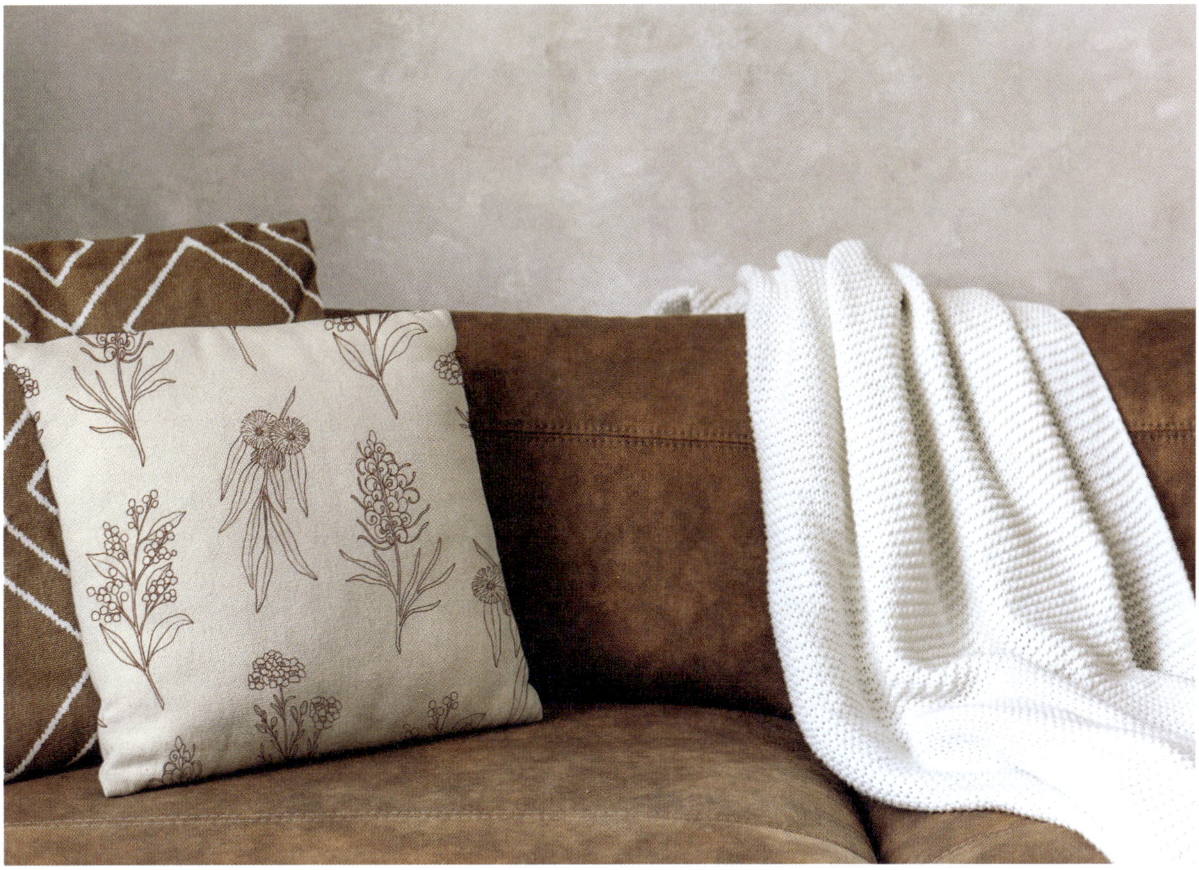

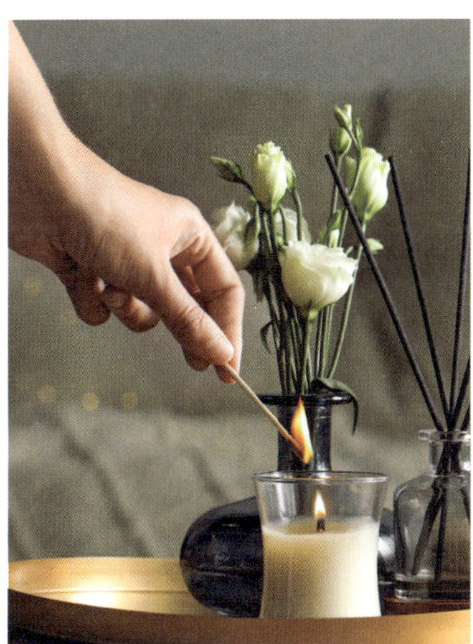

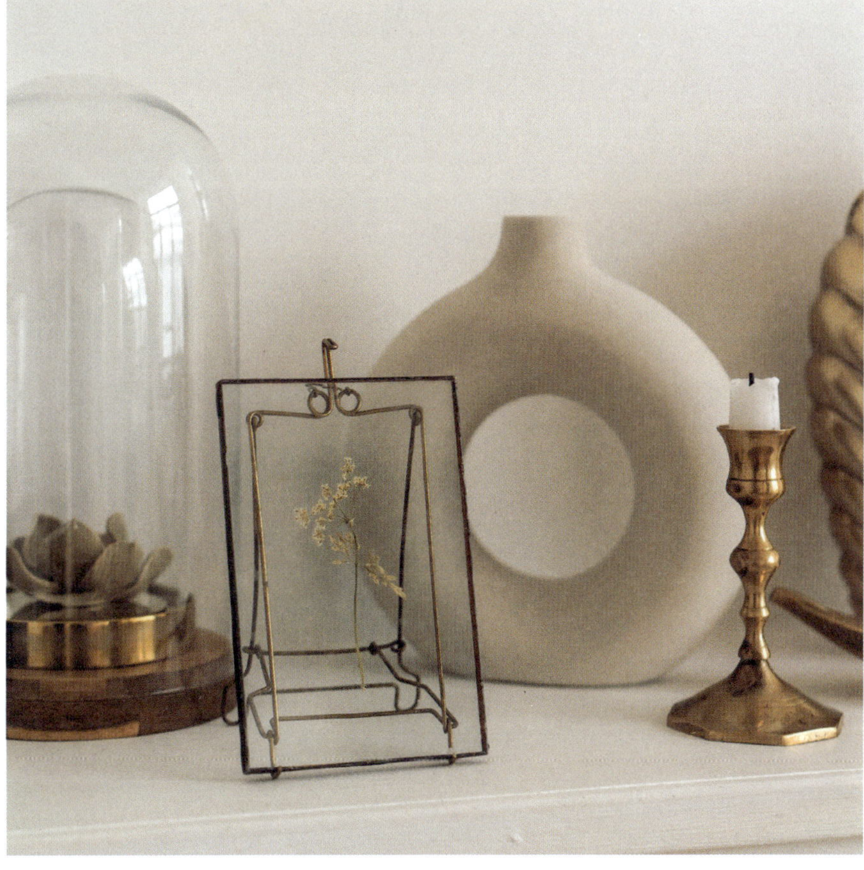

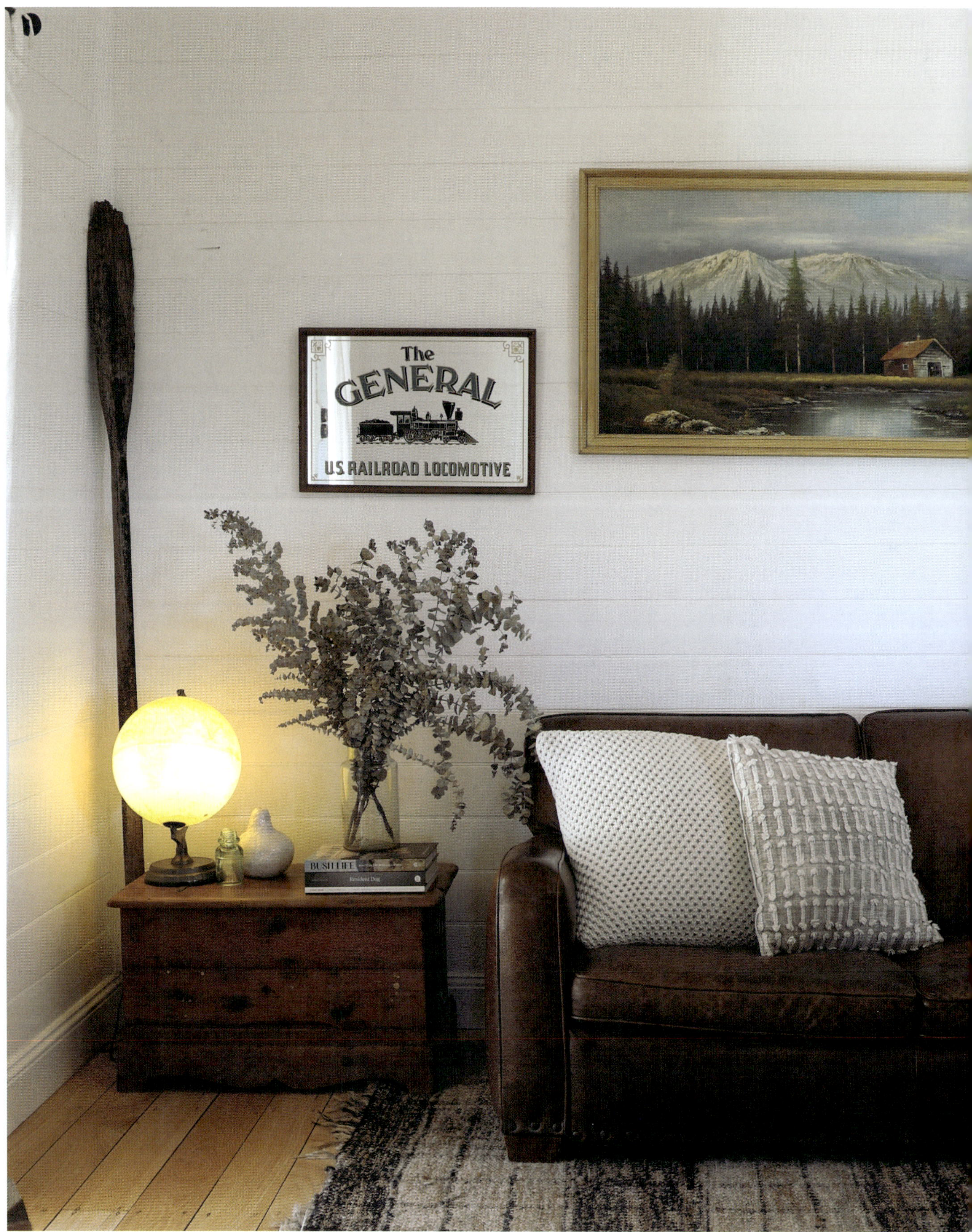
The
GENERAL
U.S RAILROAD LOCOMOTIVE
BUSH LIFE

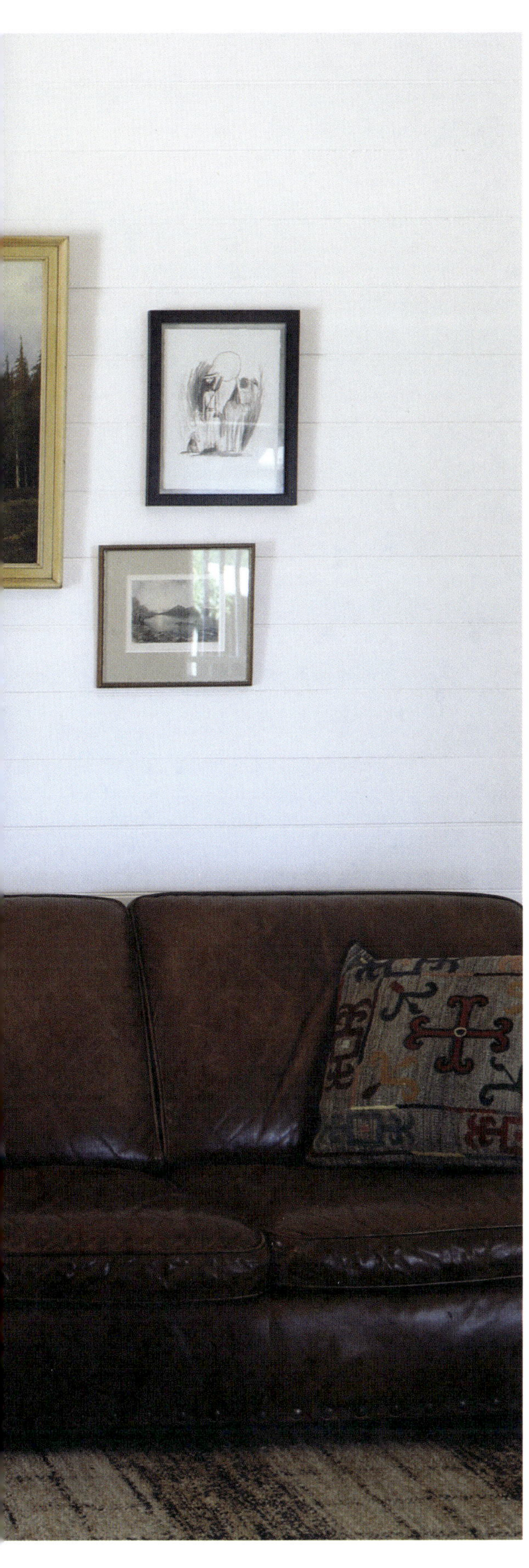

Cherished items and quirky artworks displayed against white VJ panelling help create the modern country look in this living room, but it's the well-loved, soft-leather couch that really nails the comfort and authenticity that's synonymous with the style.

Flowers fit in any home style and the best choice is always your favourite, but is there anything quite like pink roses to evoke to romance and nostalgia of the past?

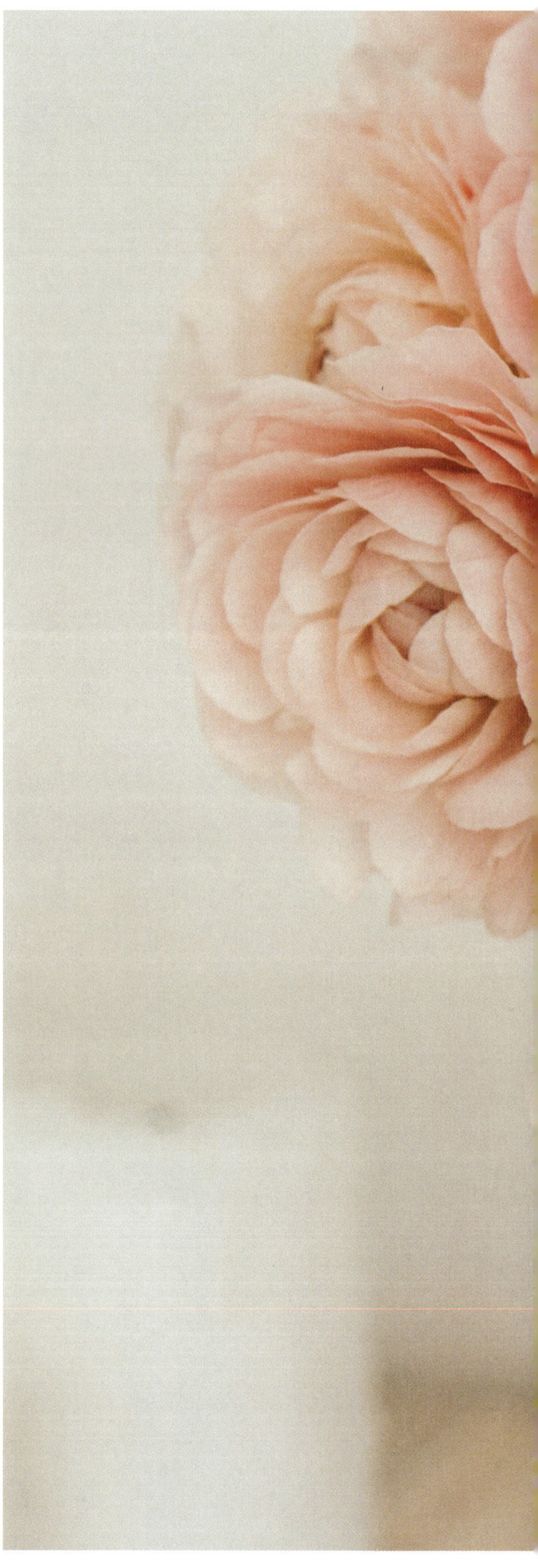

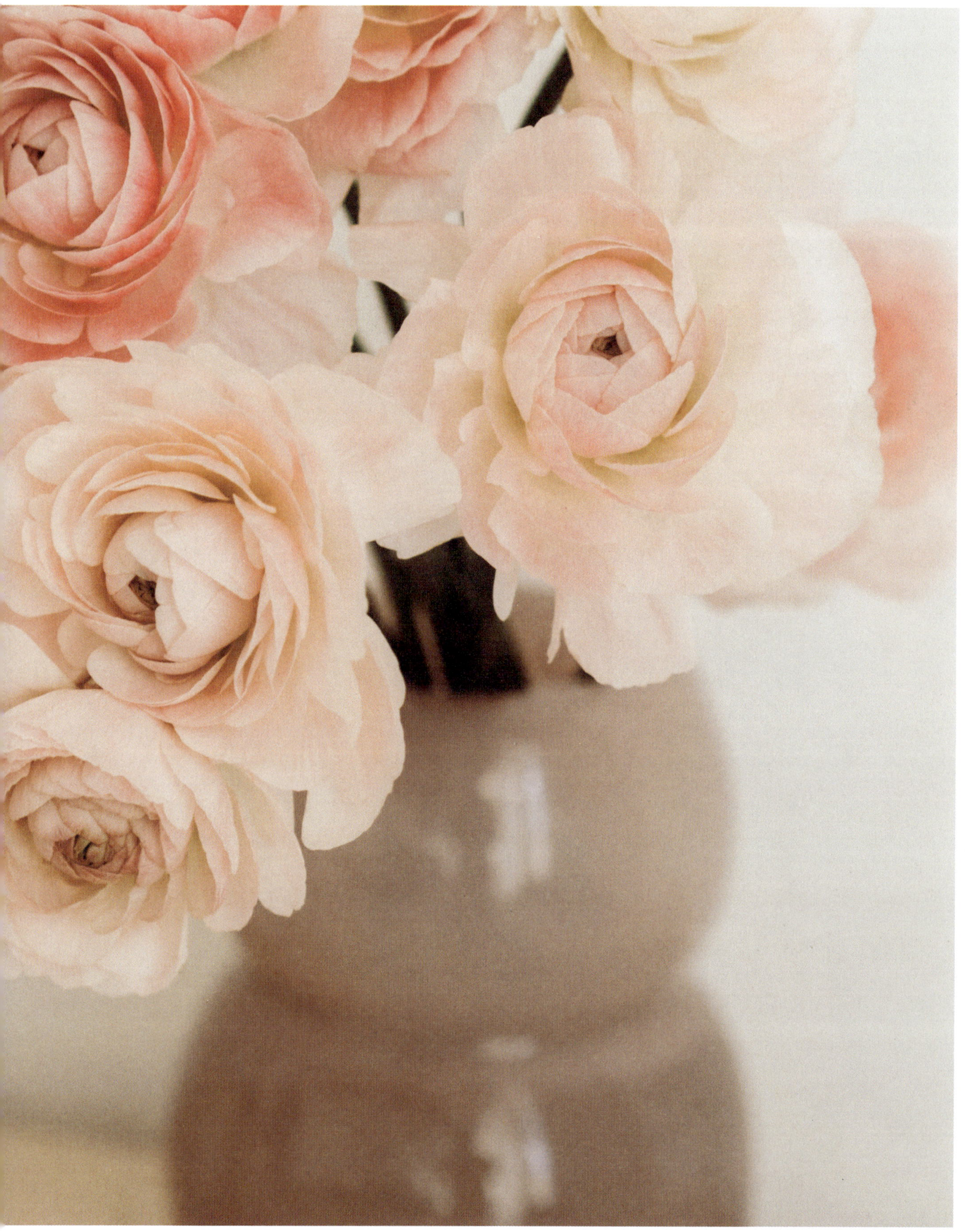

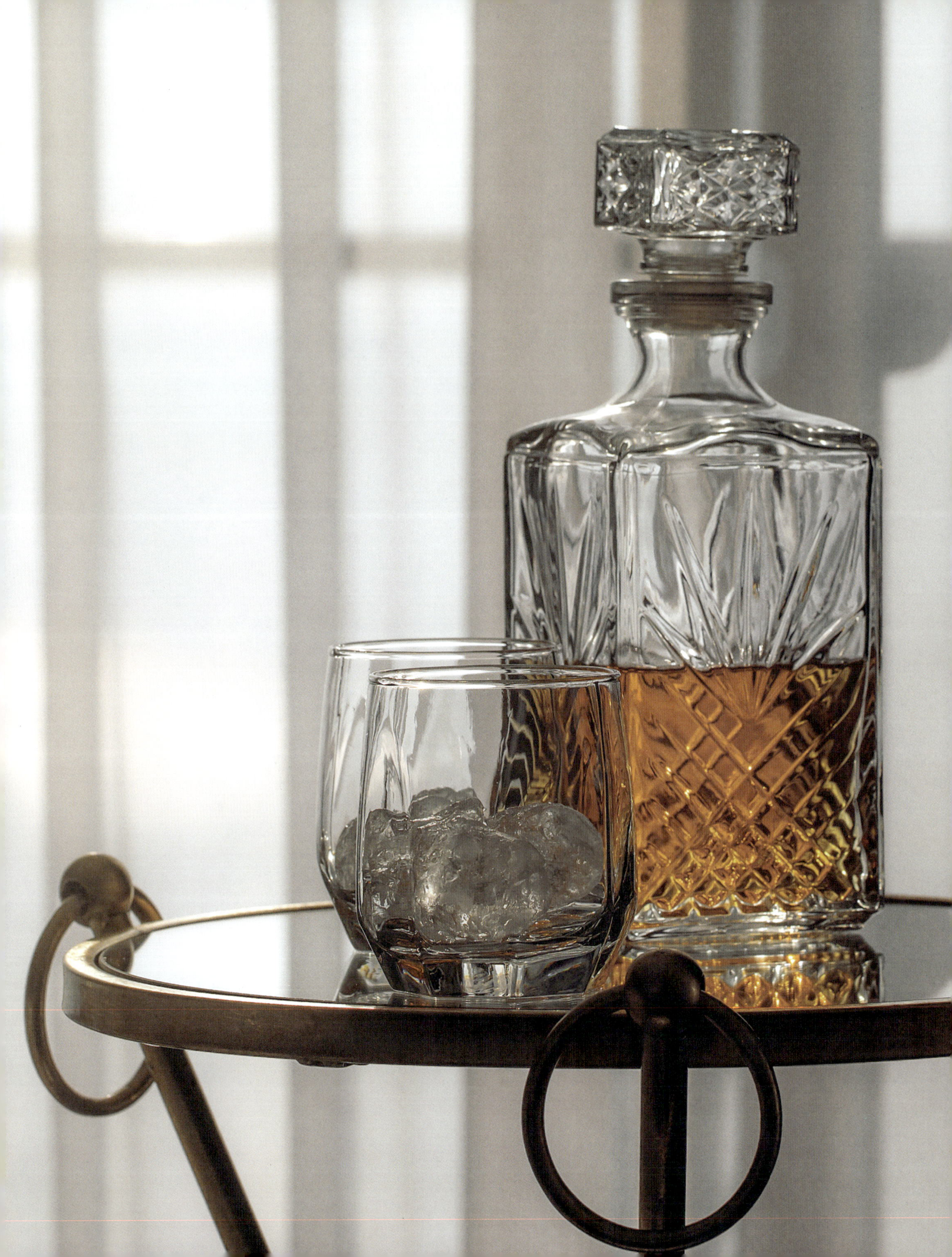

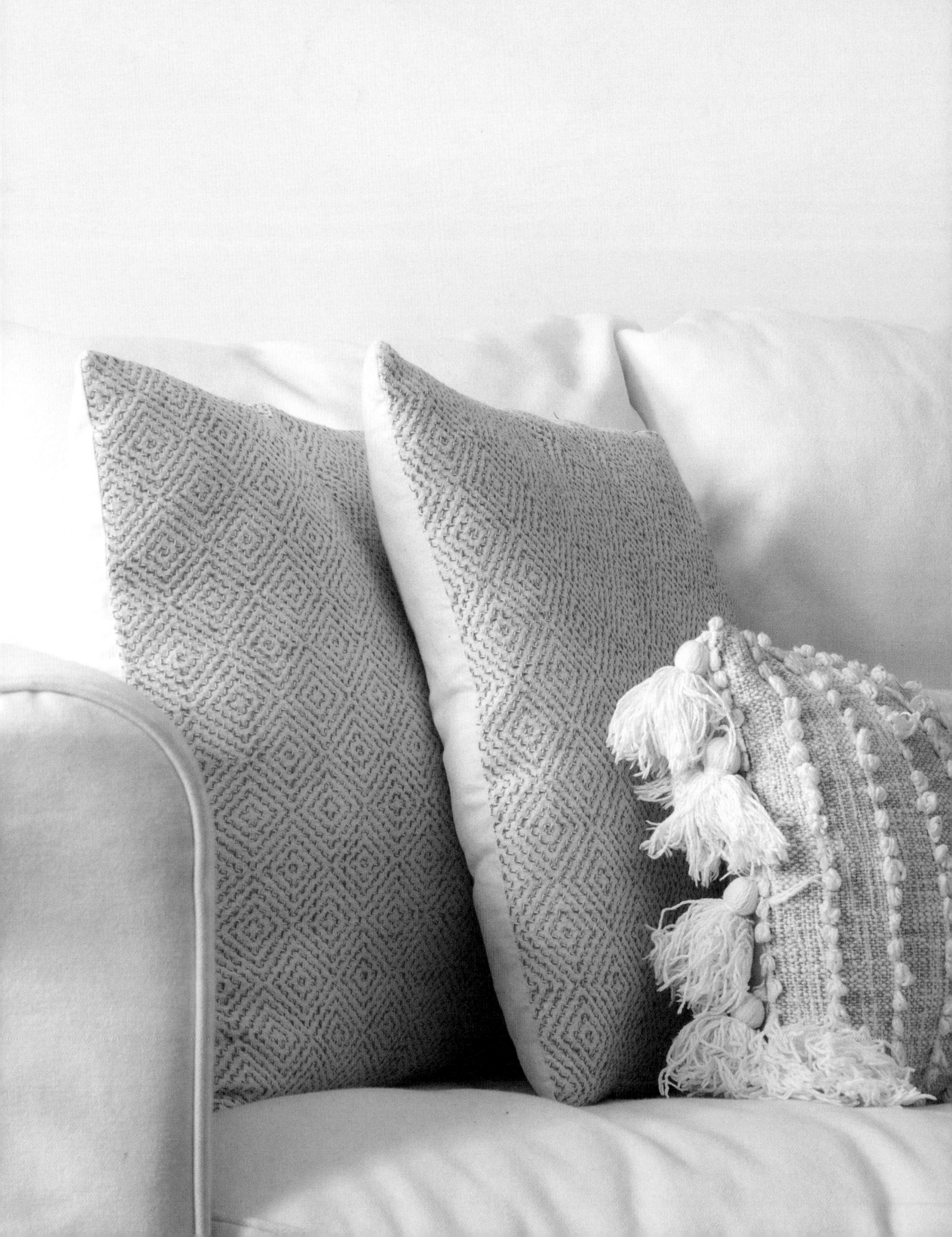

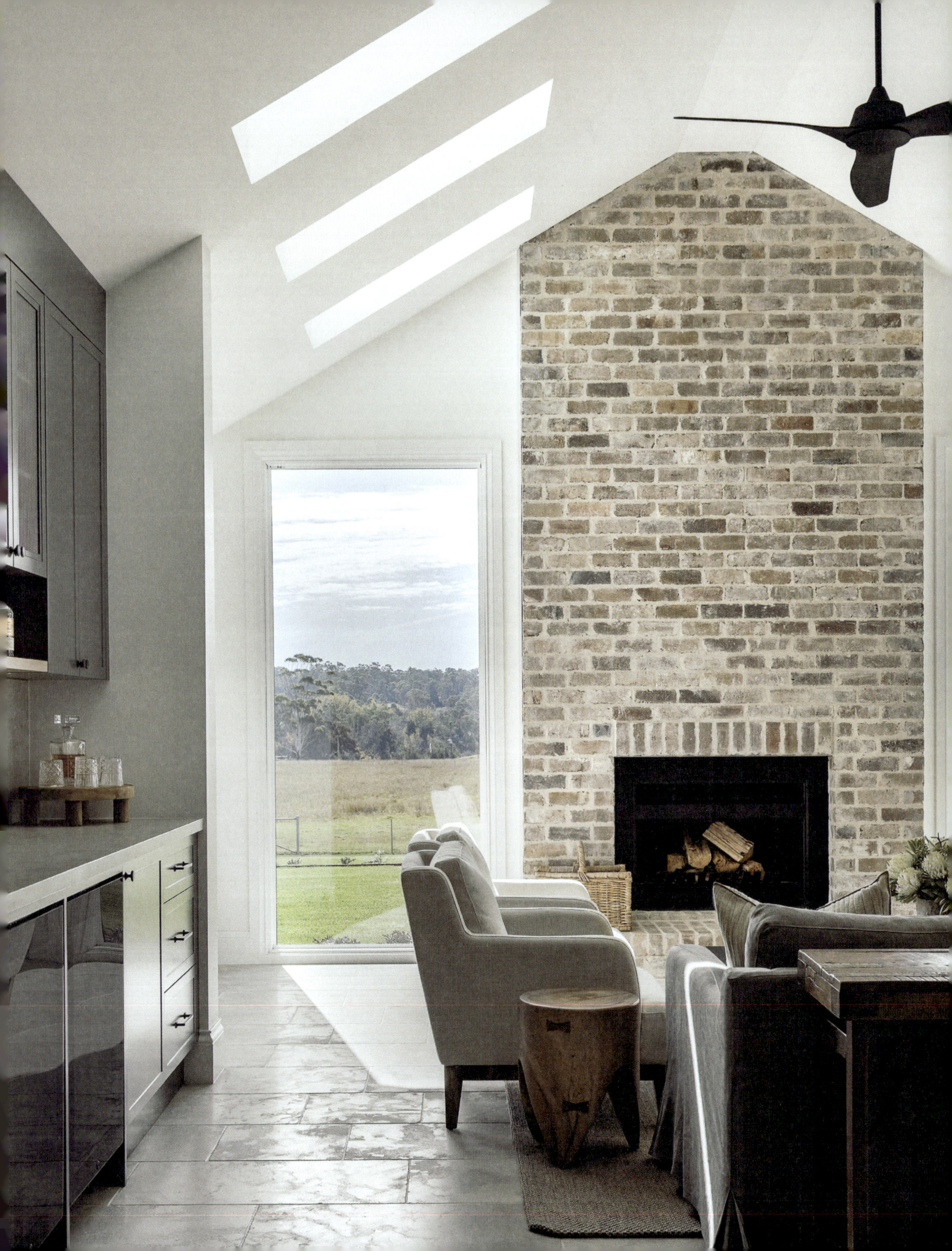

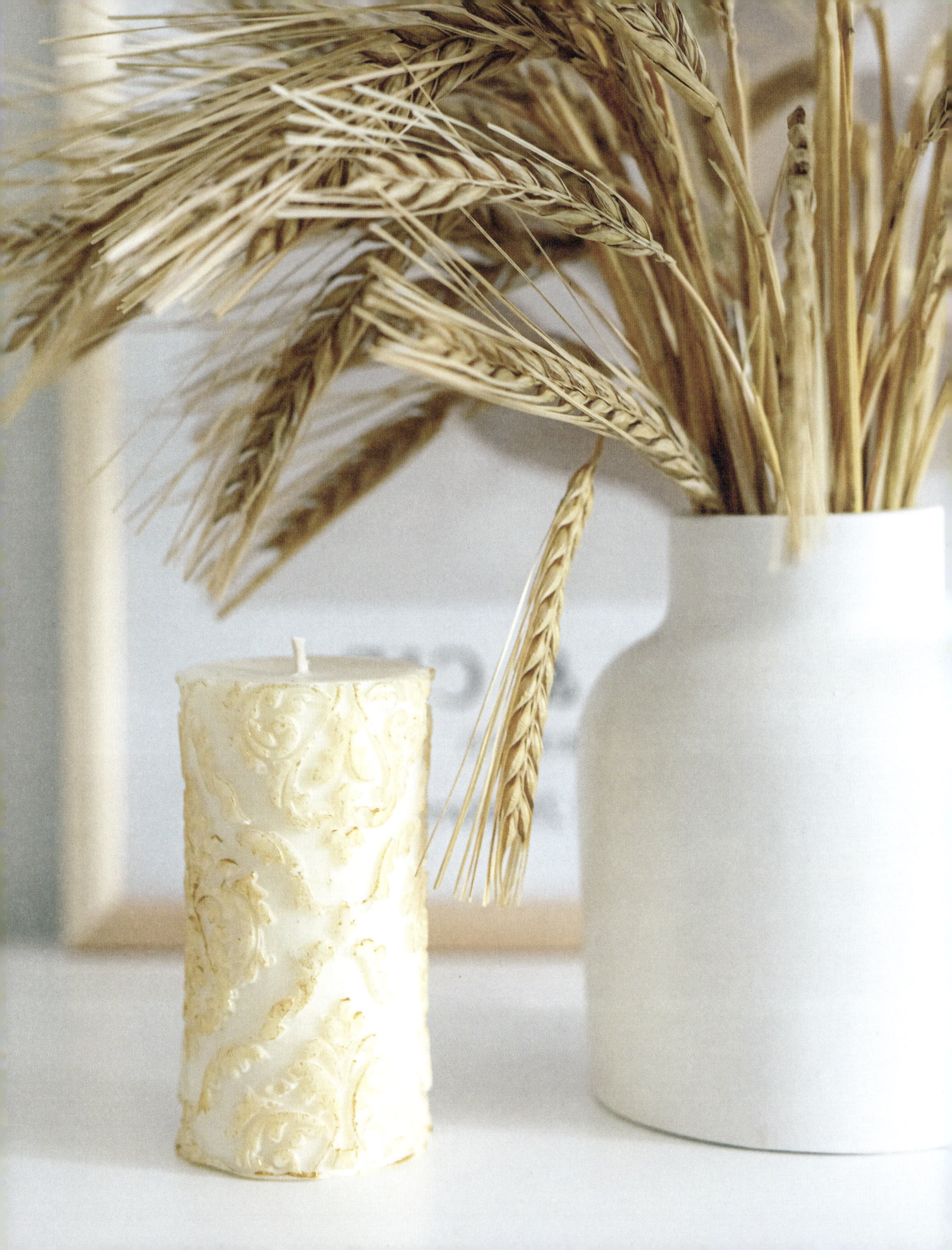

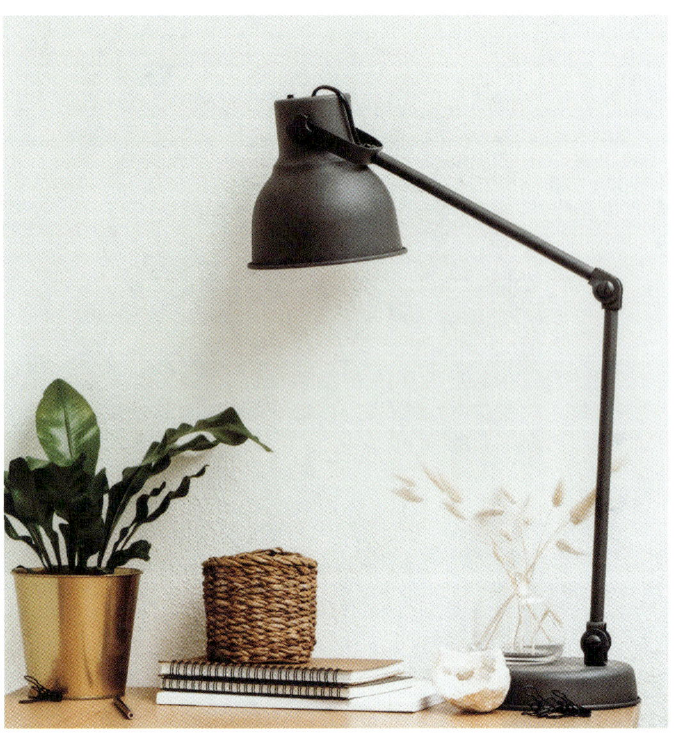

Layers of texture, muted colours and a limewashed timber trunk for a coffee table create a cool-meets-comfort mood in this relaxed living room.

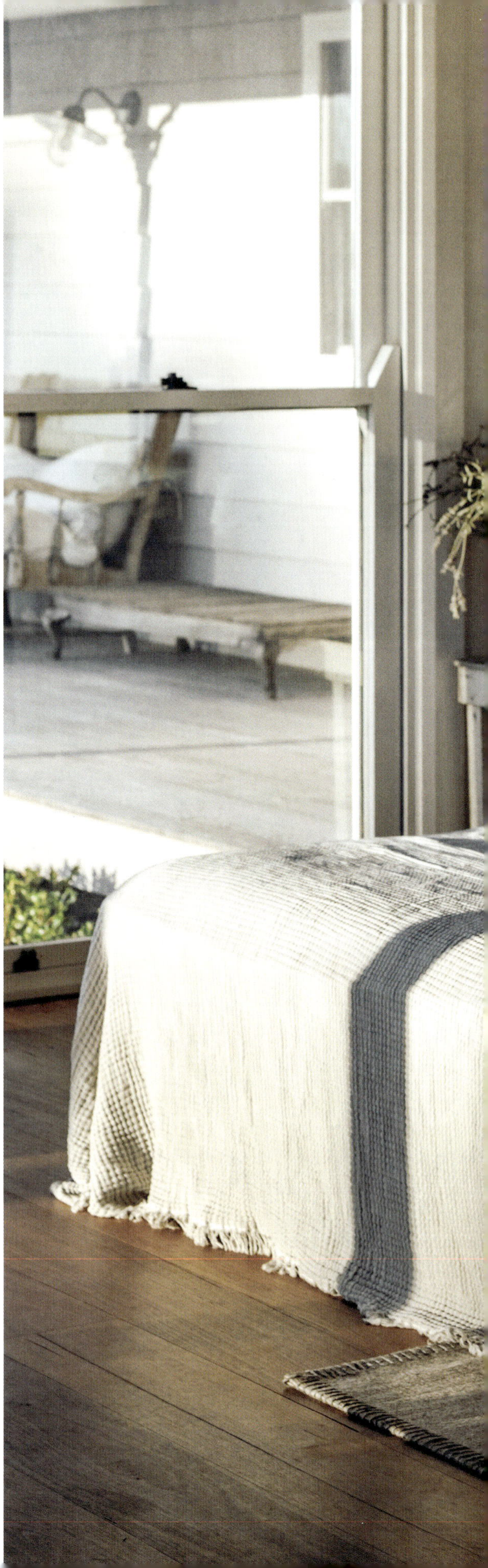

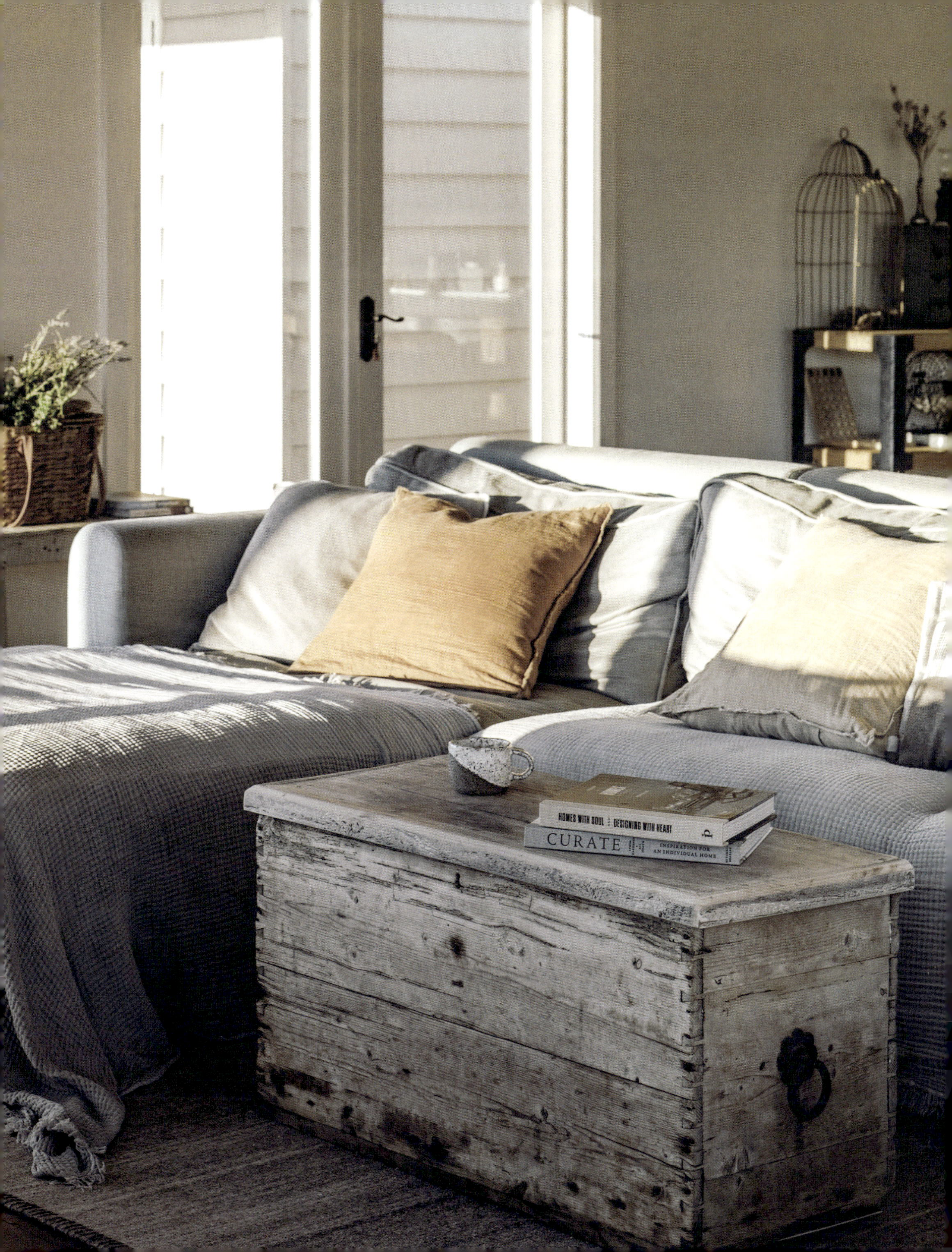
HOMES WITH SOUL
DESIGNING WITH HEART
CURATE
INSPIRATION FOR AN INDIVIDUAL HOME

The living room is the perfect place for candles – and candles are perfect for setting the mood and extending the invitation to linger a while. Vintage candlesticks in cut glass with taper candles set a traditional scene, while pillar candles in clay or stone jars or set on dishes add a more contemporary feel, and often serve up a sweet fragrance too.

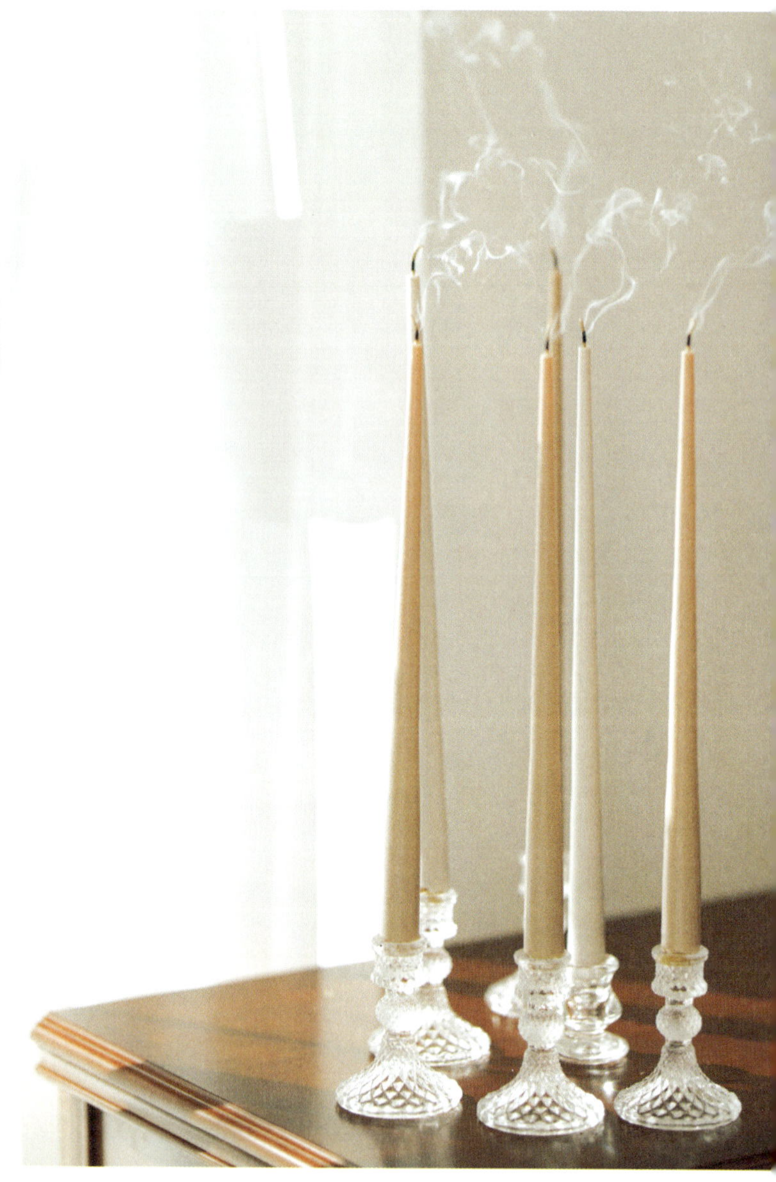

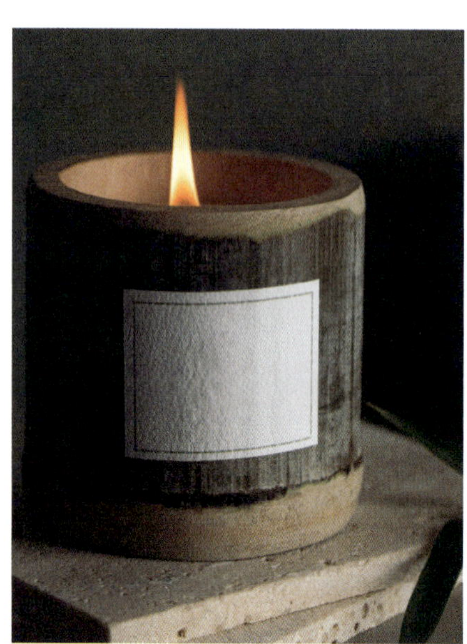

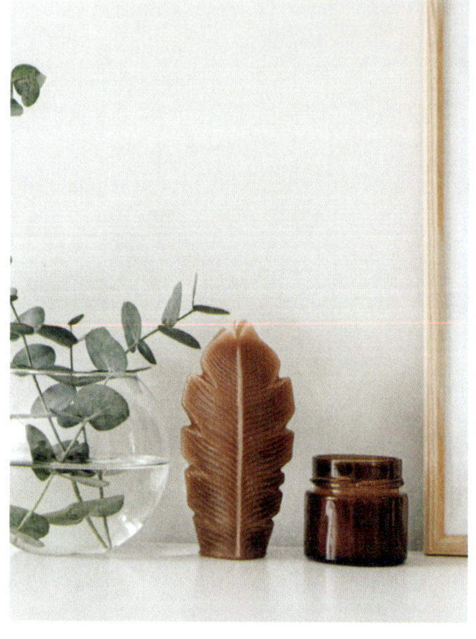

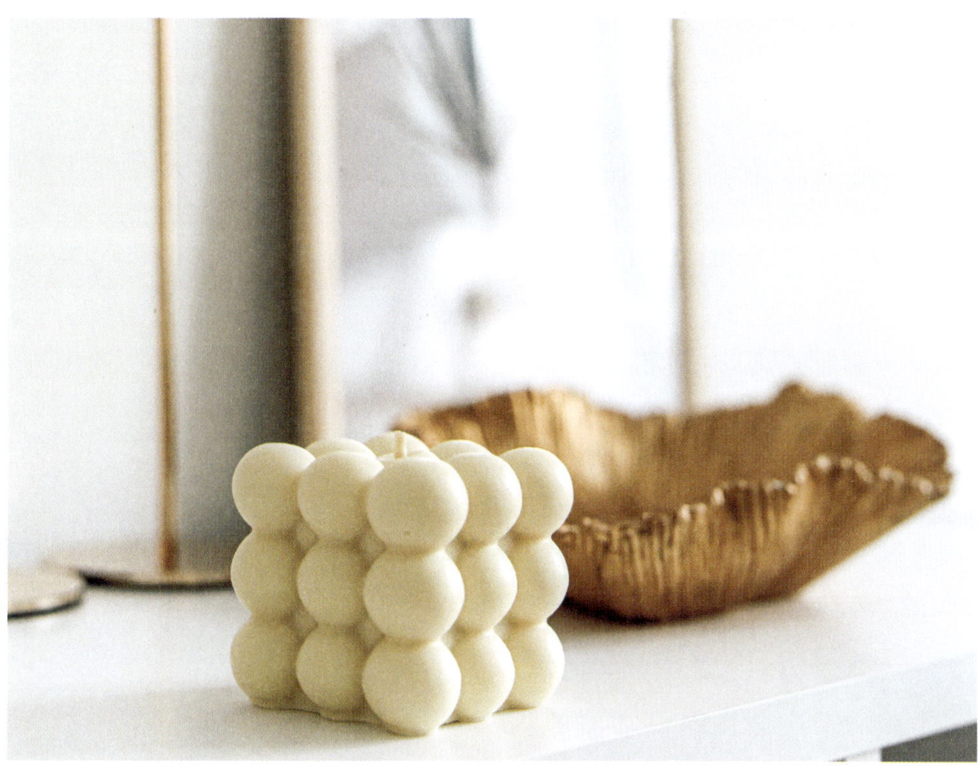

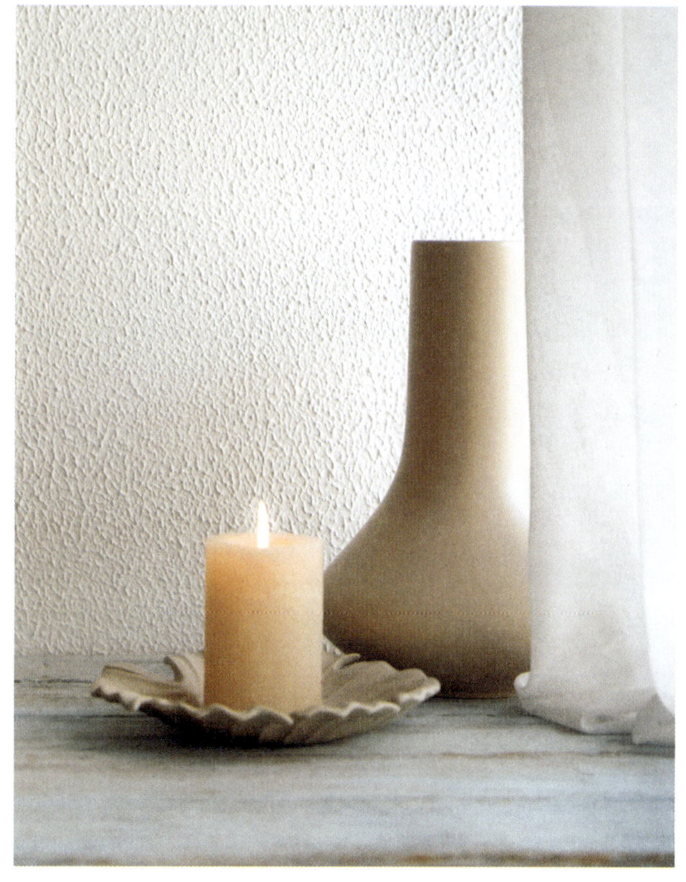

Candles in bold or interesting shapes or colours can easily double as decor elements, especially when grouped with complimentary items.

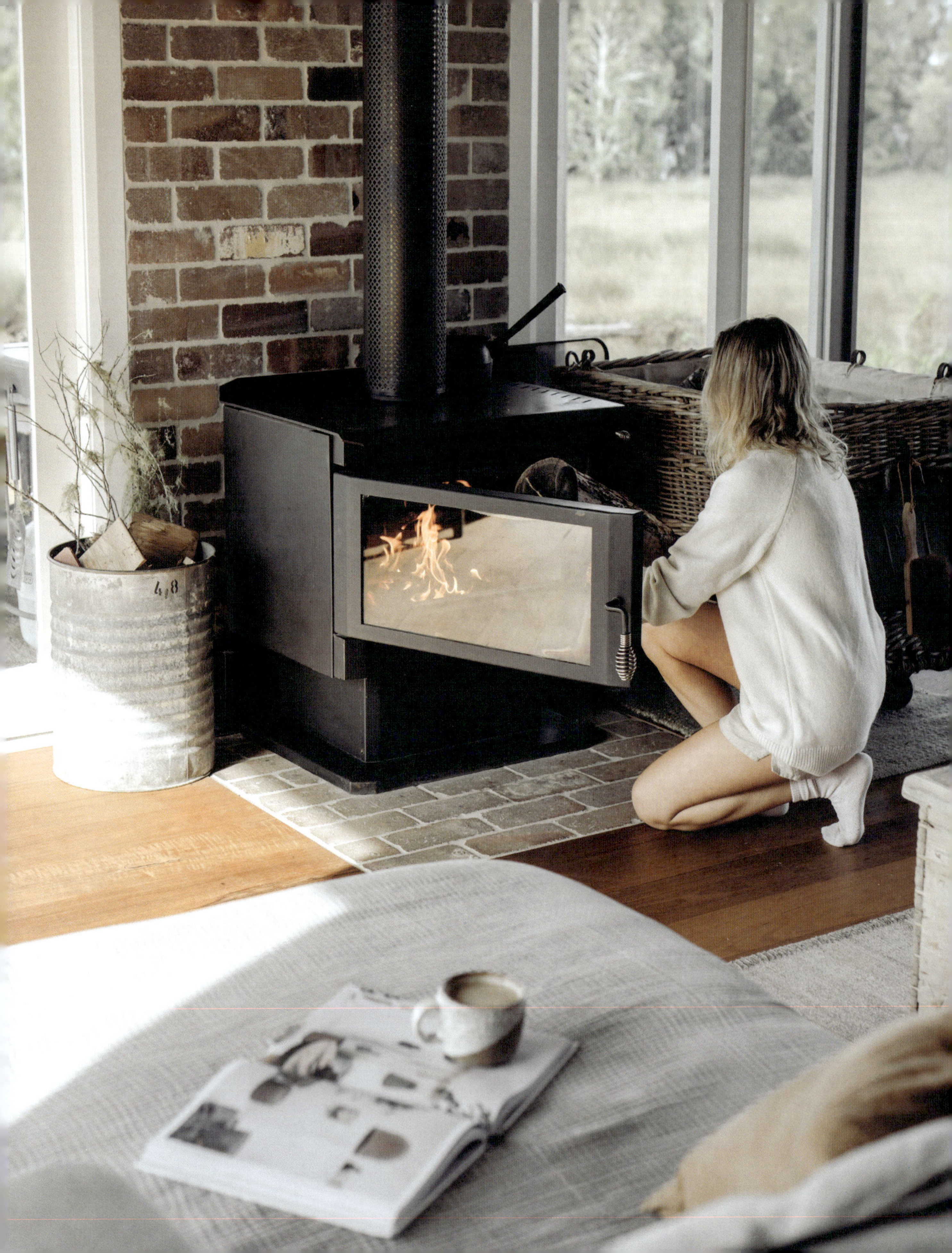
48

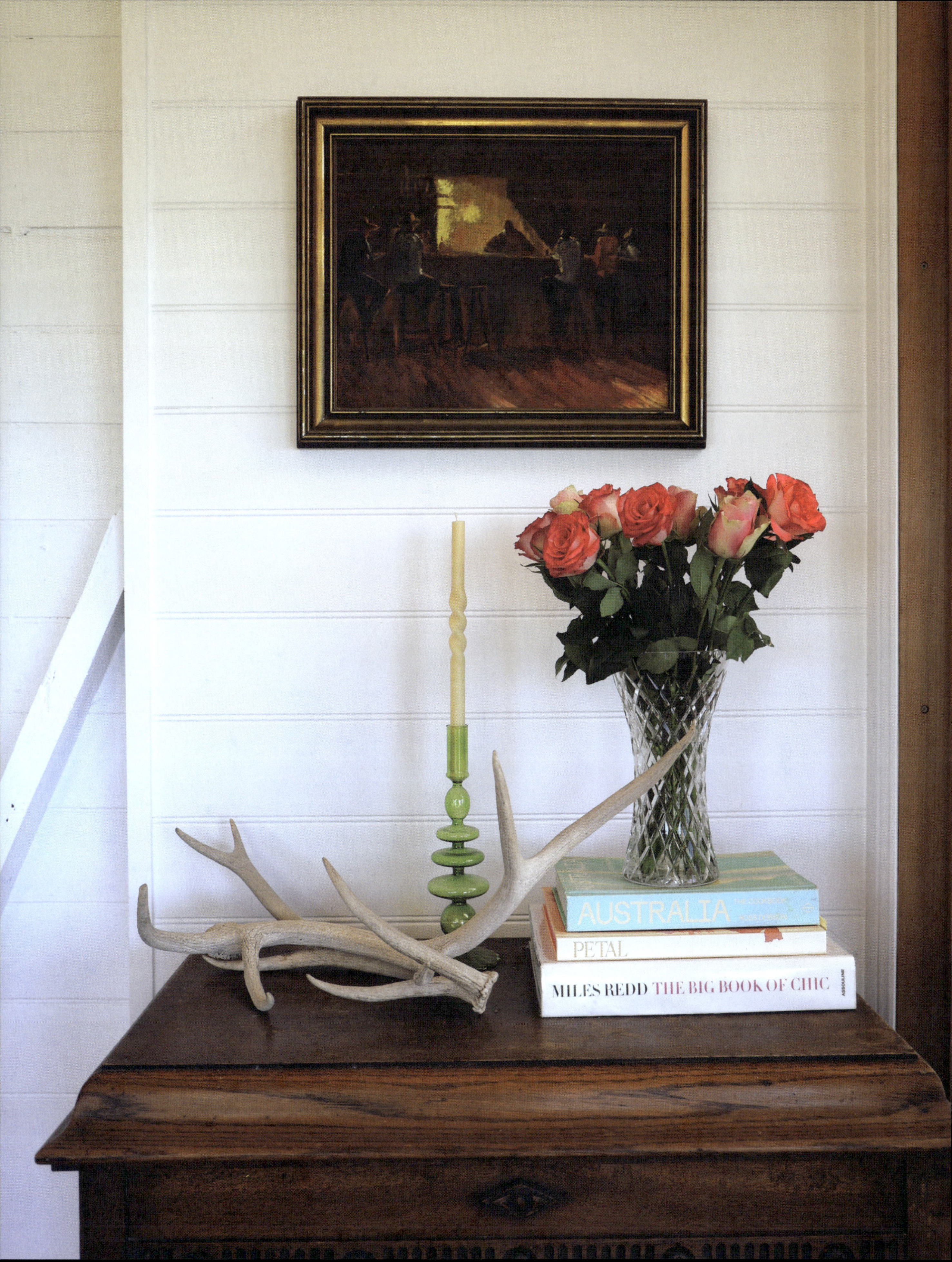
AUSTRALIA
PETAL
MILES REDD THE BIG BOOK OF CHIC

The Quick List

Cowboy boots or hats on display, providing a playful nod to the overall style

Firewood made into a feature

Soft, buttery leather sofas inviting relaxation of body and mind

Book displays on side tables and coffee tables

Easy-to-wash slipcovers providing durability in well-loved living spaces

Paintings or prints of traditional scenes to add an authentic feel

Generously sized area rugs to help unify spaces

Storage trunks that double as coffee tables

'Moments' created for pausing to reflect on your treasured books and other display items

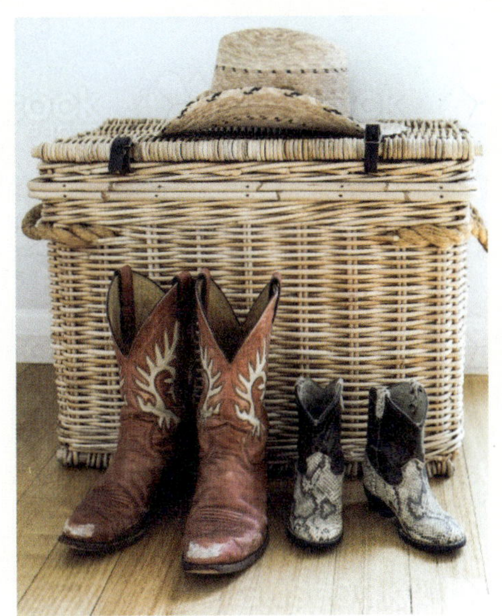

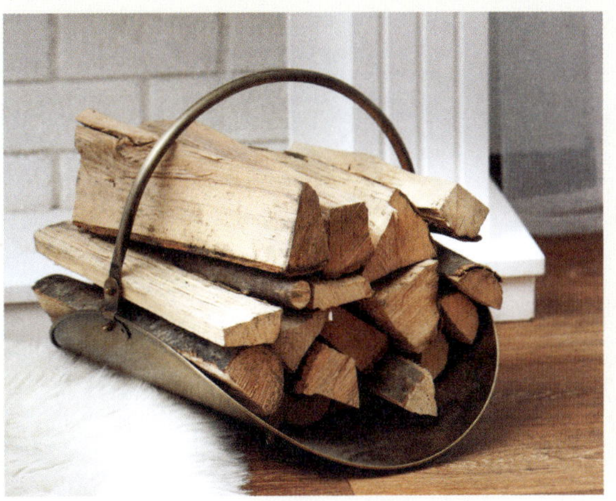

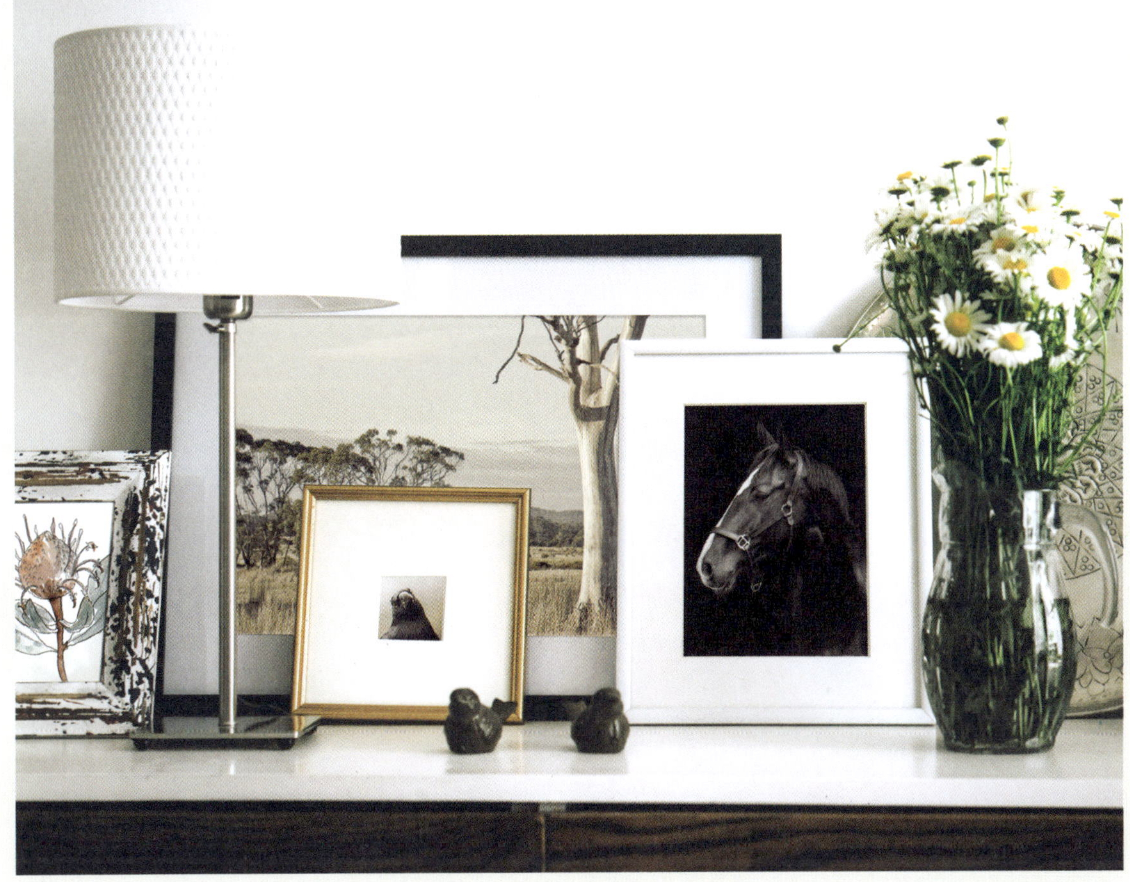

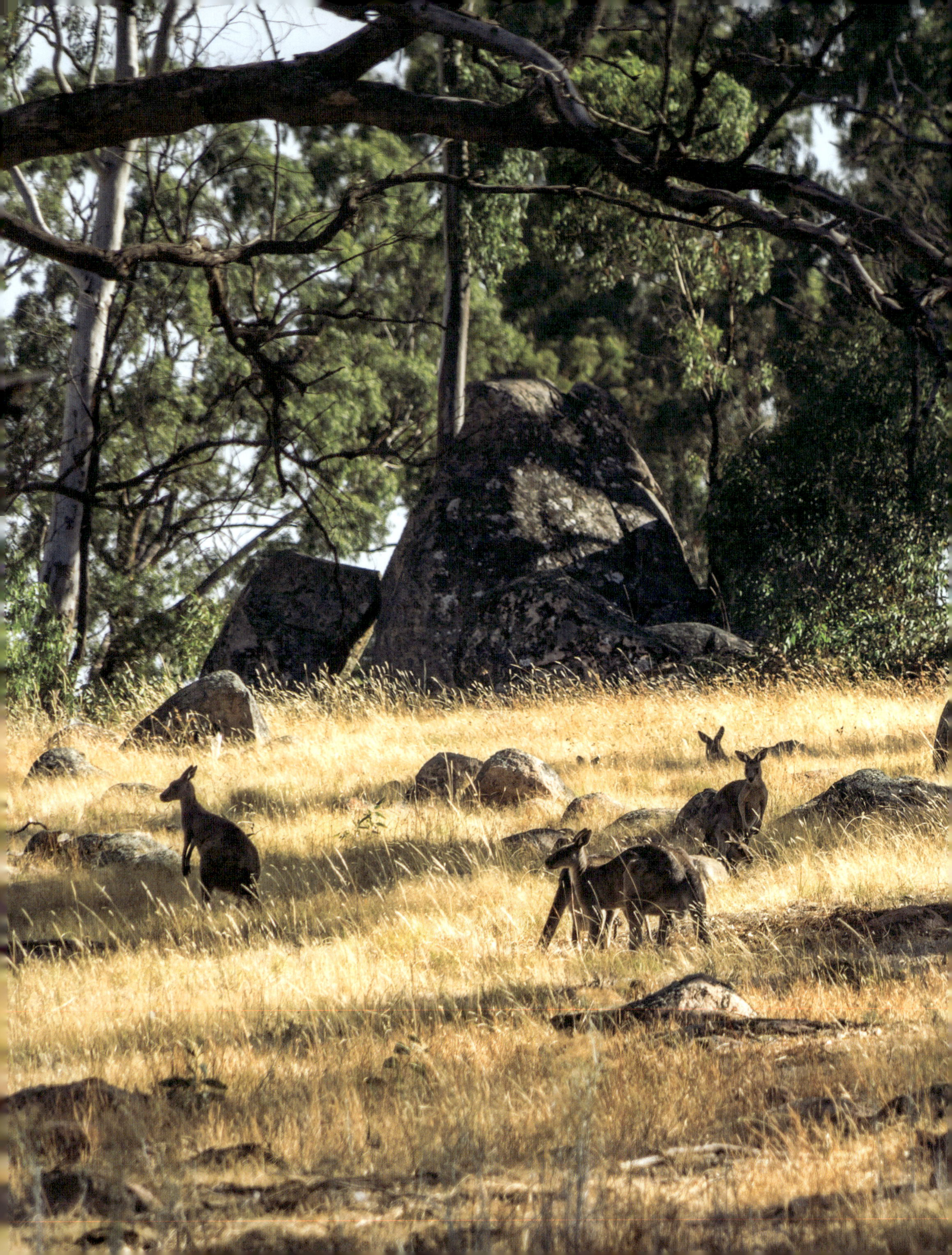

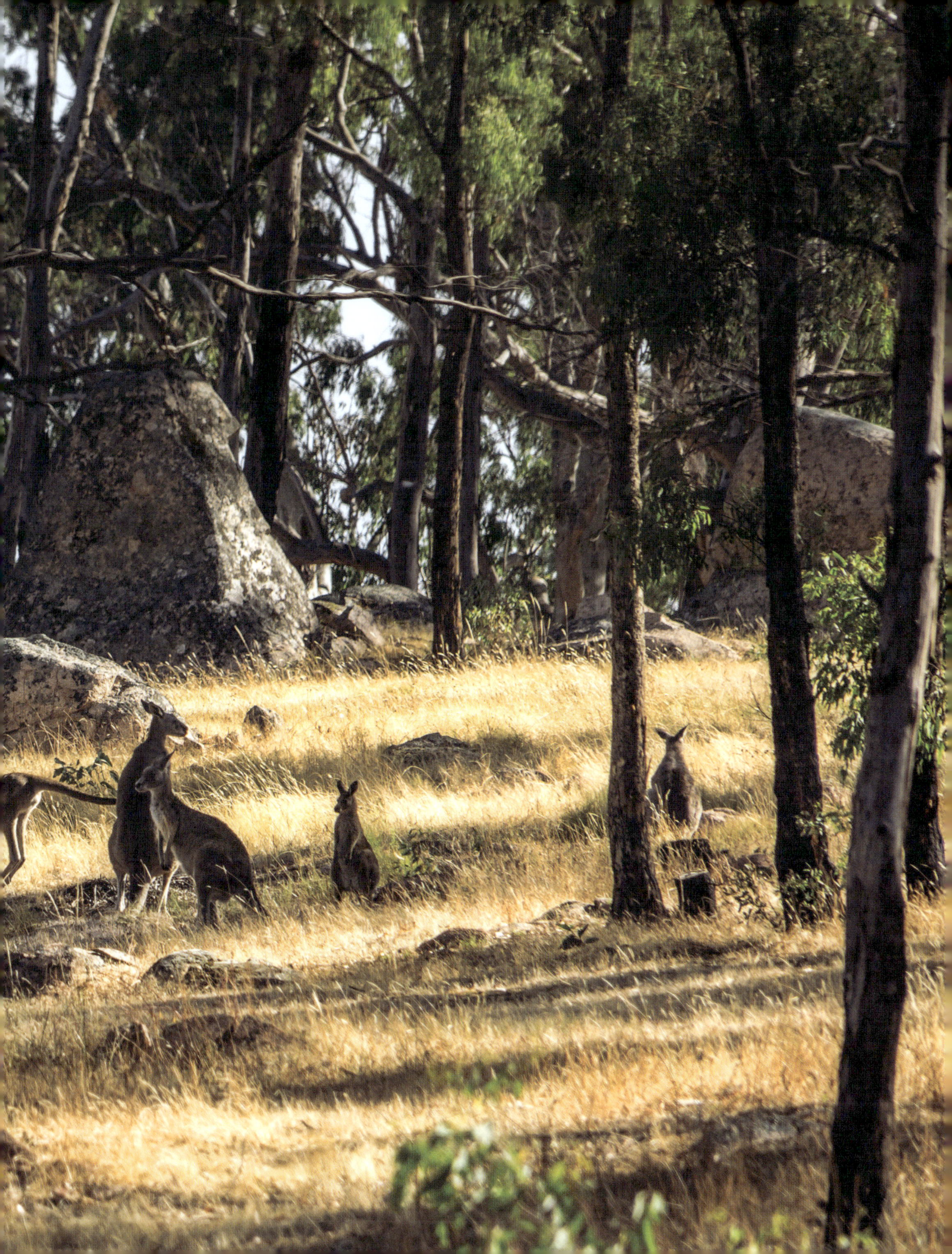

chapter four

sleeping

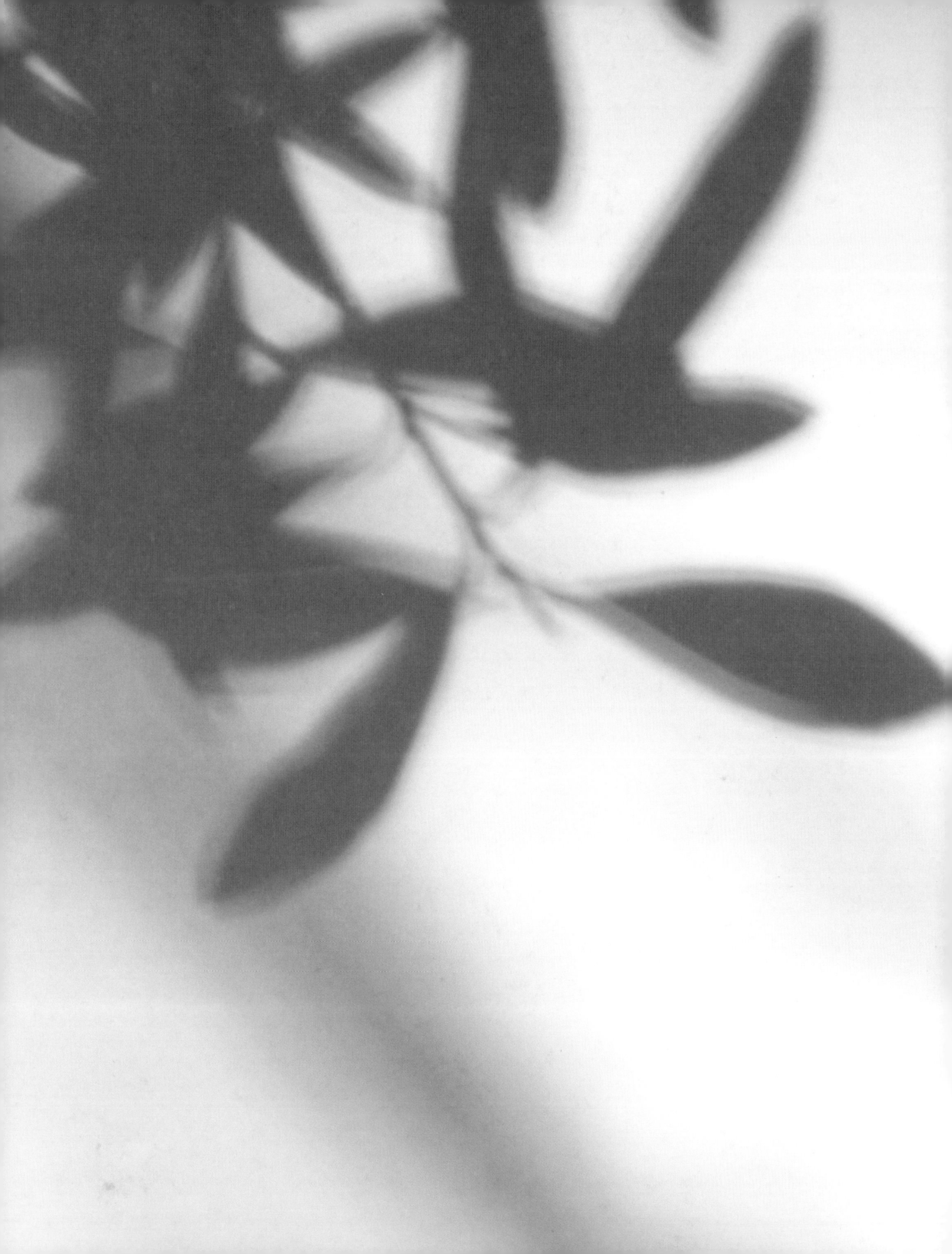

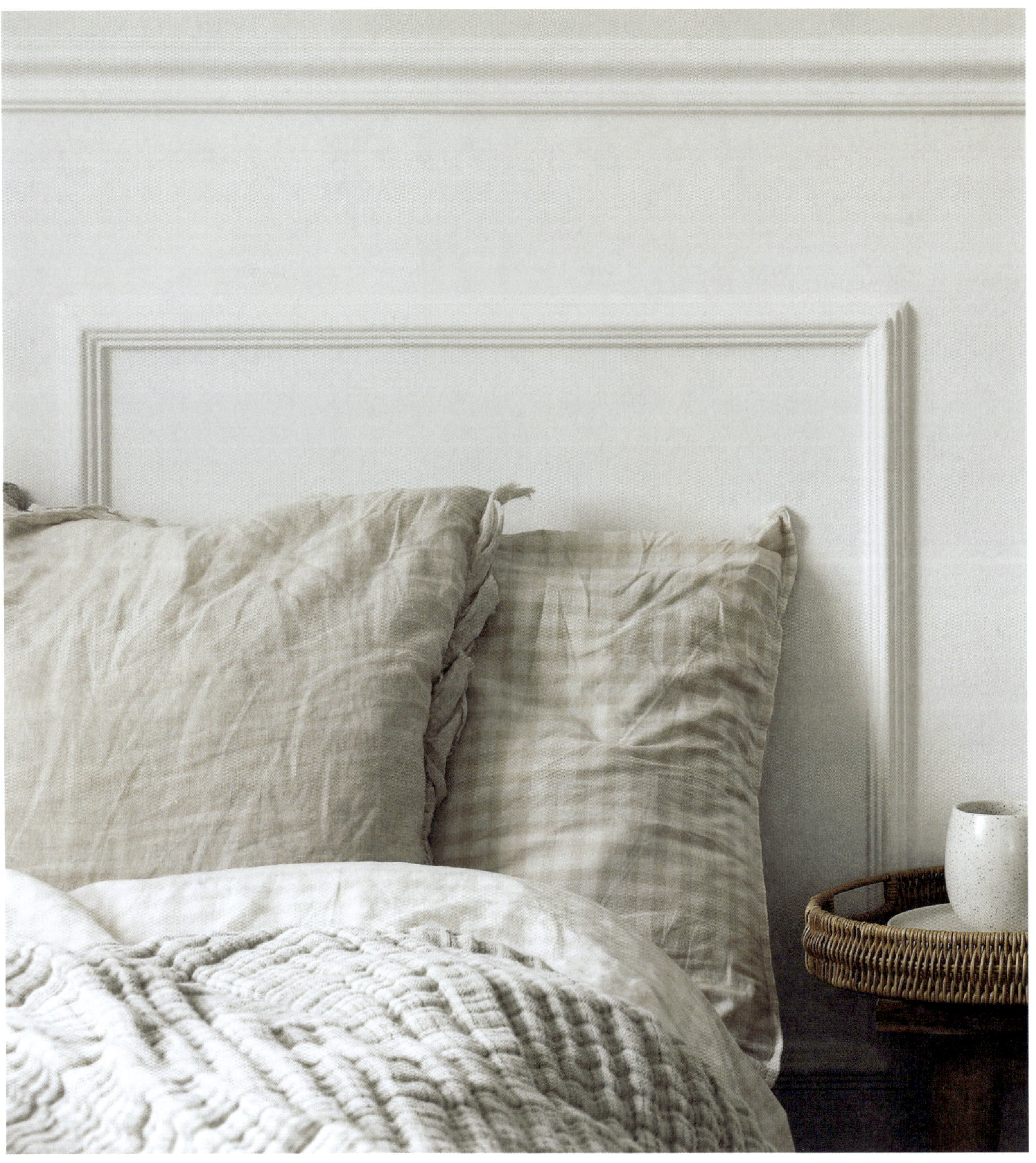

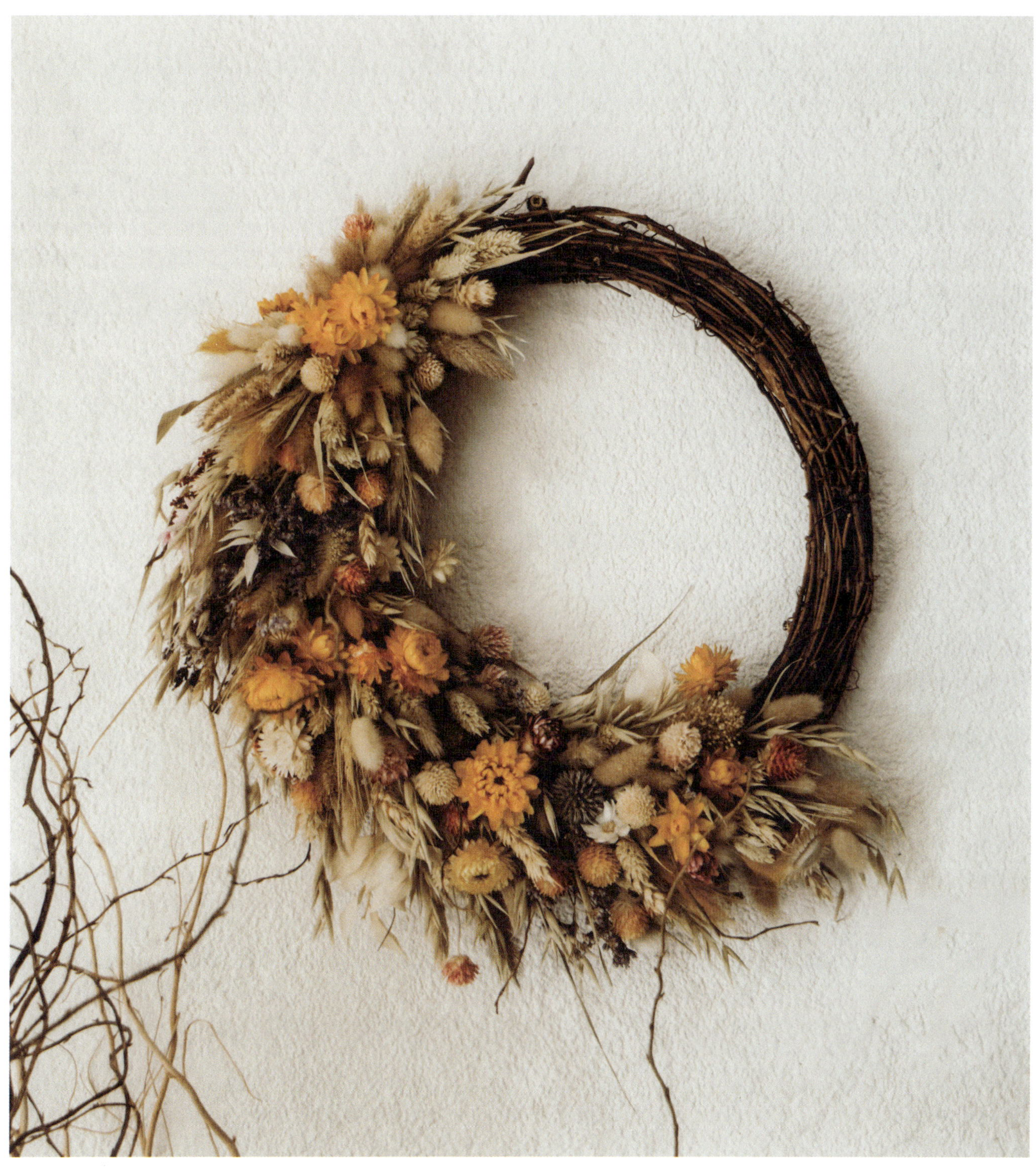

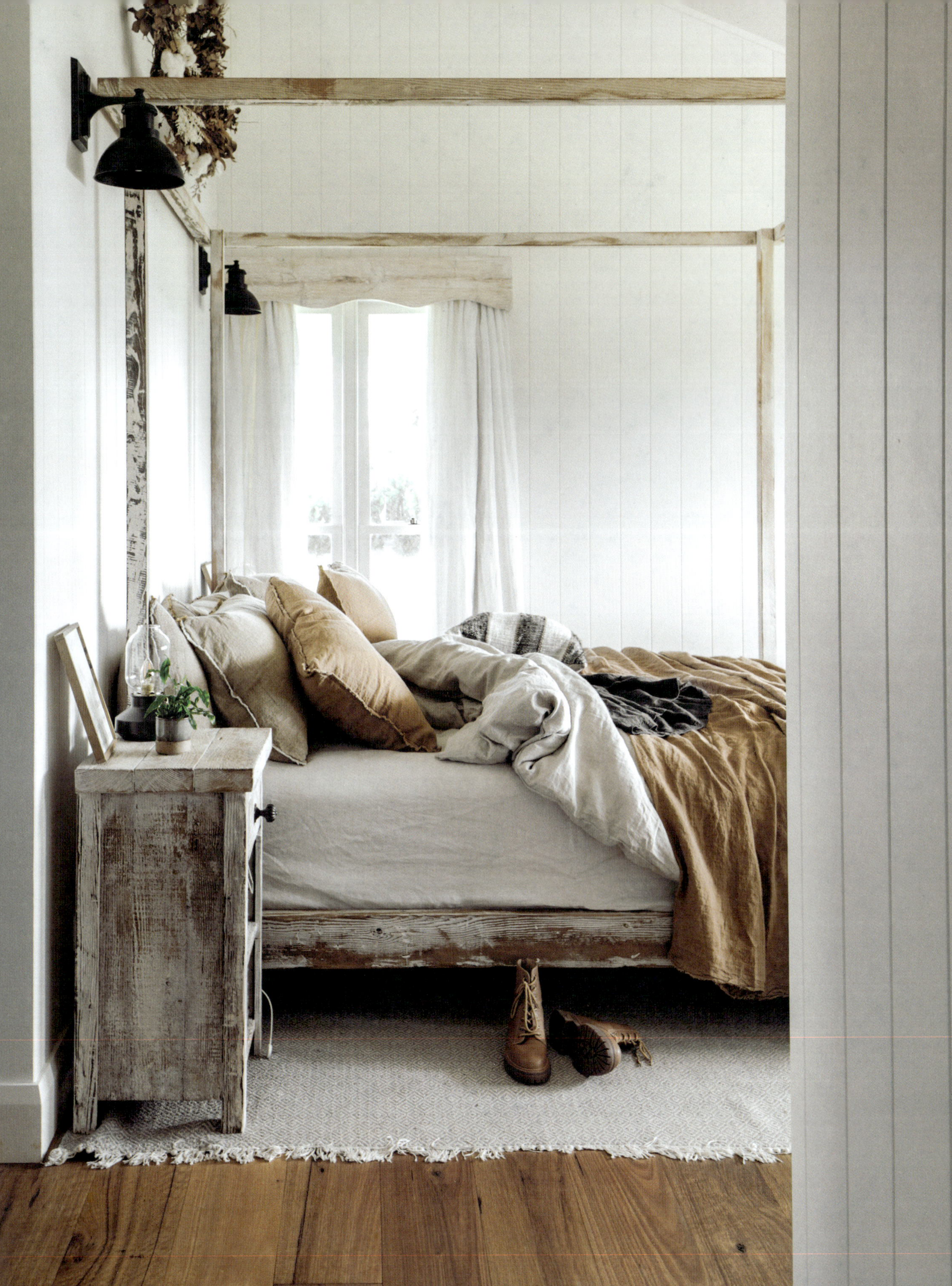

Where we rest and sleep is important. Ideally, it's a haven, providing rare peaceful moments away from work or the kids or both. It's an end-of-the-day moment to ourselves.

A bedroom in the modern country style will contain many elements common to any well-styled bedroom, including maximum use of natural light, layered soft furnishings, well-considered mood lighting, cute personal touches and the best bed linen you can afford.

Create a cohesive look by extending the key styling elements from the rest of your home, while allowing the bedroom to be the place where you add a little extra flair to express your personality. Family photos, dairies or journals, beloved items of decor or flowers, a quirky bedside light or alarm clock are all perfect styling choices.

The centrepiece of any bedroom – the bed – is always going to be an important styling decision. Traditionally a cast-iron, farmhouse-style bed would be a gimme for country style, but in the modern variation of the style that's not the case. Keep with the theme of natural materials, such as wicker or timber (consider softer timbers or finishes such as the limewash shown here), mixed with metal elements and you won't go far wrong.

In the bedroom, soft palettes of greys, greens and blues help create a relaxing vibe. Floral accents are popular, either in the furnishings or with flowers on display, fresh or dried. Candles, similarly, create a nod to the past but can be displayed in simple contemporary holders with scents like eucalyptus or lemongrass keeping the air fresh.

In the kids' rooms, vintage teddies or toys are a super-sweet way to evoke days gone by, and fit the style perfectly.

For maximum cosiness in the bedroom, don't forget plenty of pillows, cushions, throws and rugs, essential underfoot on timber floors.

TOP FIVE

1.

The right bed

2.

A calming colour palette

3.

Natural light and
feature lighting

4.

Personal touches

5.

A pure focus on comfort

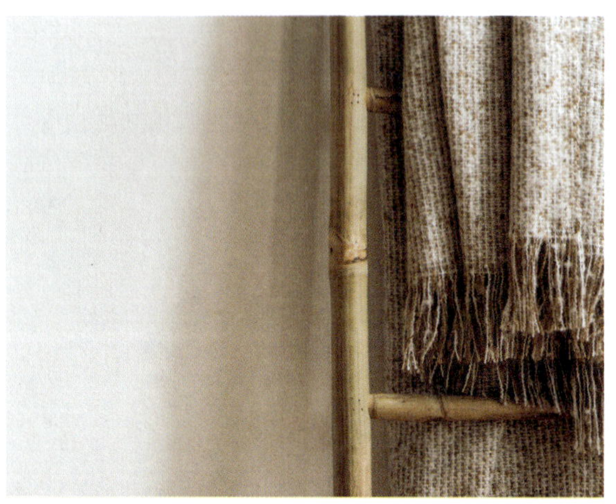

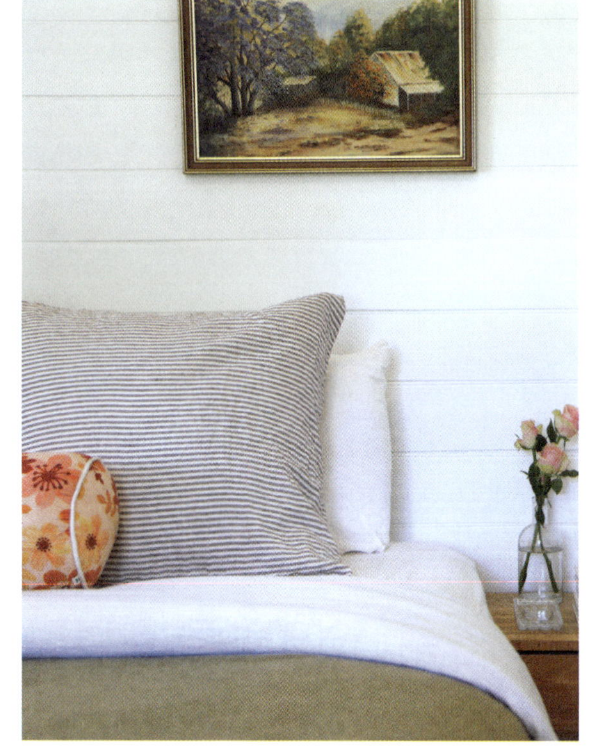

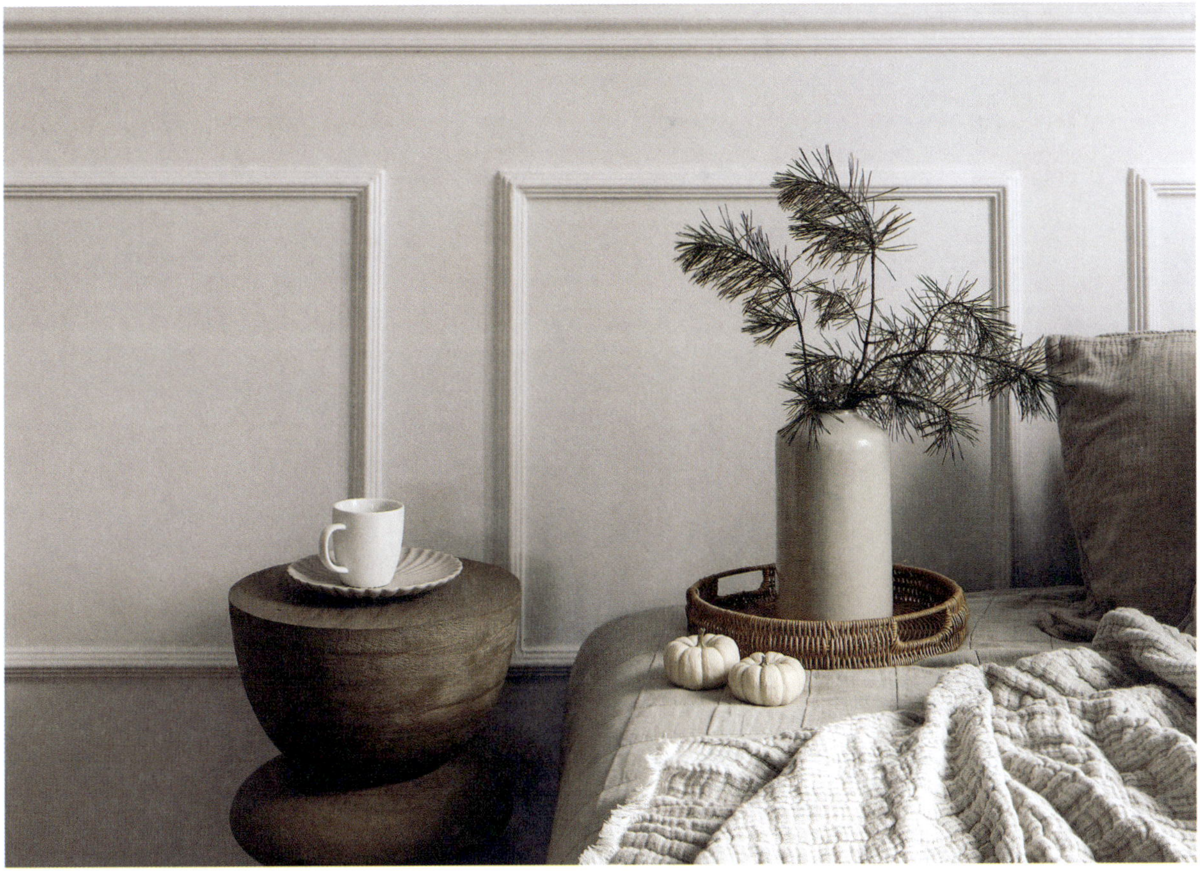

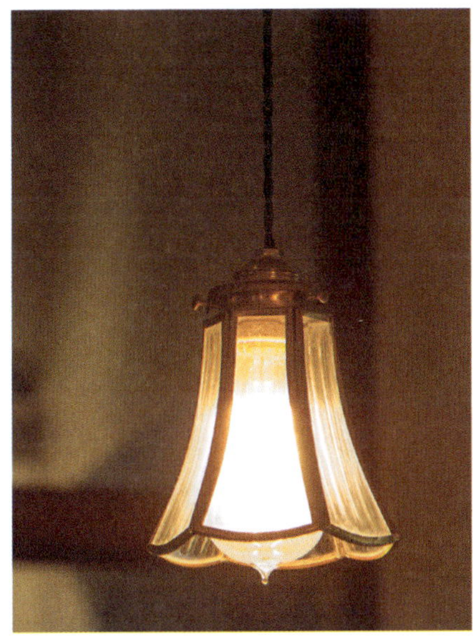

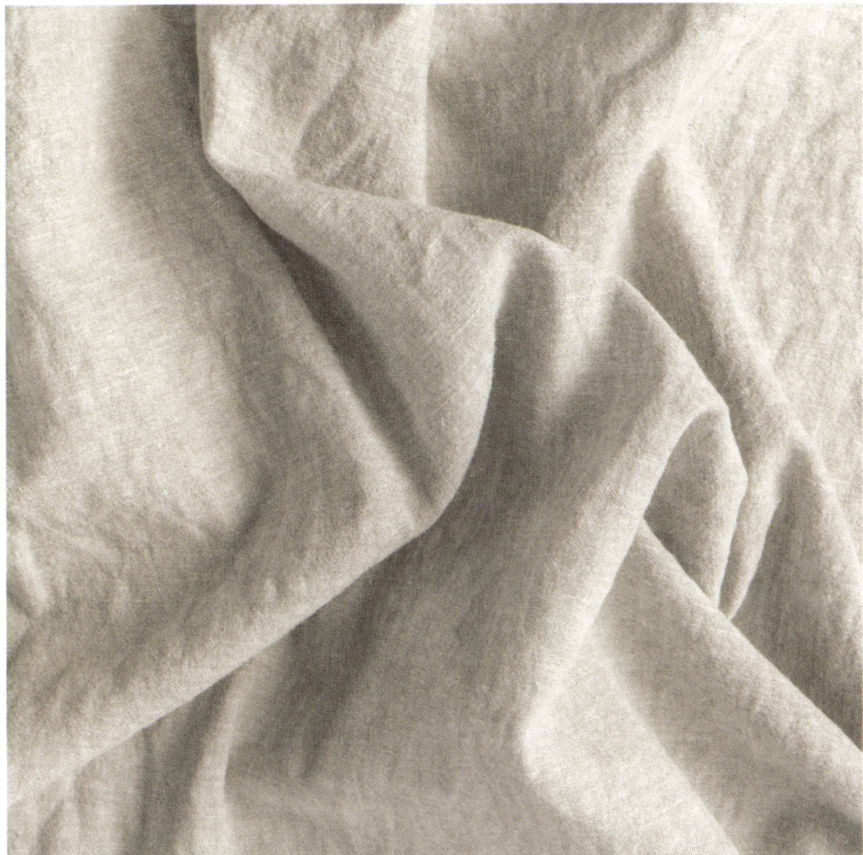

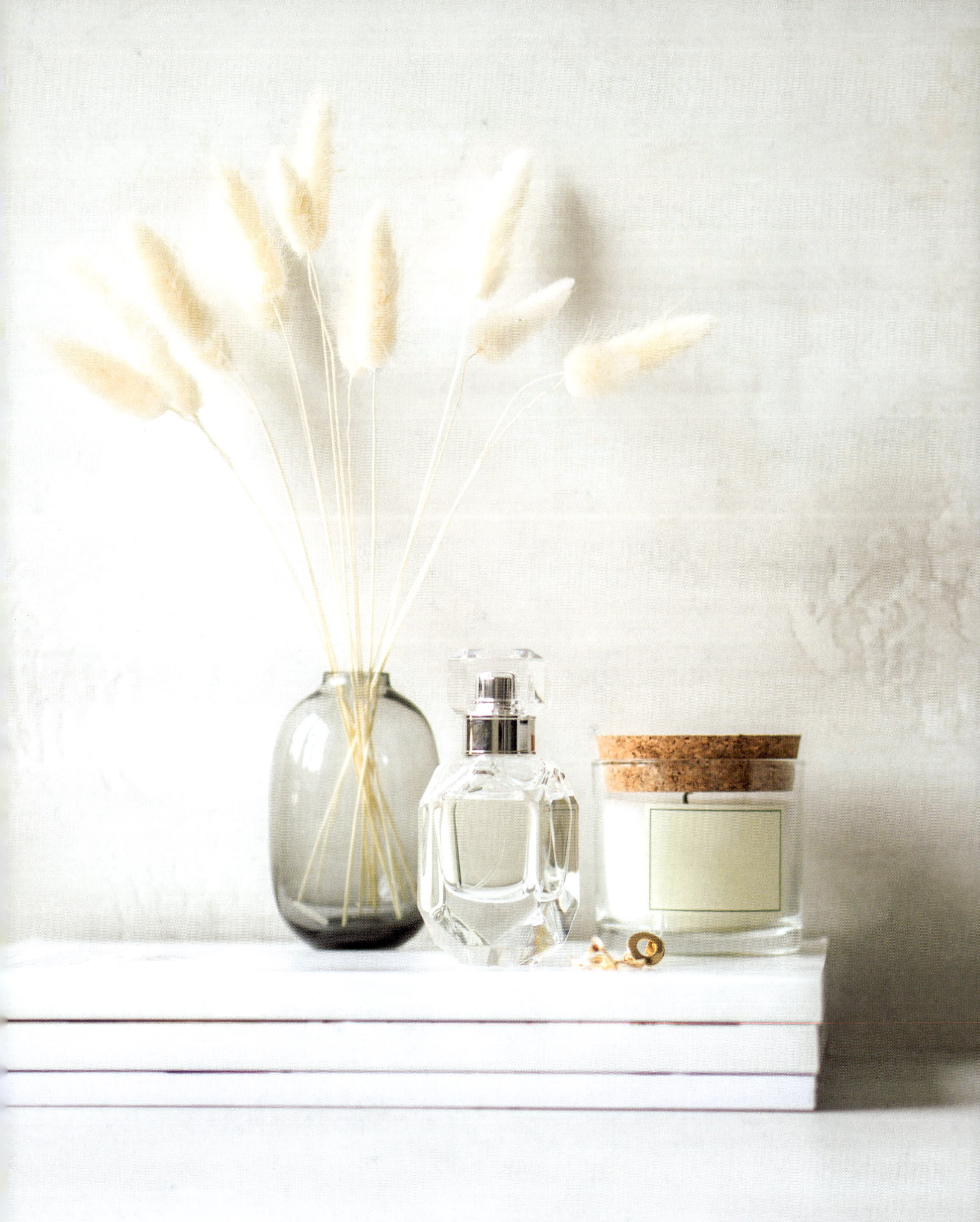

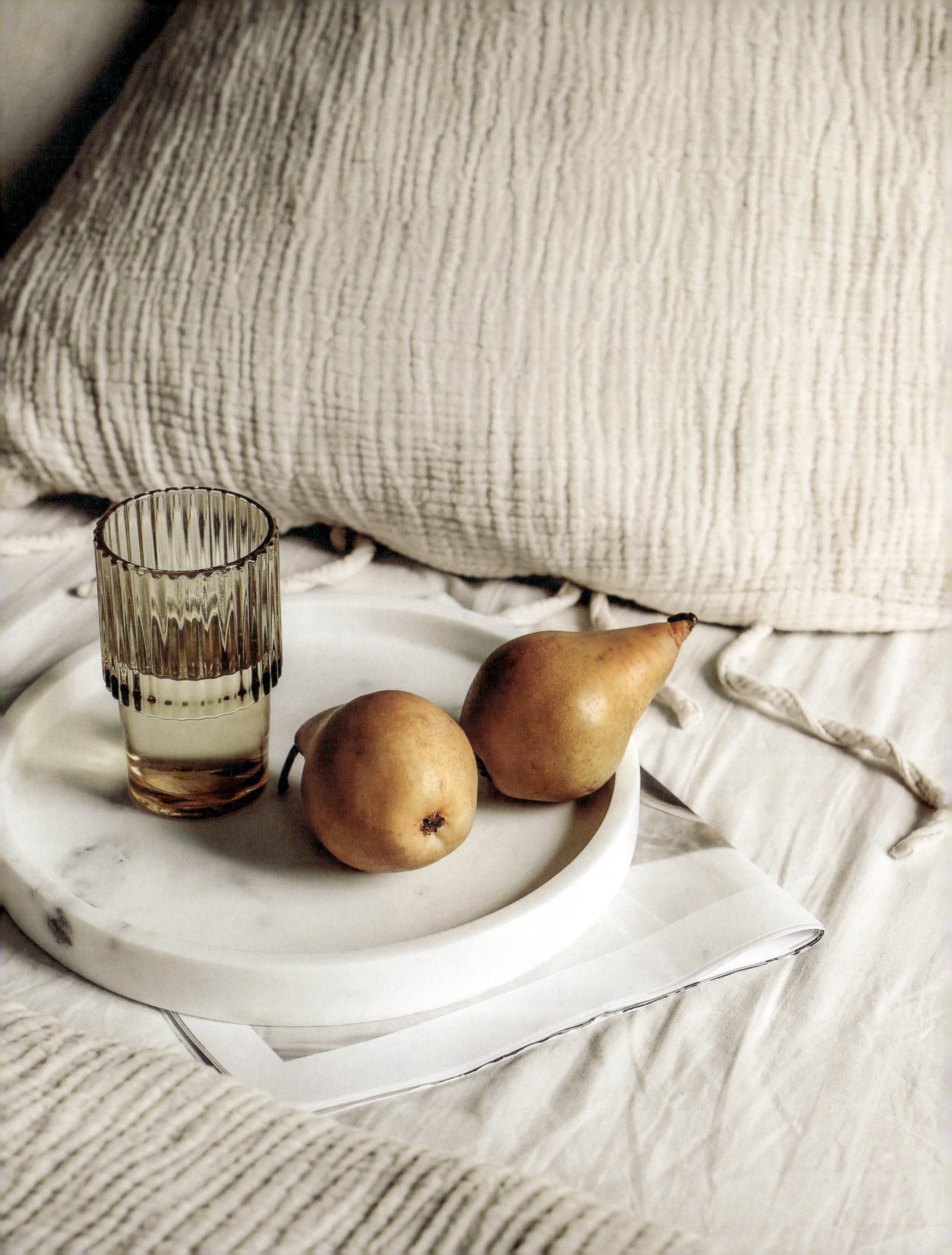

Create a sweet and simple bedside display with the help of a couple of well-chosen coffee-table books. A vintage candlestick holder and glassware complete the look in this scene – but whatever your treasured items are, they will look special in this spot.

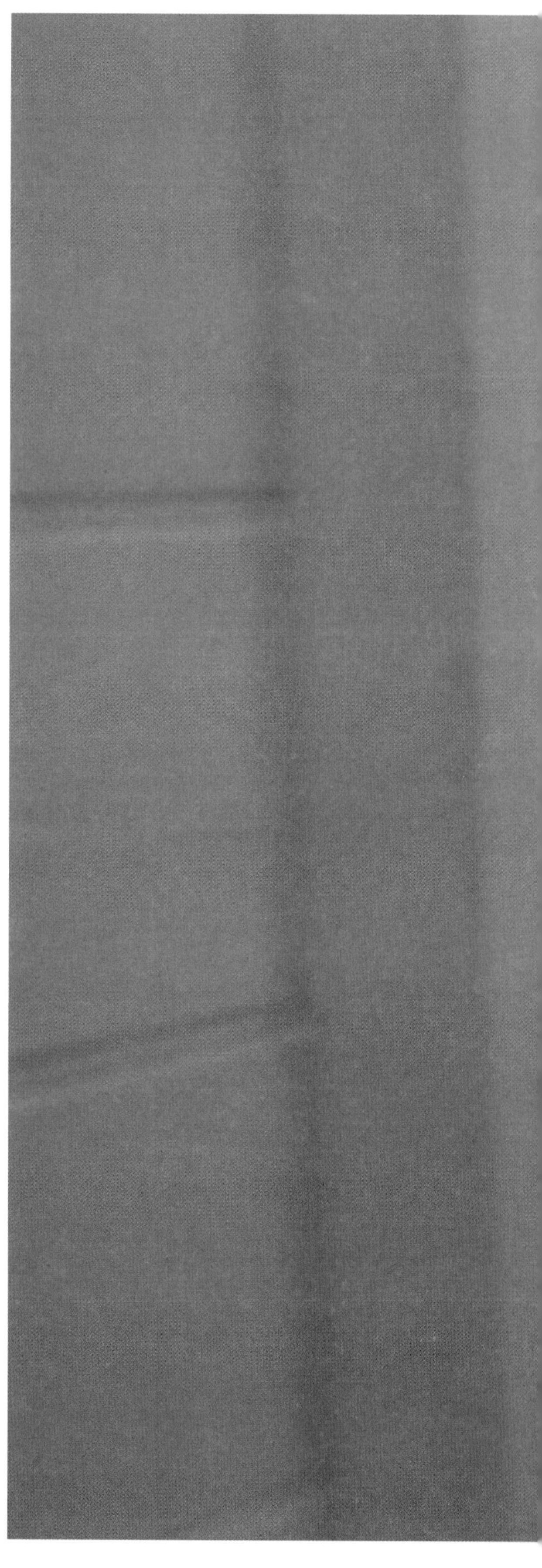

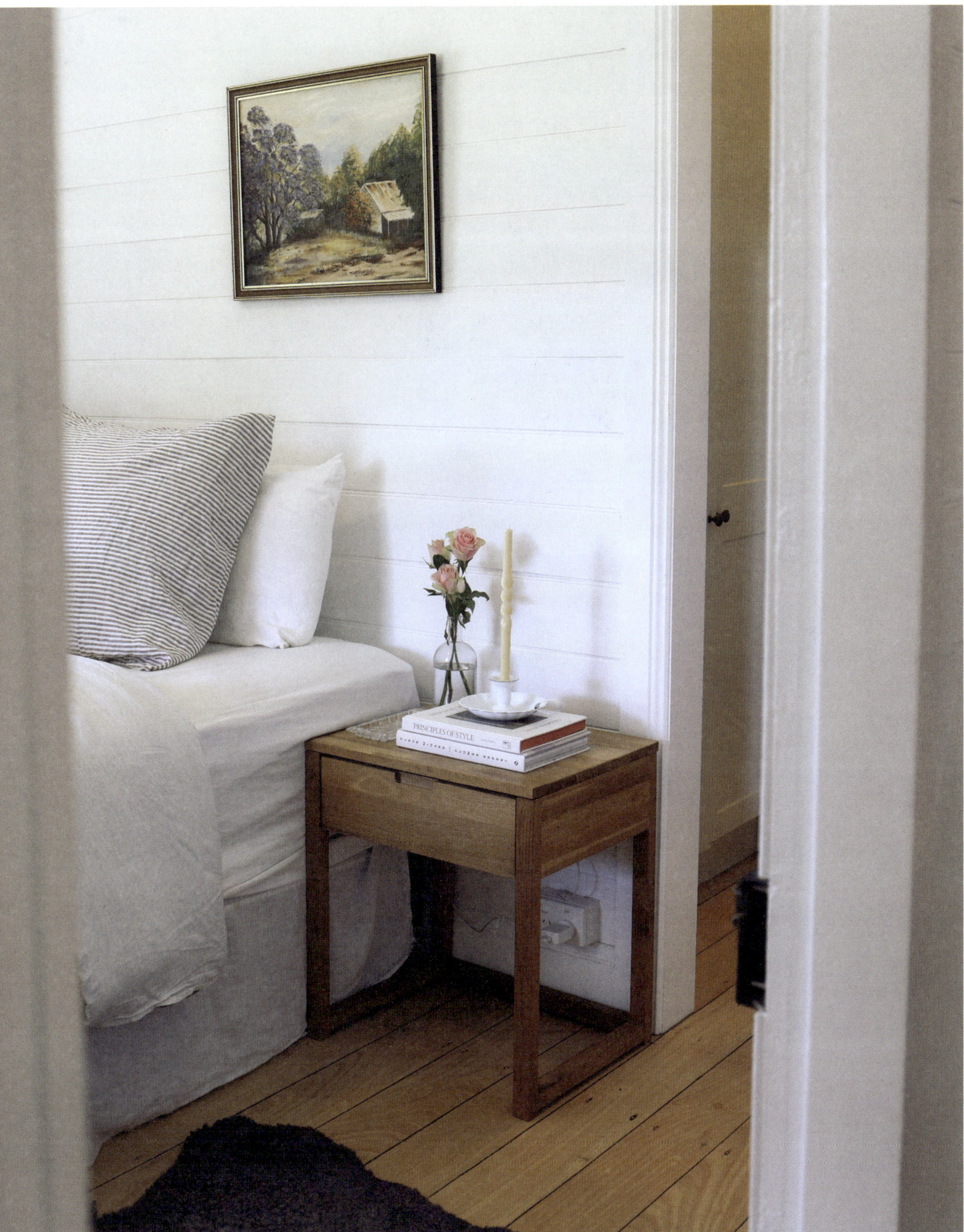
PRINCIPLES OF STYLE

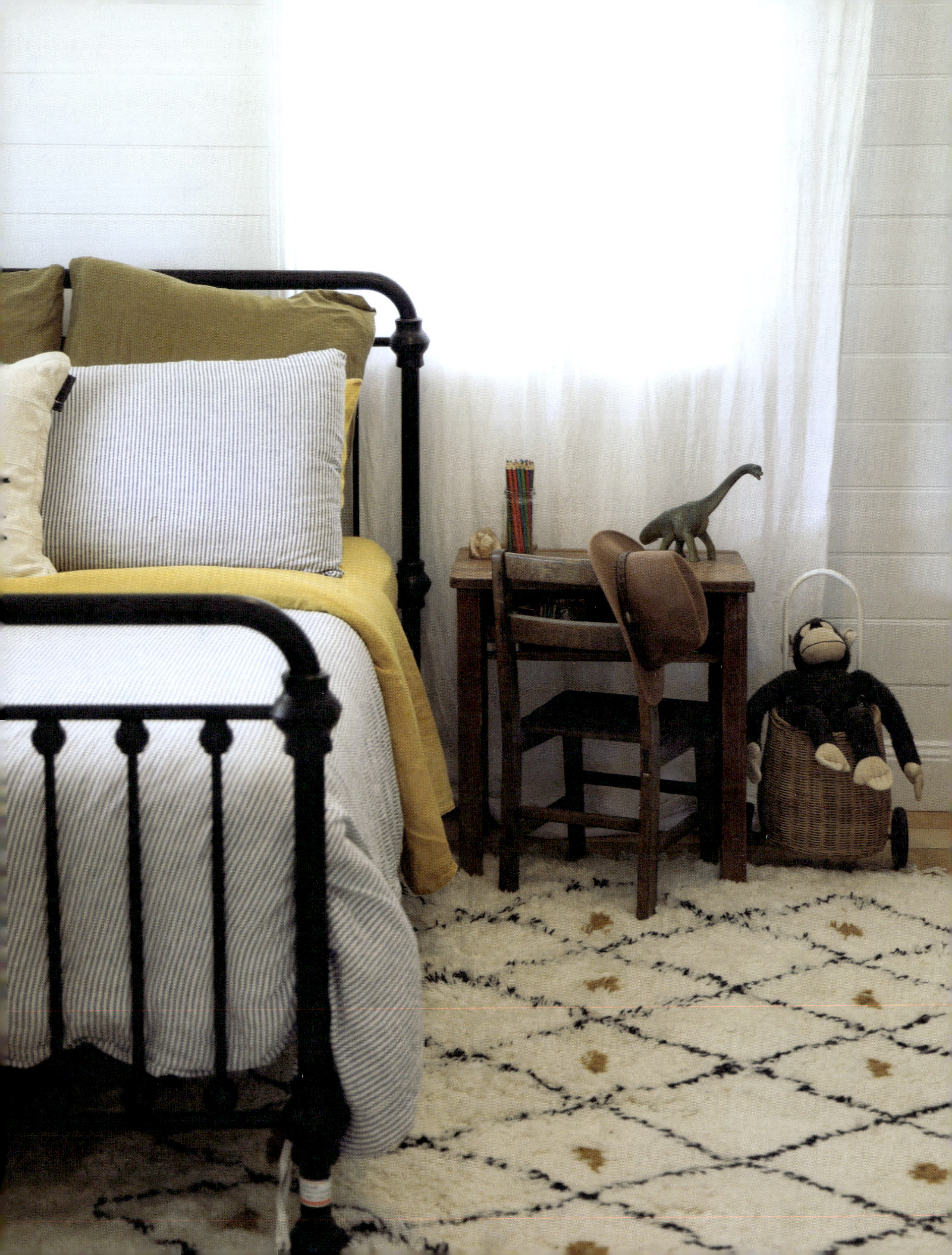

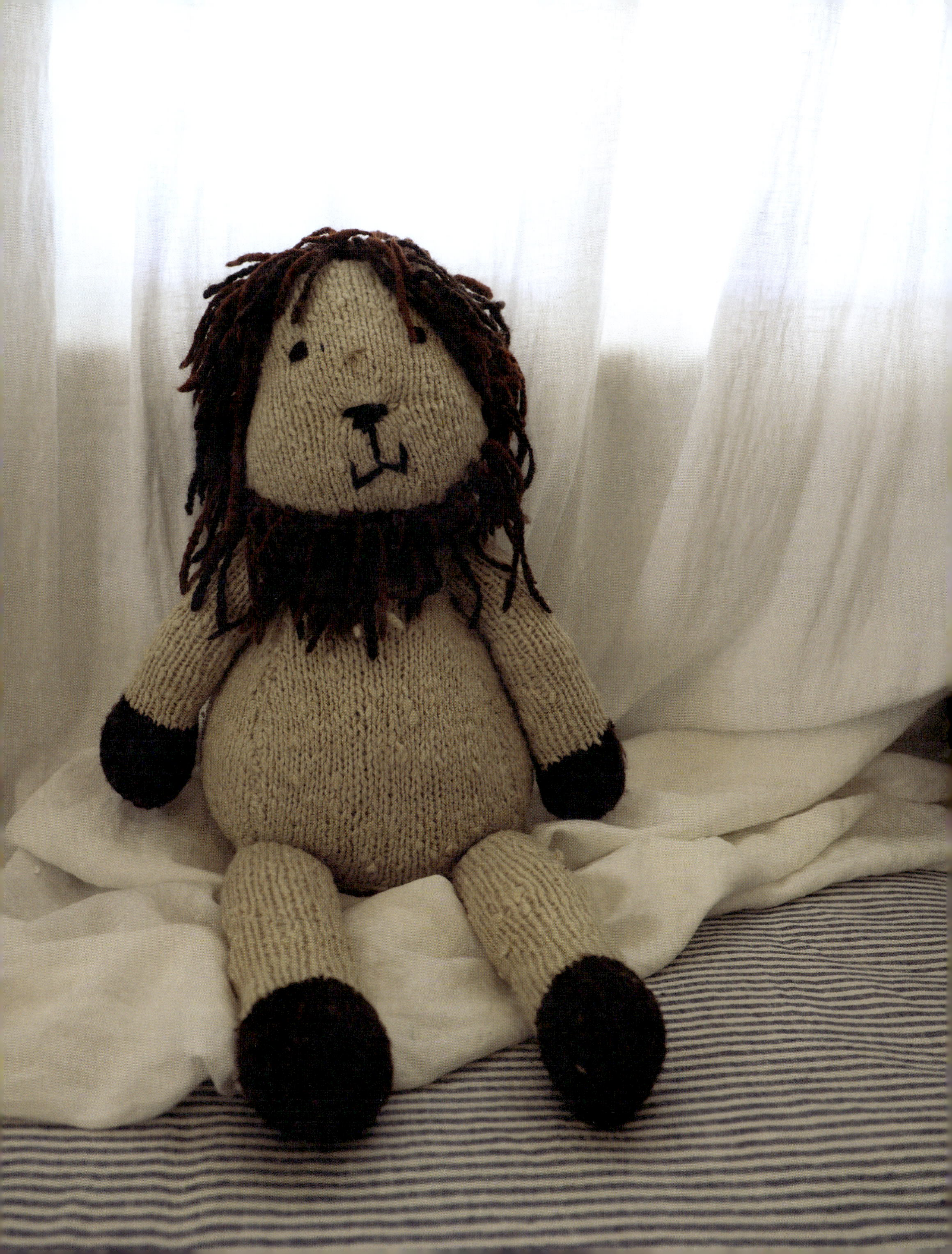

Kids' bedrooms provide a particularly fun styling opportunity when it comes to the modern country look. Vintage teddies (or new teddies made in the style of) bring cuteness and character in equal measure.

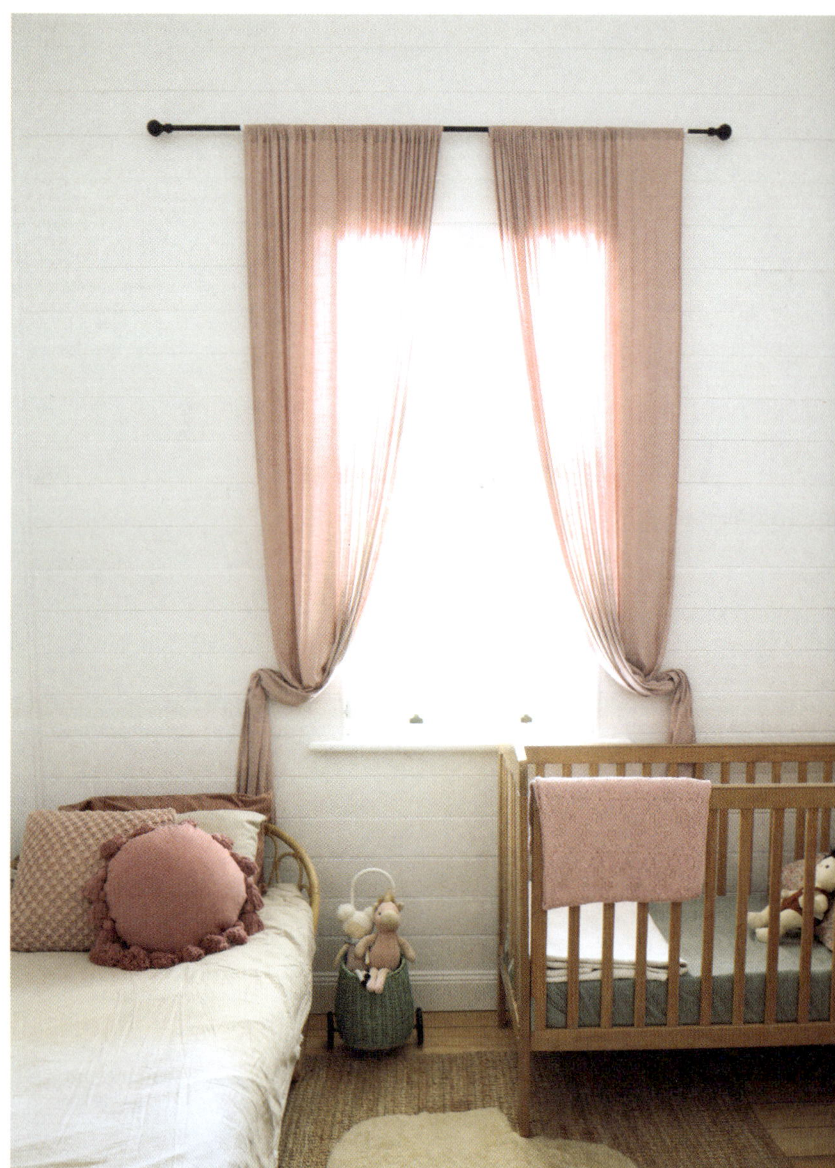

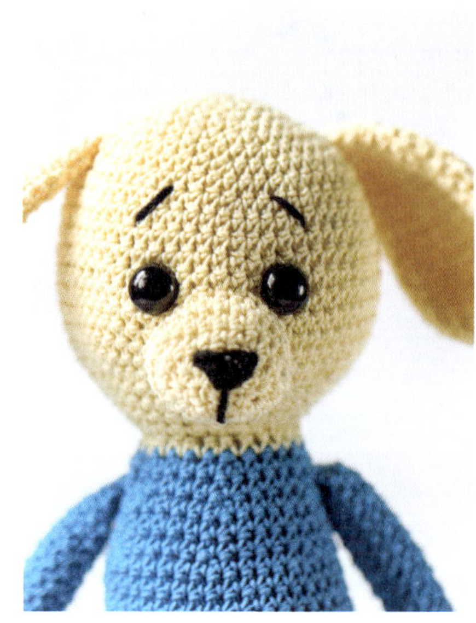

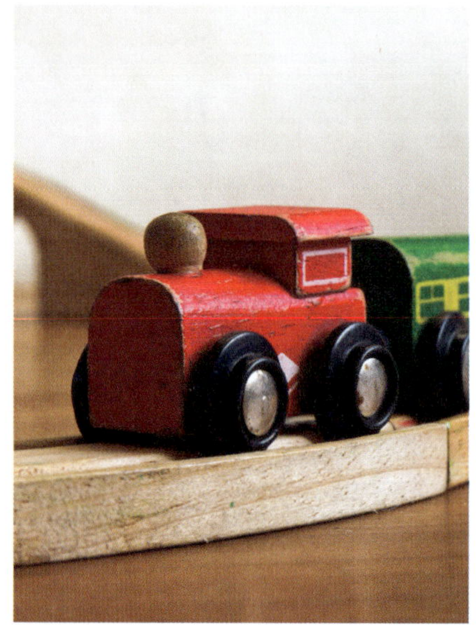

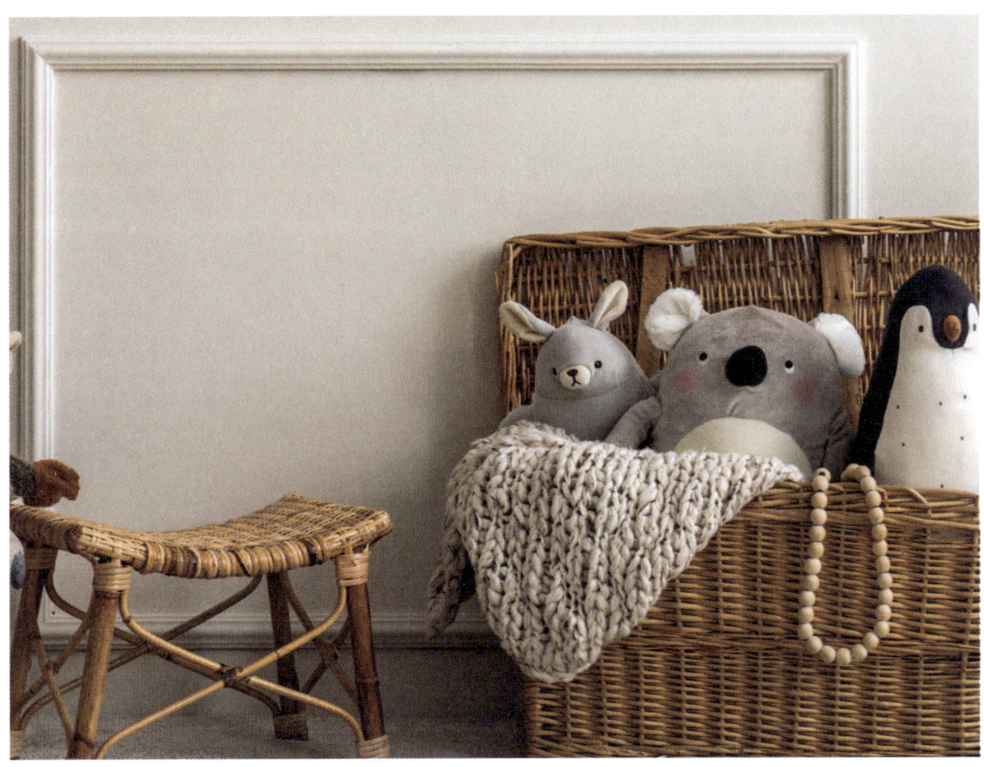

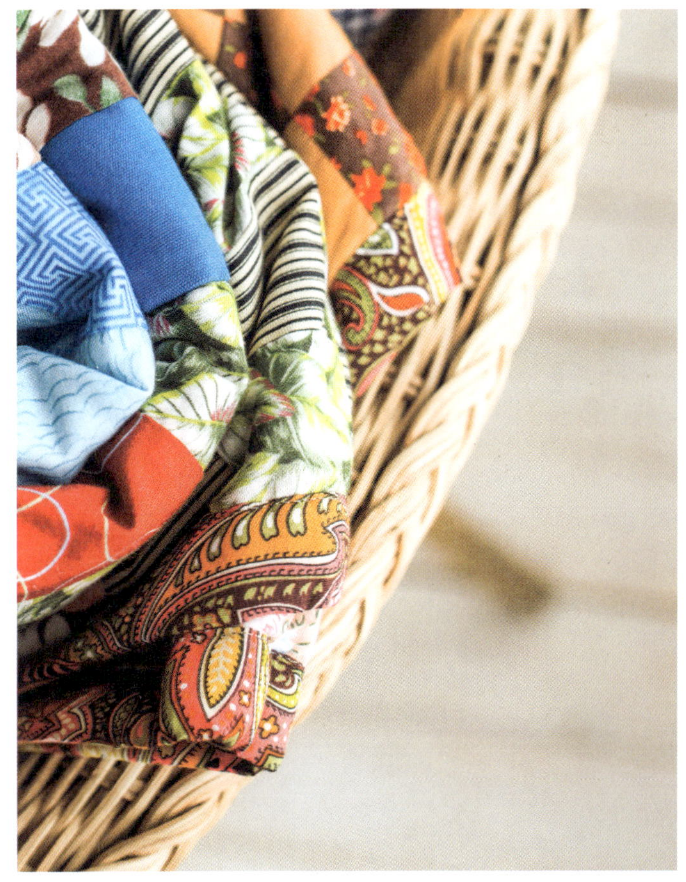

Mini coloured wicker baskets are perfect for storing little ones' little things. While vintage toys (purchased in antique shops or, if you are lucky, handed down through the family) look sweet and add an air of authenticity, they tend to be hard-wearing too.

'Friends, like flowers, make life more beautiful.'

MICHELE FARABEE

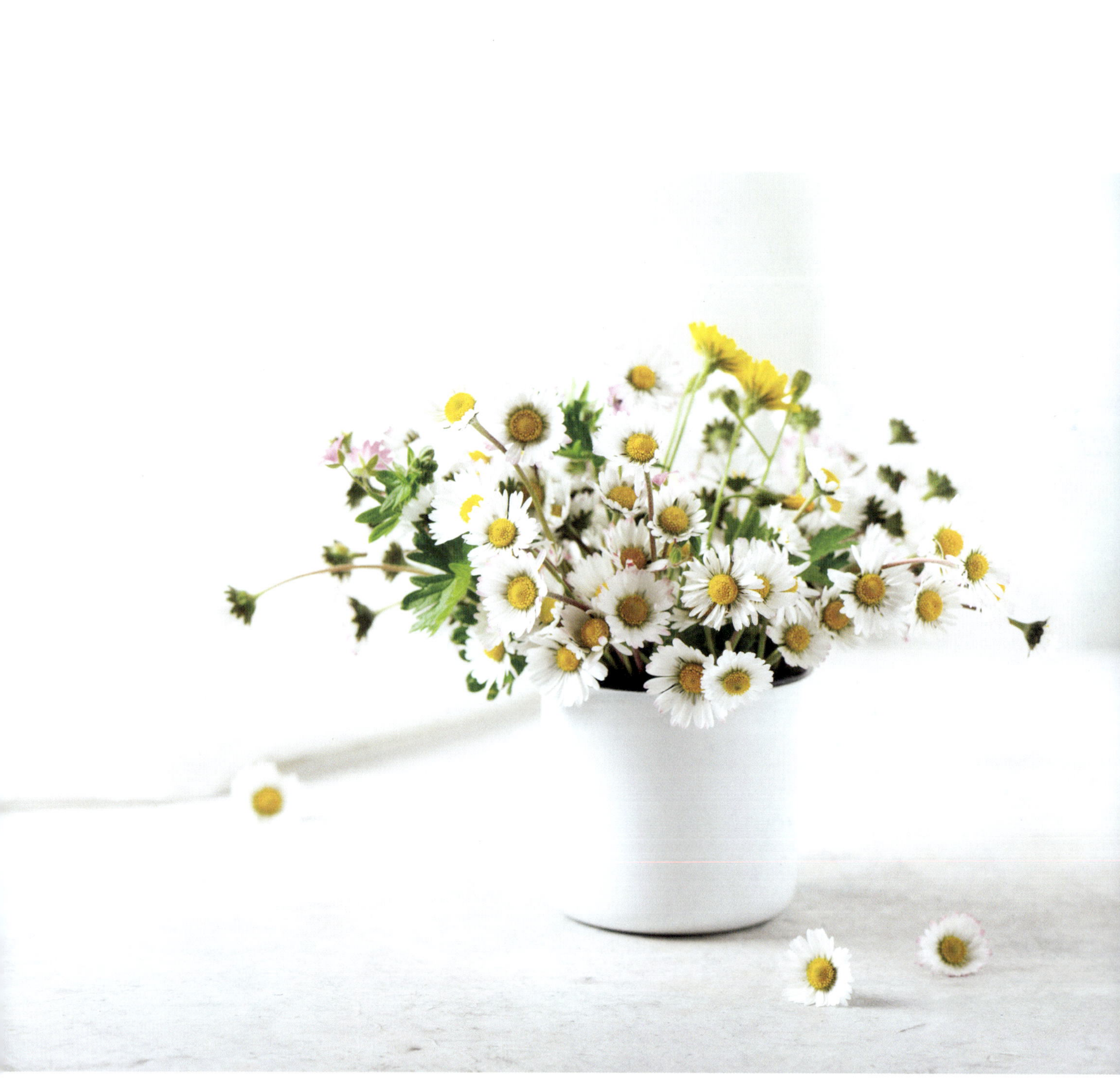

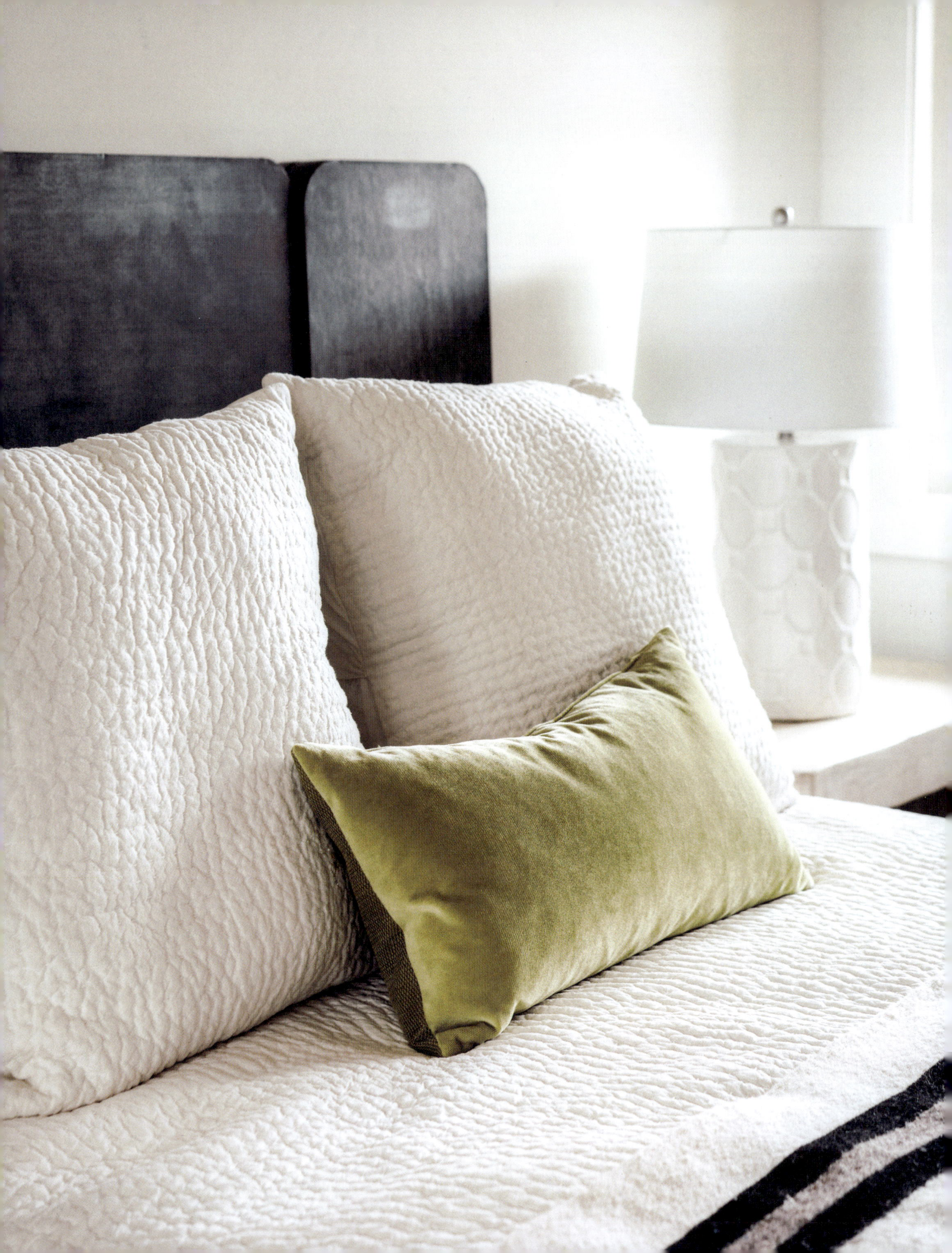

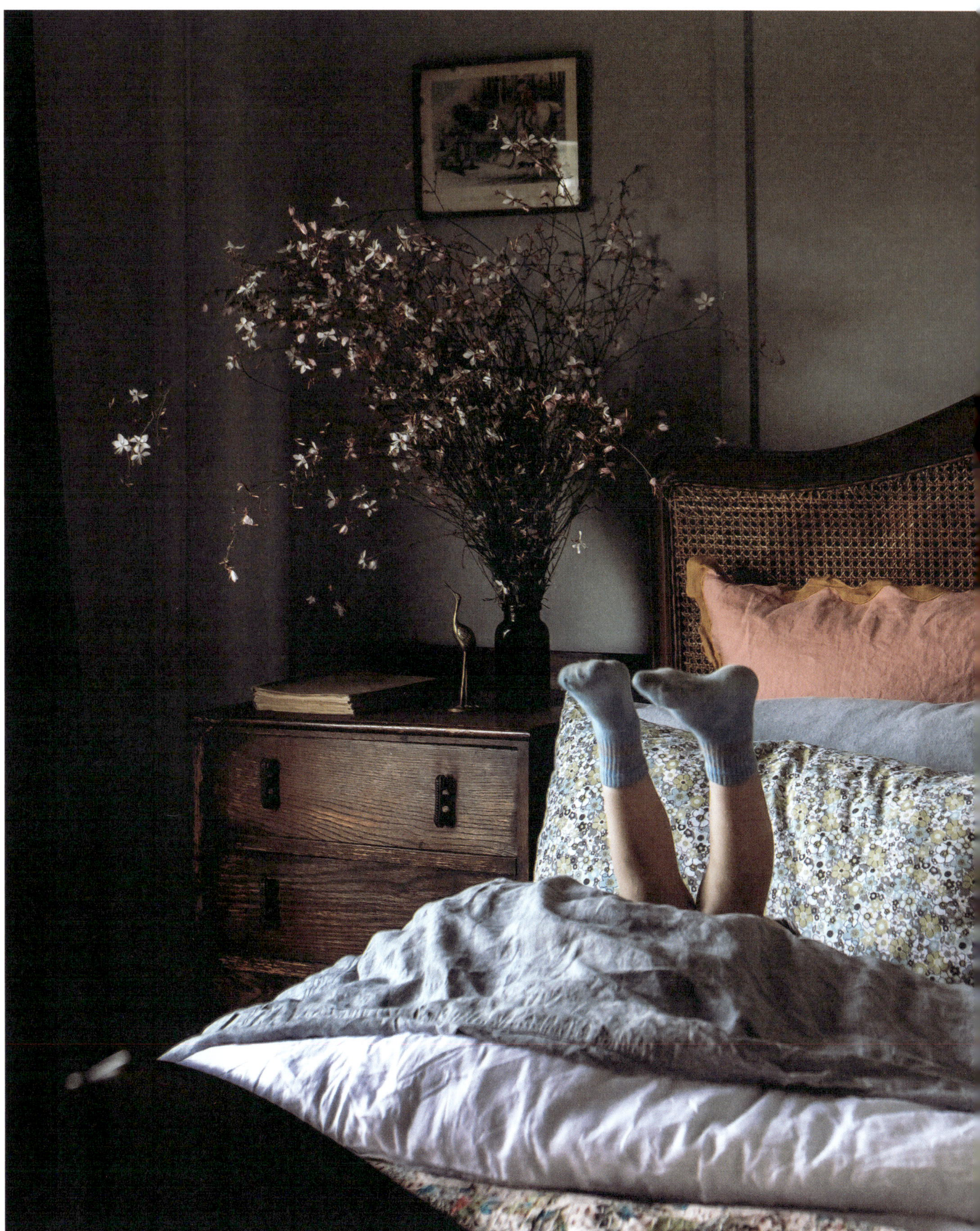

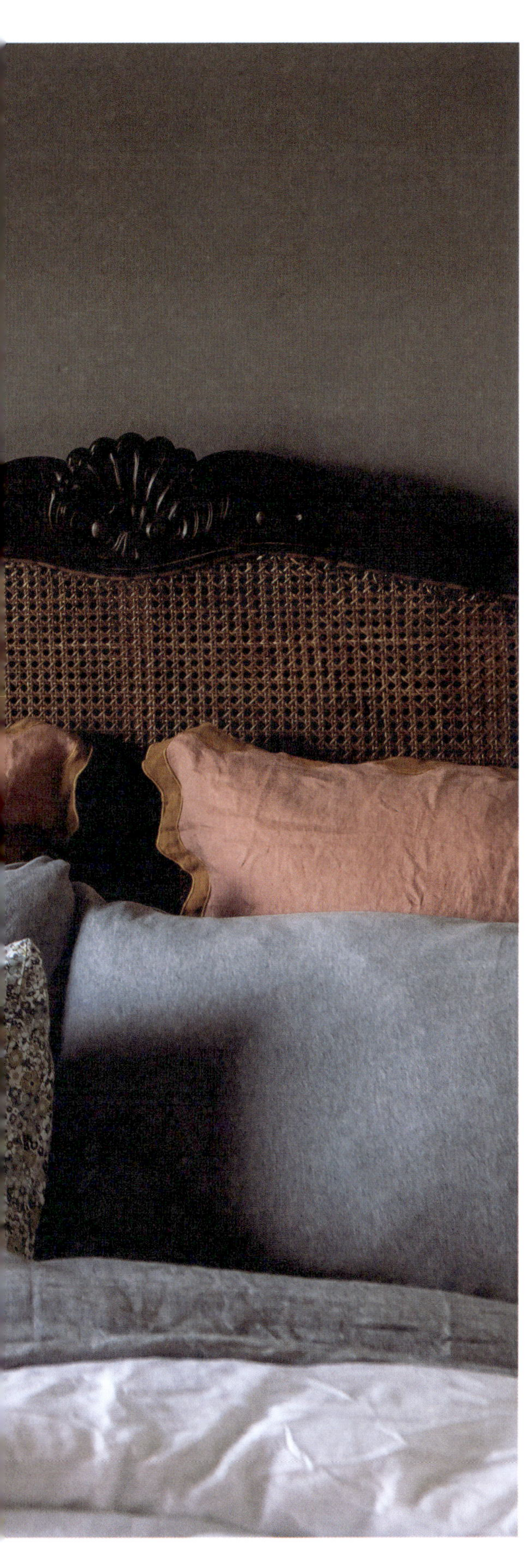

The wood and wicker headboard featured in this country-styled bedroom is a choice that's well complimented by the rich ochre and blue tones of the linen. A mere hint of floral (just one pillow) helps to edge the look of this bedroom more in the direction of modern than traditional country.

The Quick List

Wrought-iron or wicker bed

Vintage toys and teddies in kids' rooms

High-quality bed linen (the best you can afford)

Warm, earthy colour choices for bed linen

Stacks of books on bedside tables

Extra throws and cushions for comfort

Simplicity in styling – not too much

Spot lighting for bedsides and to illuminate dressers and wardrobe areas

A touch of floral pattern, but no more

Gingham and/or stripes

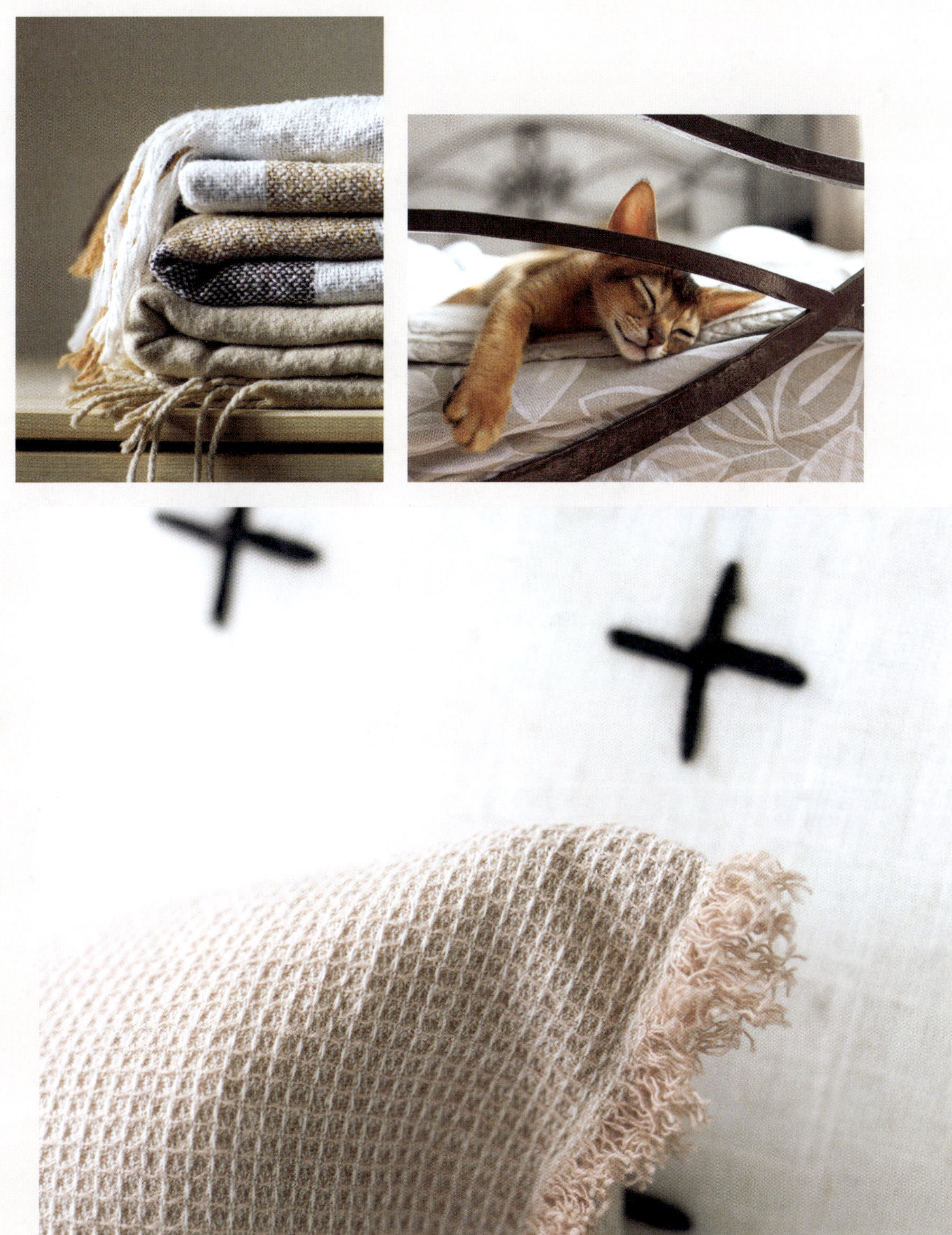

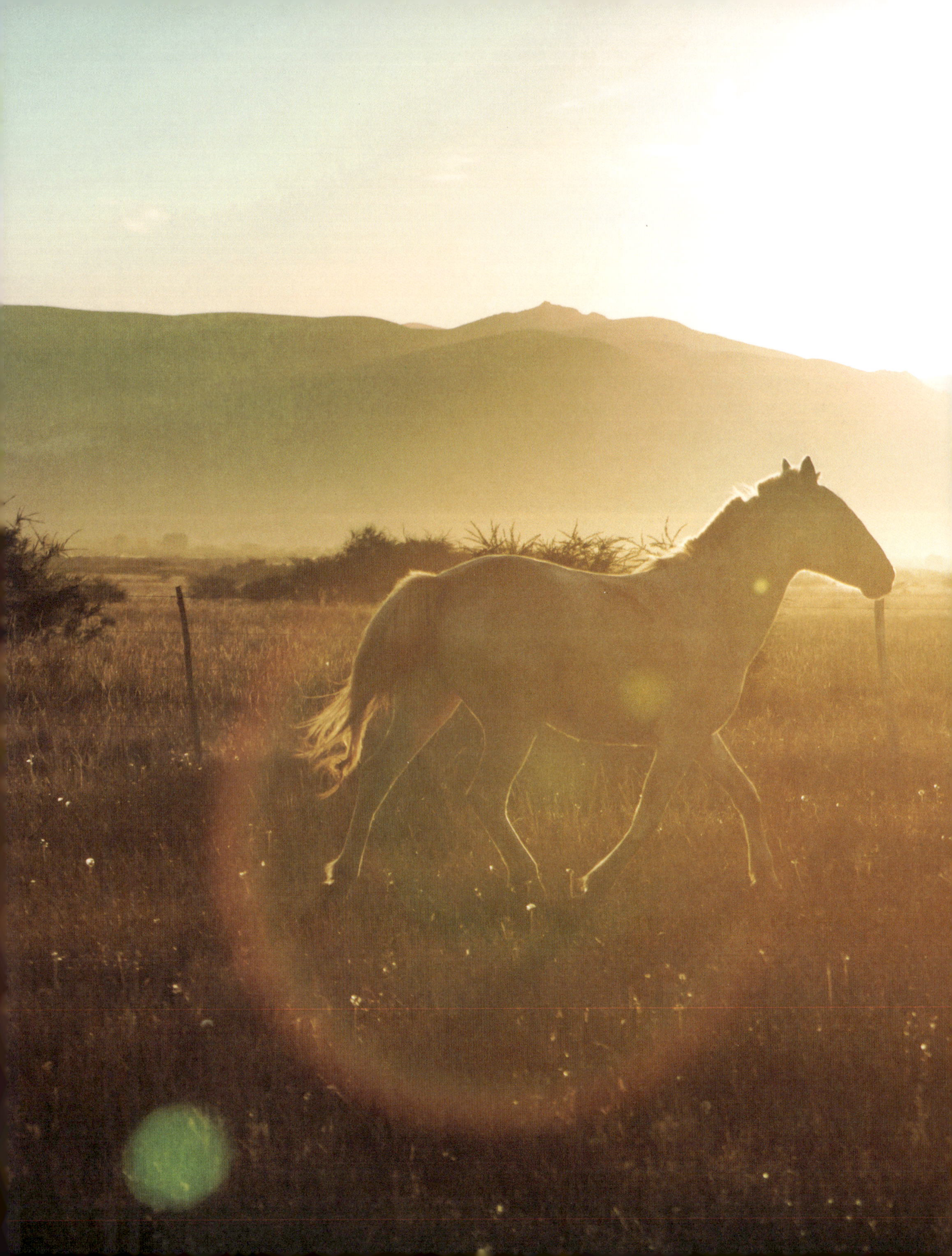

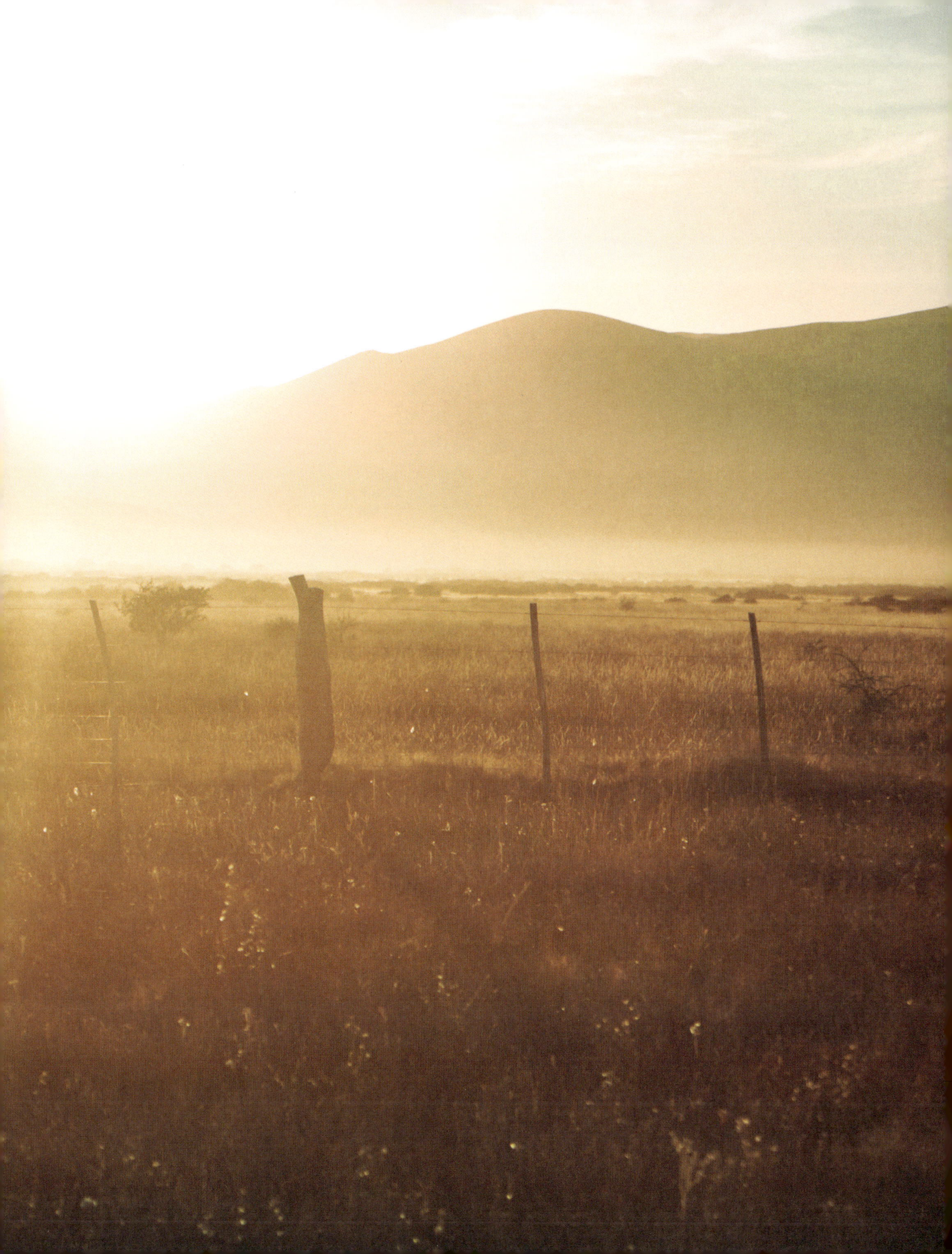

chapter five

eating & drinking

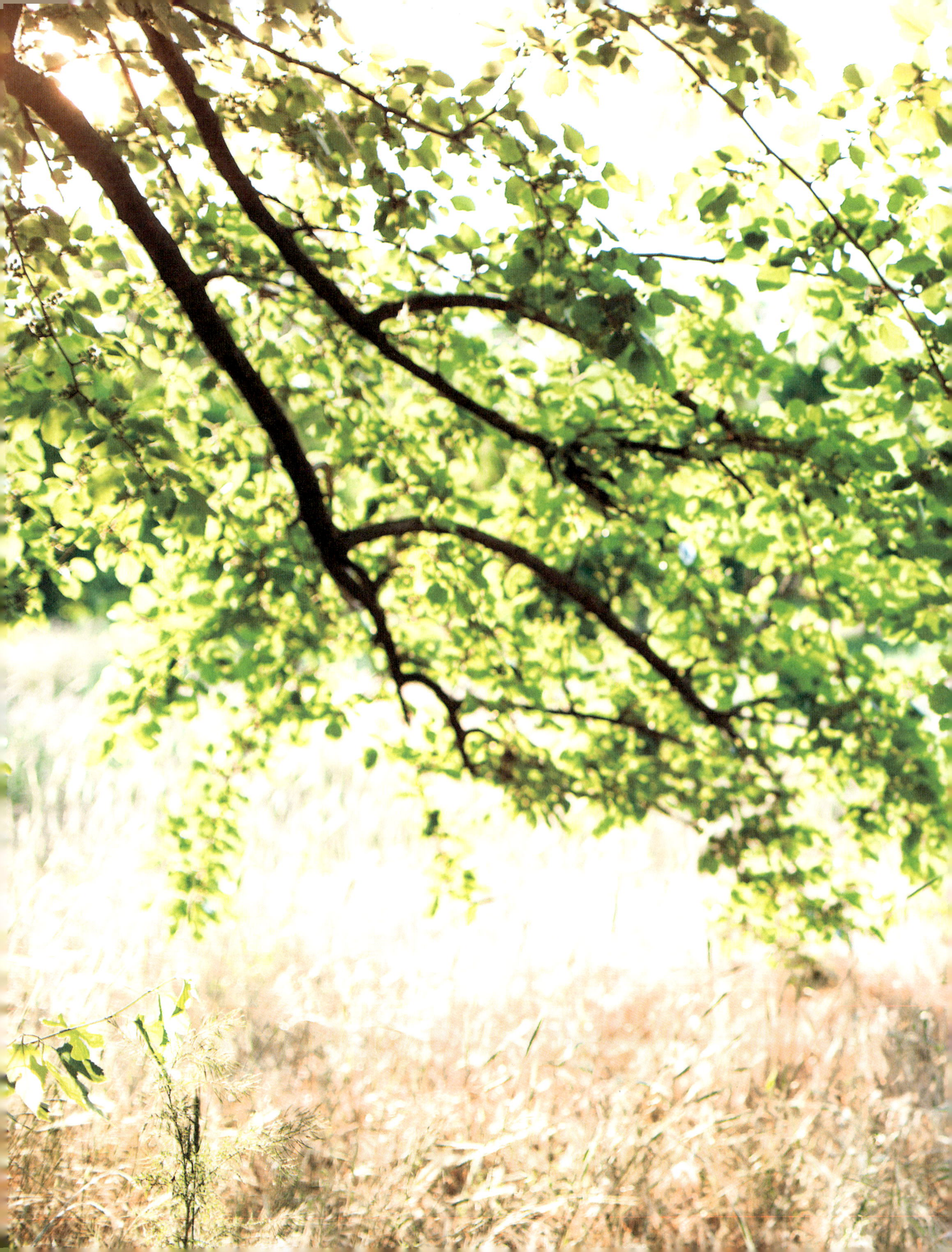

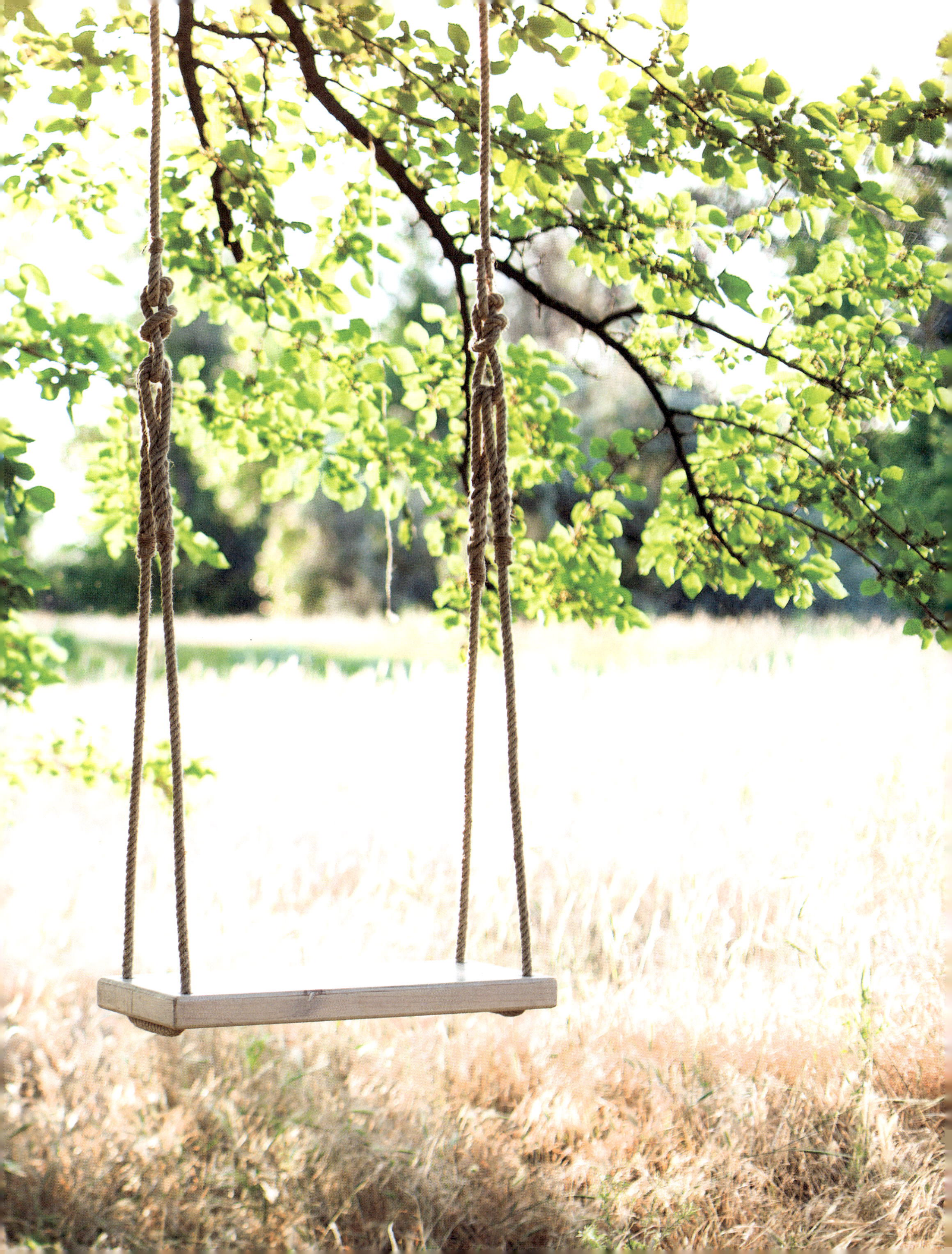

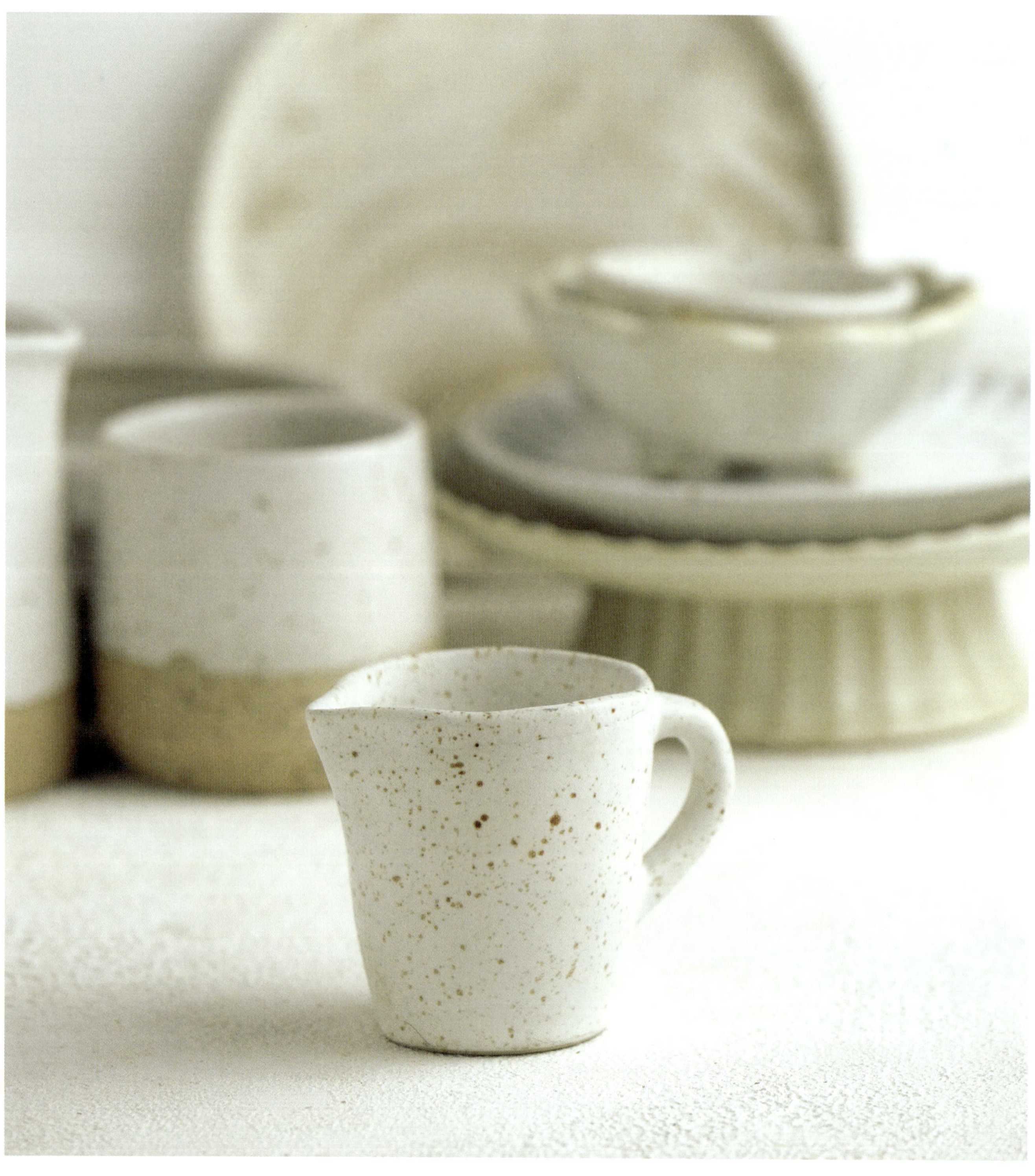

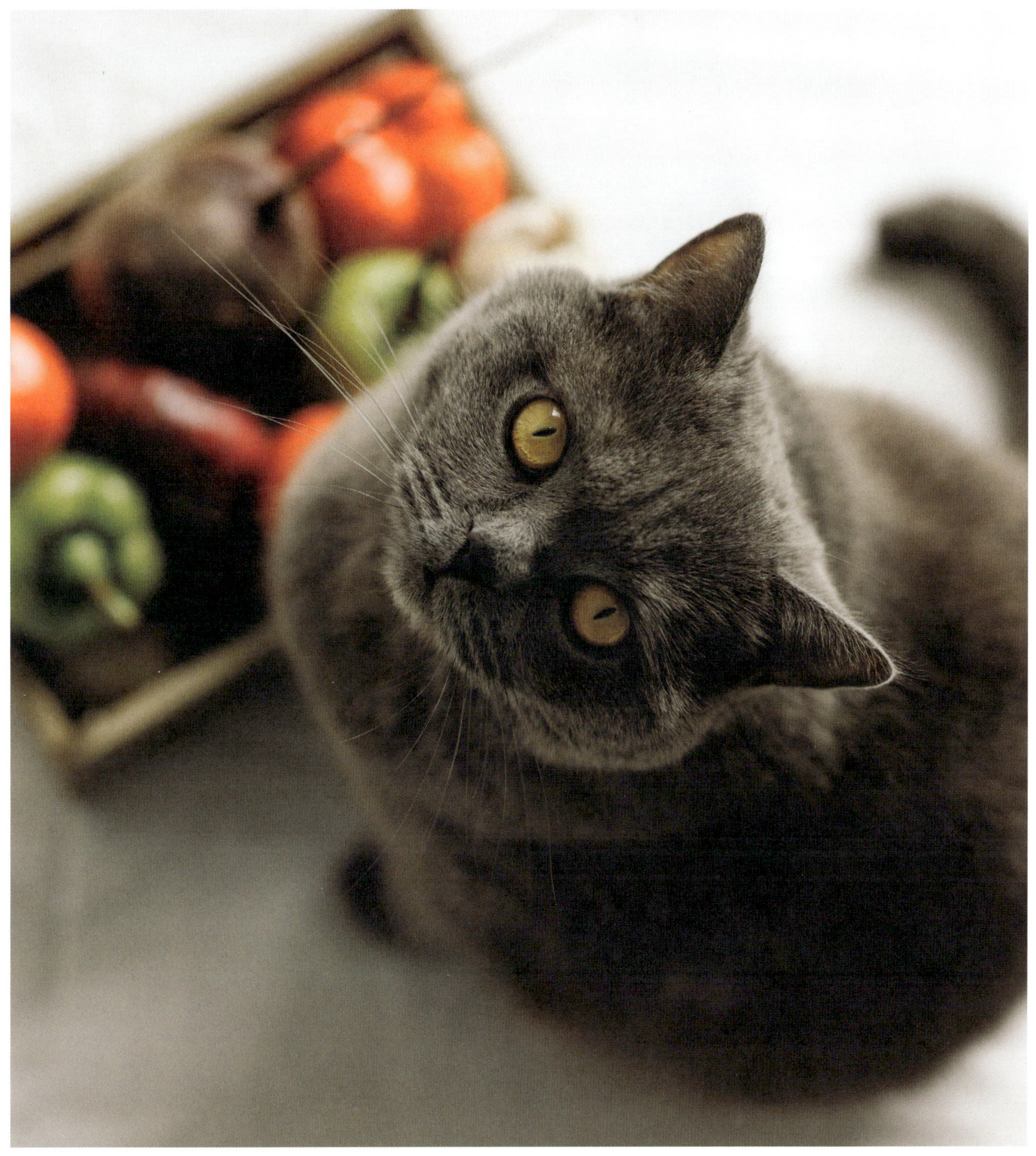

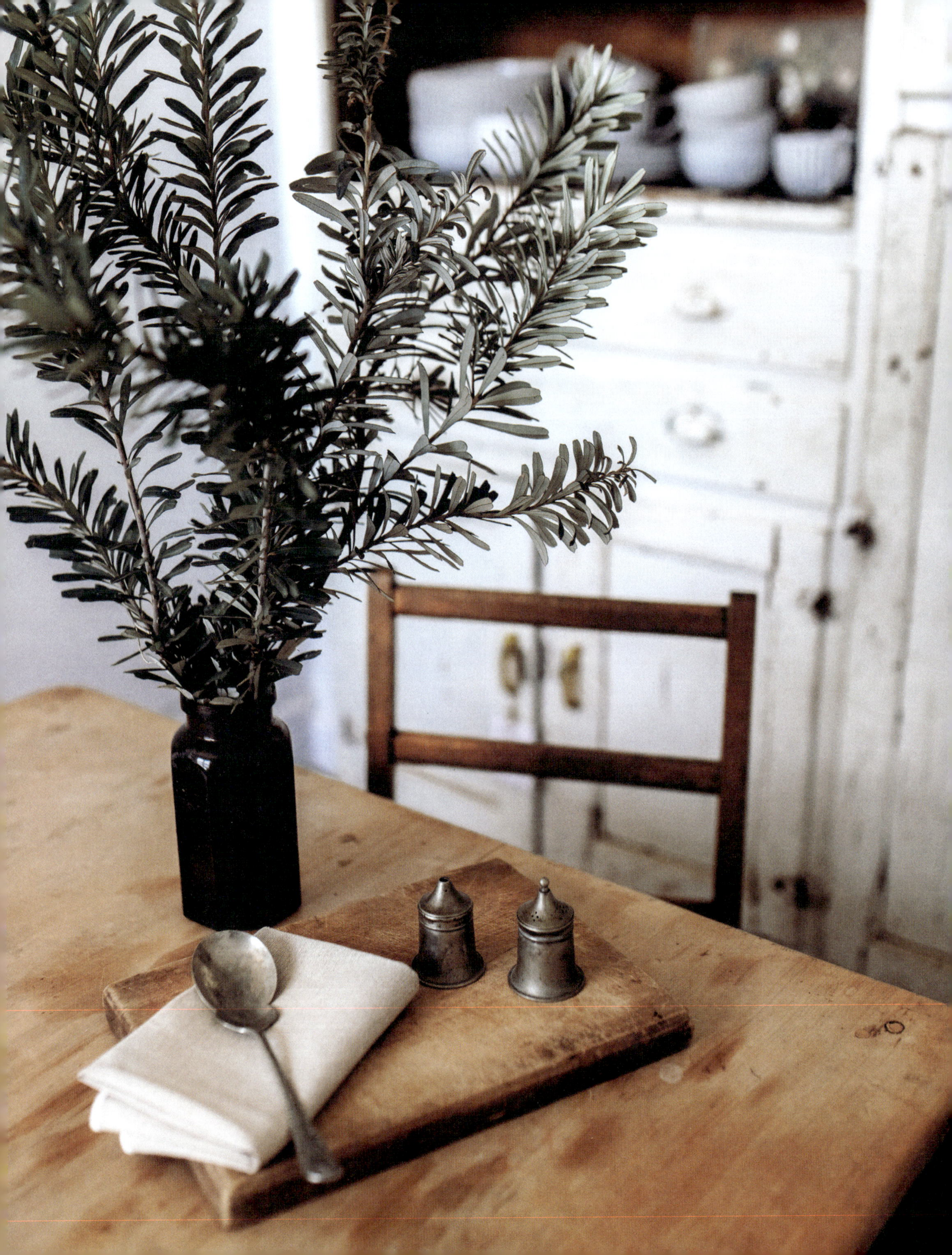

Whether you live in a historic homestead with sweeping rural vistas from the kitchen sink or a new-build in the modern country style, you'll probably be striving for the same thing: functional, easy kitchen spaces, leading into spacious and relaxed dining areas.

Modern country homes lean to the contemporary in kitchen styling, with marble benchtops offset by brass tapware and farmhouse sinks, providing a clean execution of the traditional country style.

Renovated Queenslander-style homes may retain some of the original timber cabinetry and benchtops, and feature stand-alone elements, such as a wooden kitchen dresser, on which cute collections of vintage crockery, eggcups, silverware and glasses reside. If you've got it, flaunt it: use those open shelves to display your beautiful items, as this will add character and flair to the space.

It is important to get the right balance between clutter and character in the country-styled kitchen. It's tempting to display good-looking utensils, bowls, chopping boards and cookbooks – and keeping daily items to hand makes sense. But be sure to limit yourself to items that you genuinely use on a regular basis. The modern country look is 'kitchen on display' but not cluttered – it's a delicate balance so take care with it. Display only carefully chosen items that articulate your style and fit in the theme of modern country – natural fibres, earthy tones, wood, tarnished metals and, of course, flowers, fruit and greenery.

At the heart of each space is likely to be a table – an island bench in the kitchen perhaps, and a large dining table for communing with family and friends. Make your dining table your centrepiece – it's a place for joy and connection with others. Be expansive (as big a table as space reasonably allows) and choose chairs for comfort as well as style – hopefully you'll linger there a while.

TOP FIVE

1.

Functional items on display

2.

Central, relaxed dining spaces

3.

Open shelving

4.

Balanced textural elements

5.

Carefully curated displays

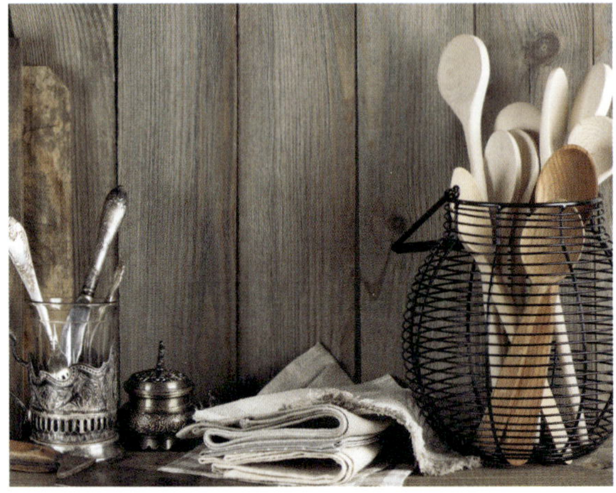

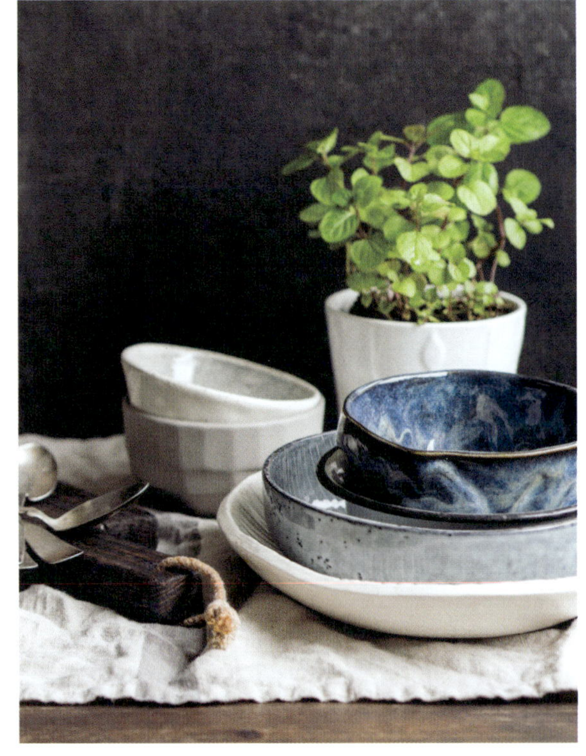

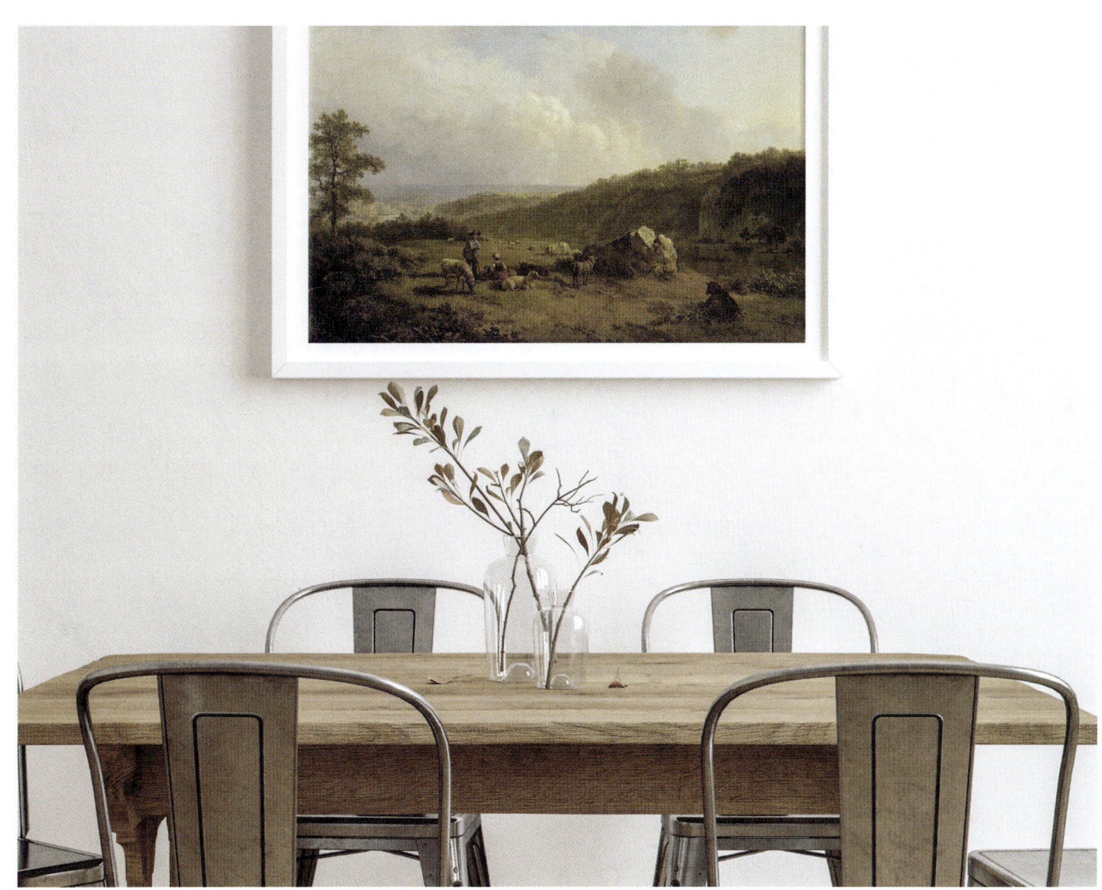

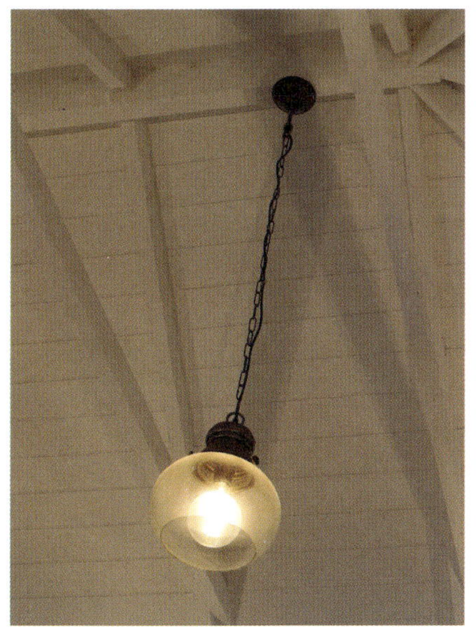

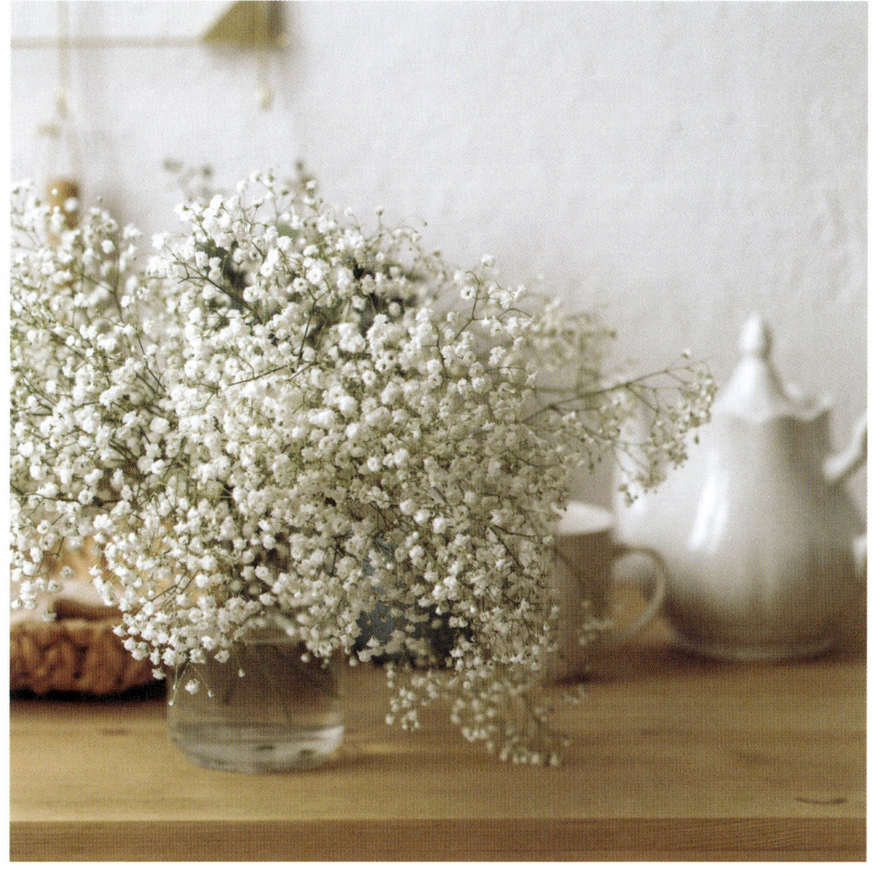

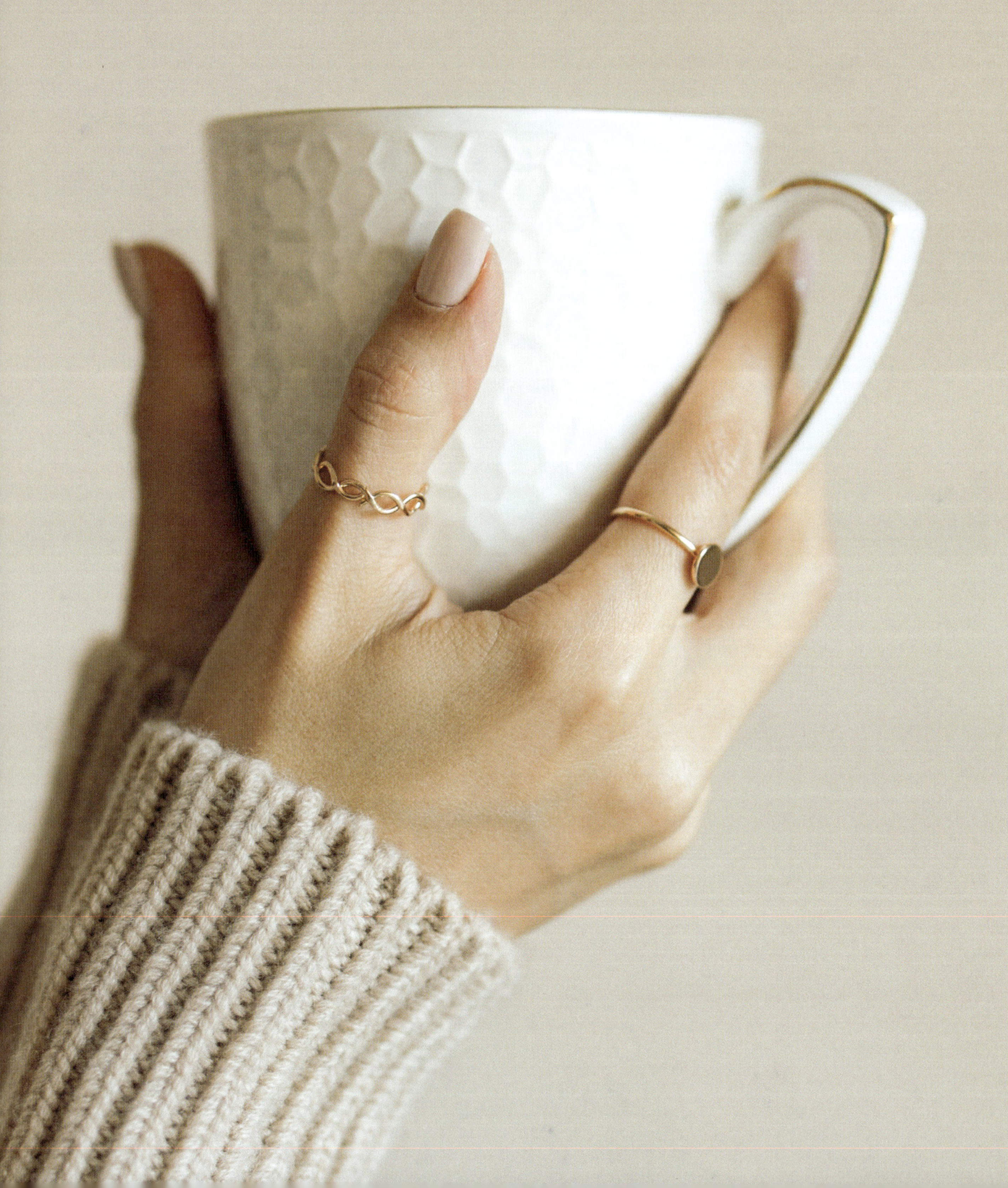

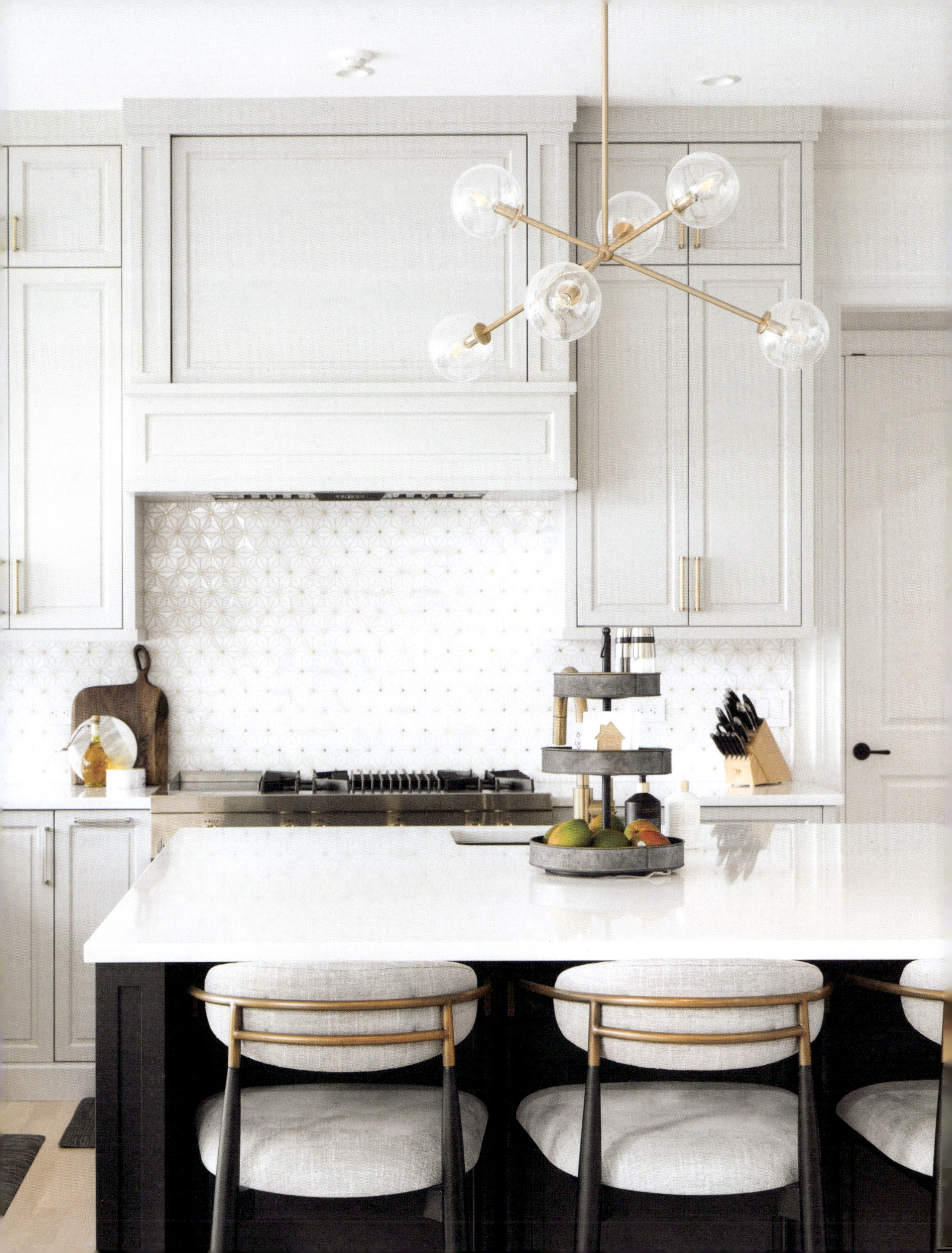

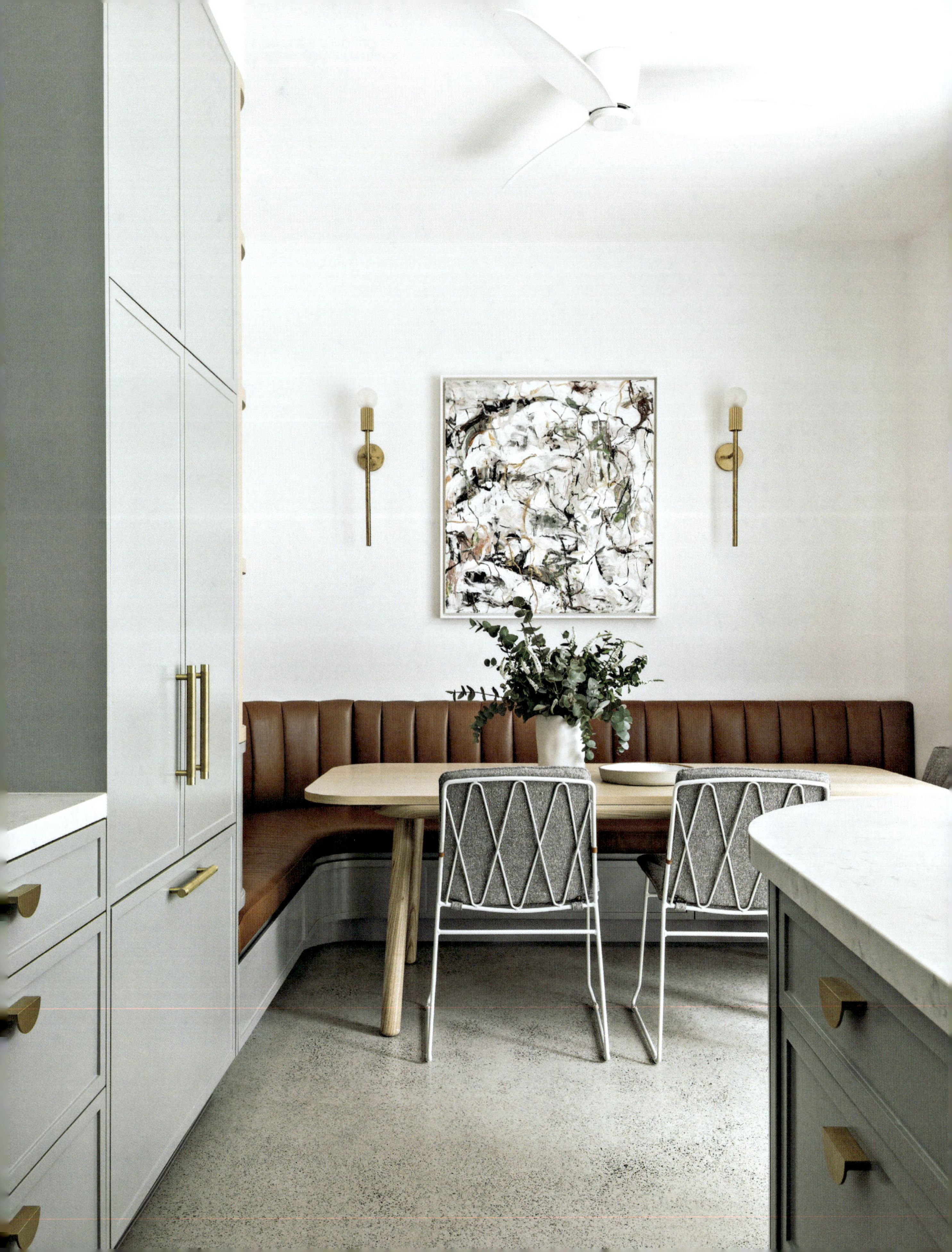

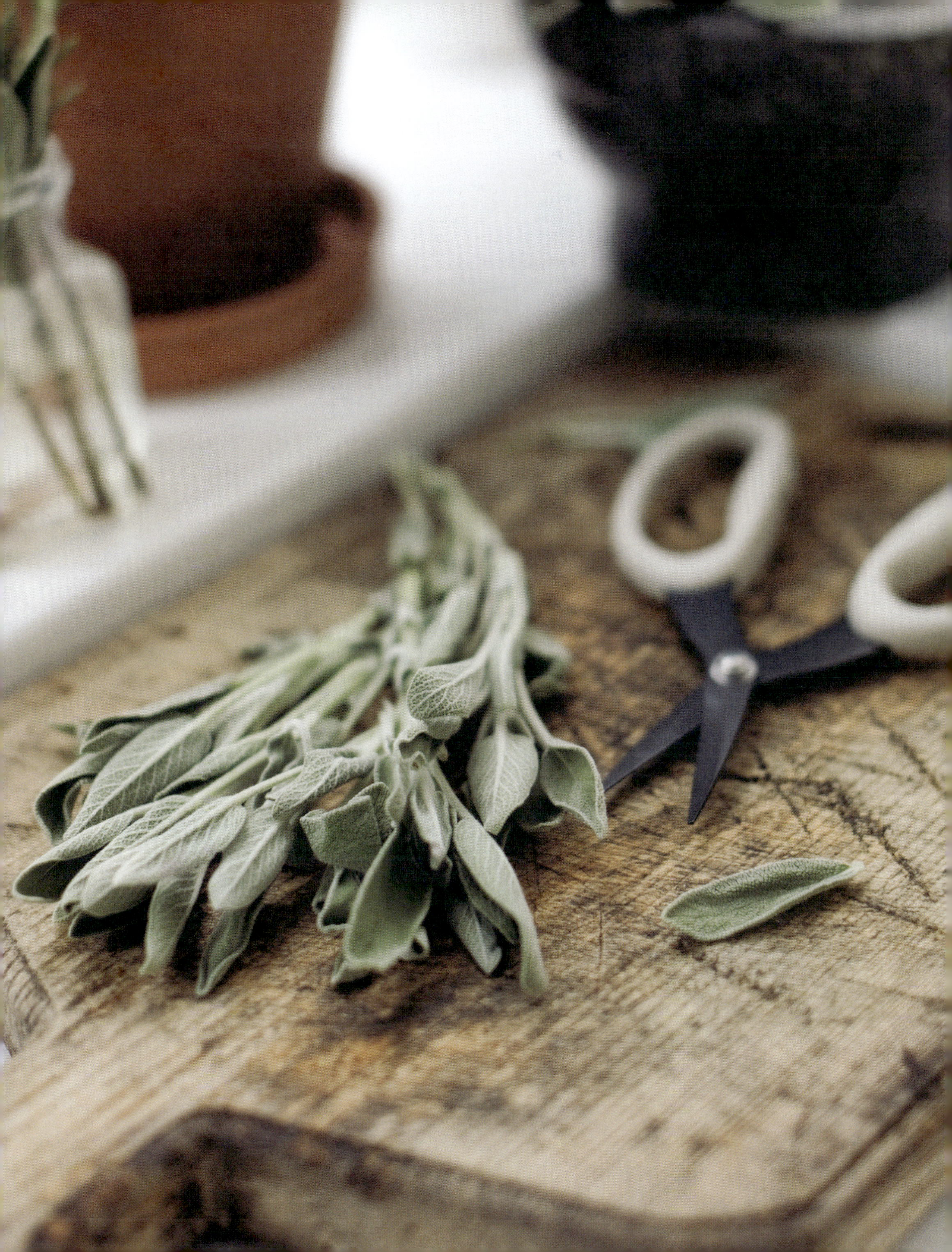

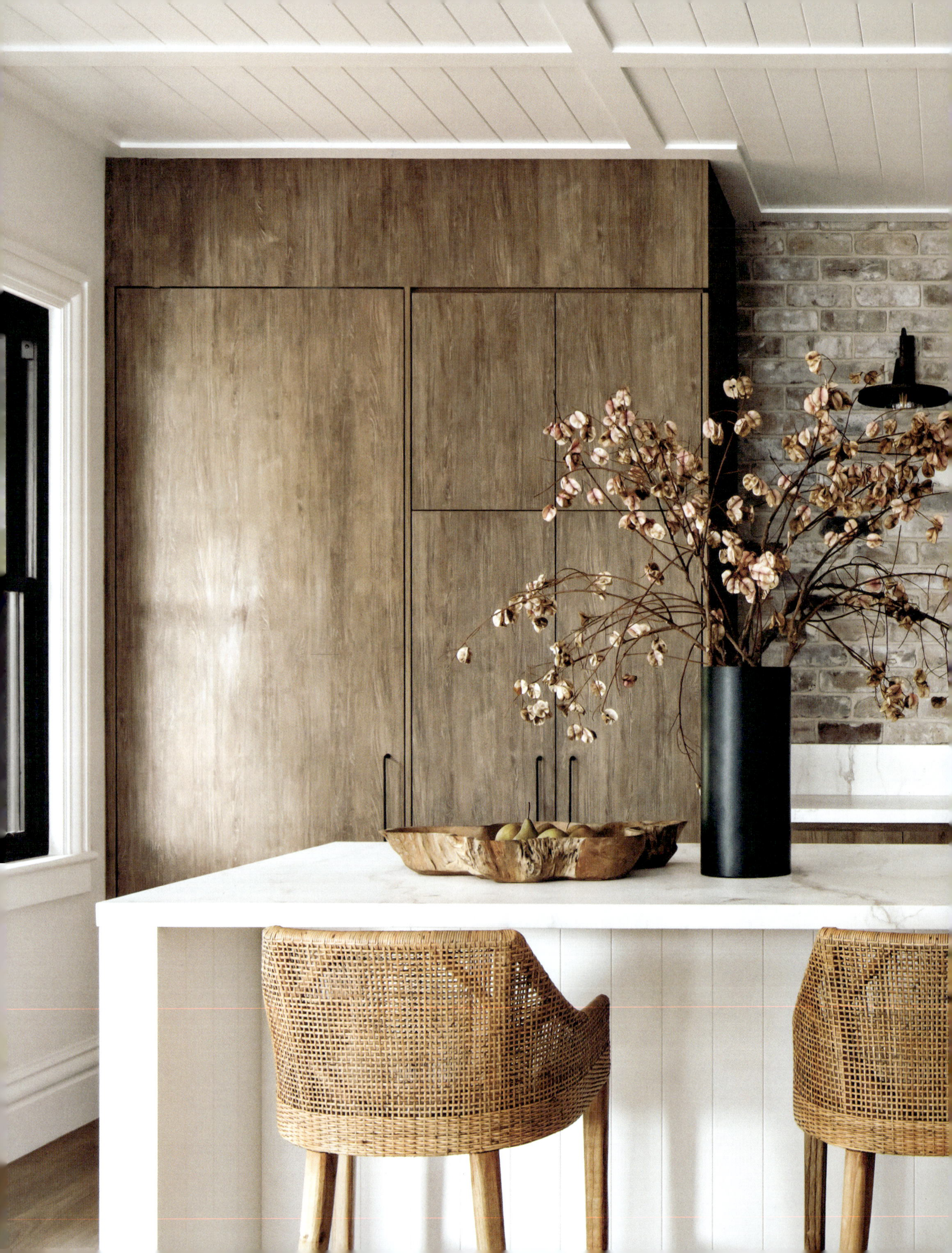

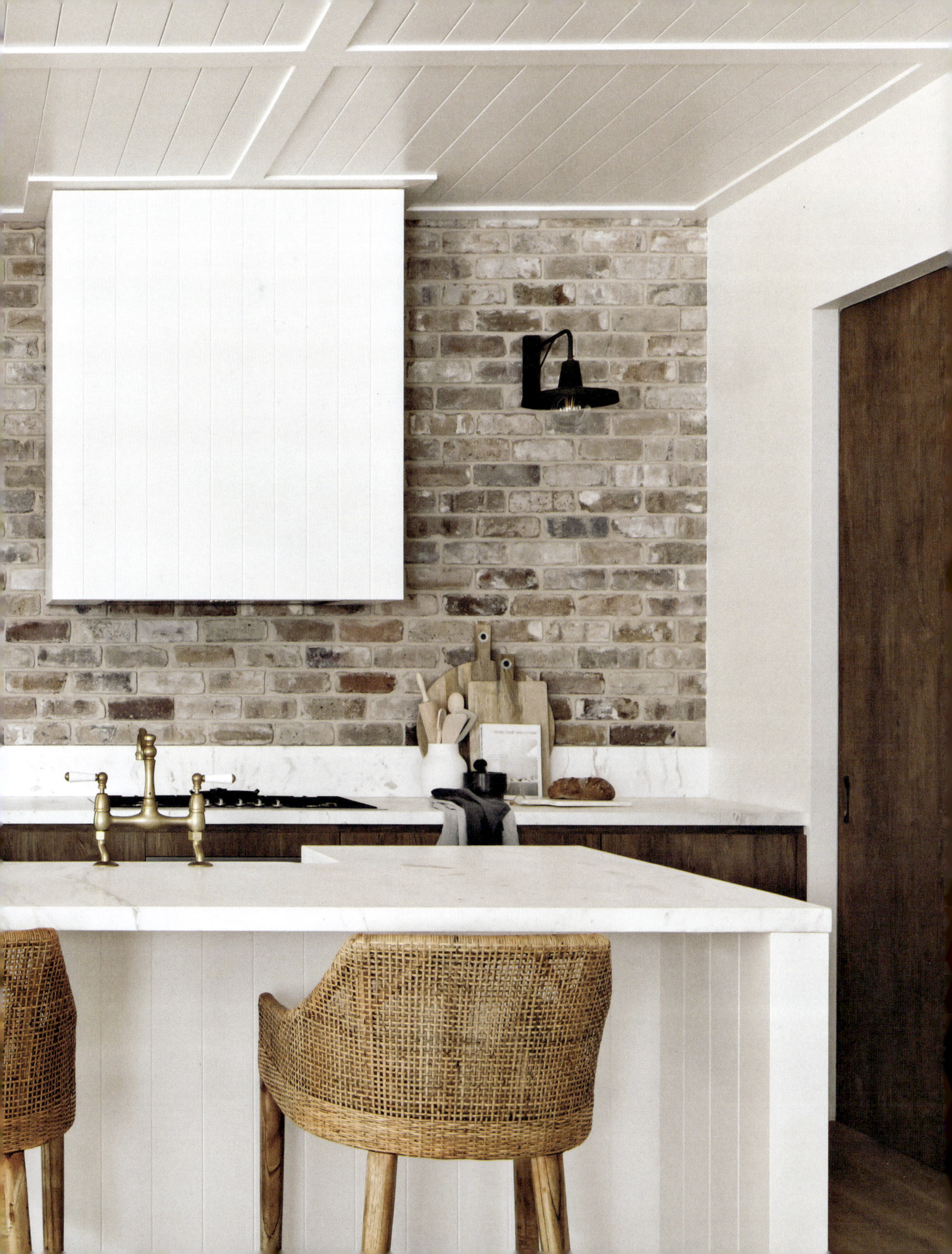

The traditional farmhouse sink has seen a renaissance in recent years, and is now a popular interior design choice. Offset by brass tapware with an aged patina, and styled with wooden, wicker and white decor, it clearly articulates the message of modern country style.

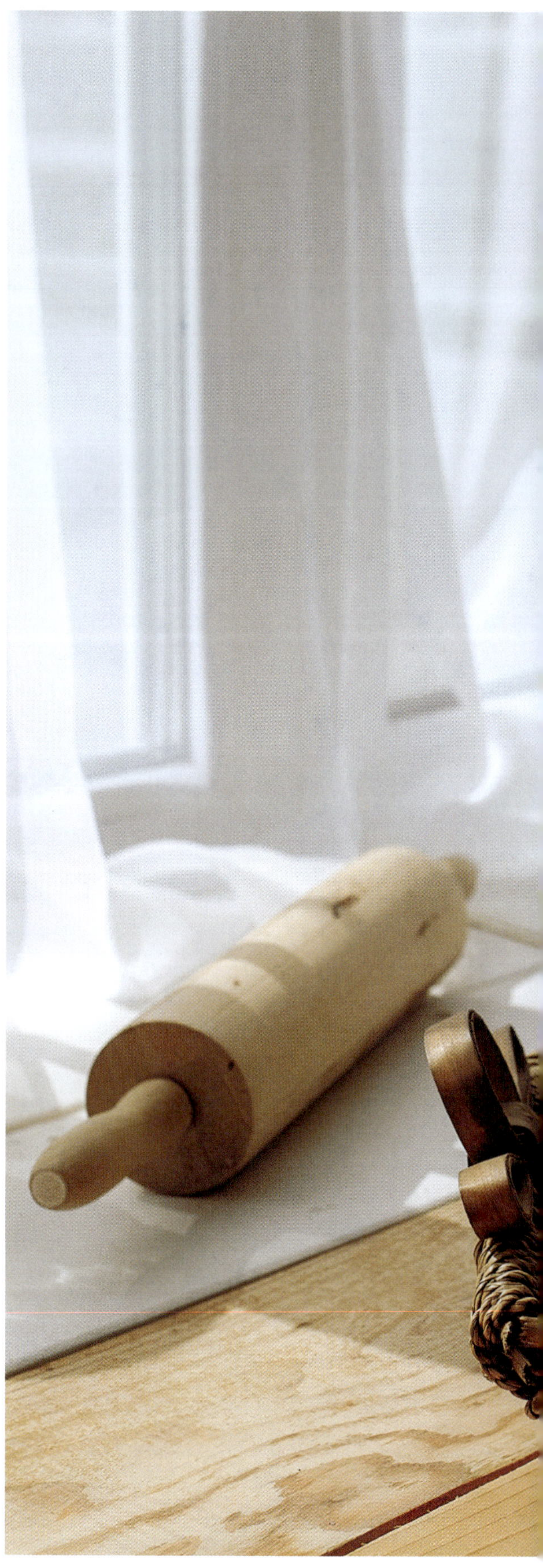

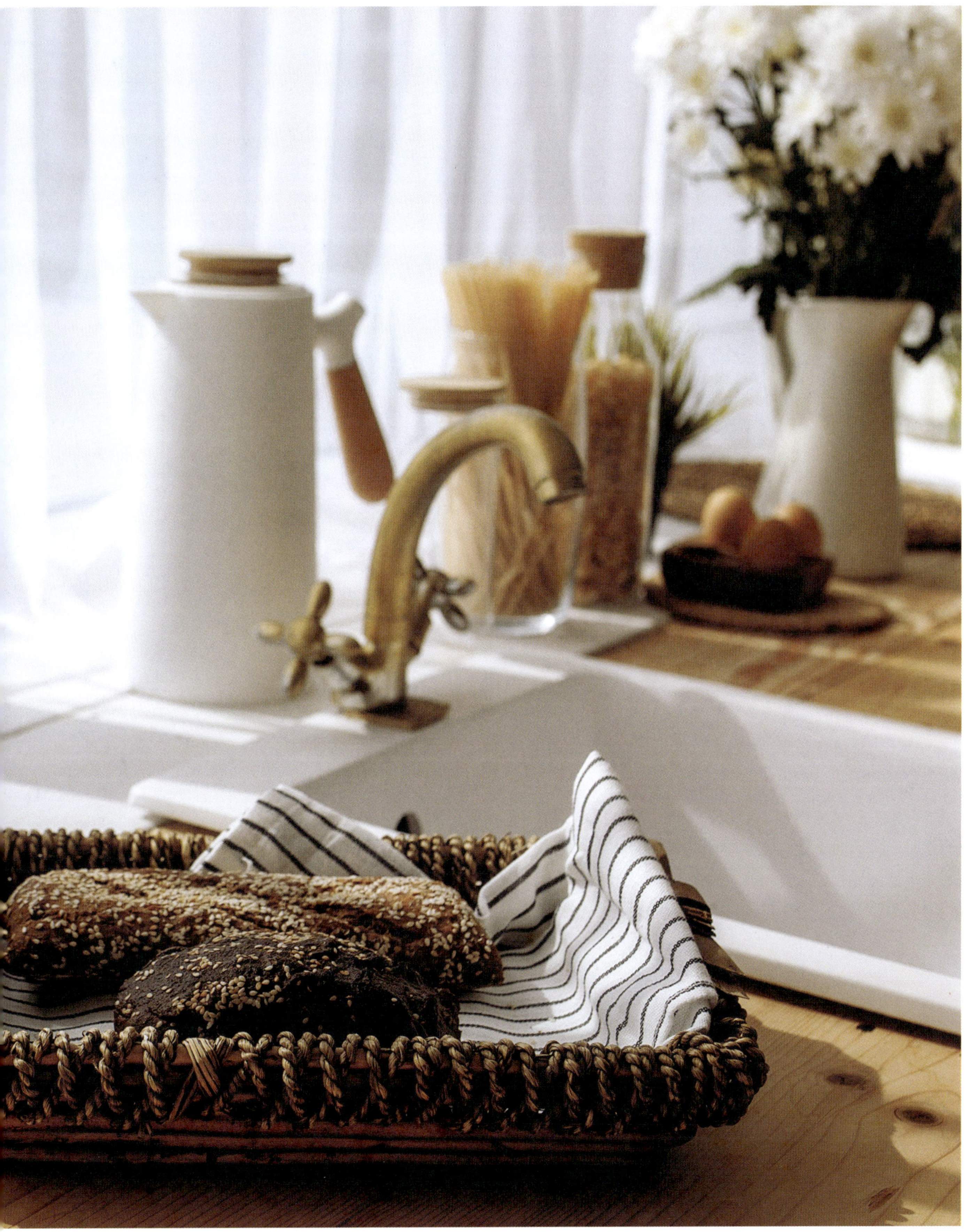

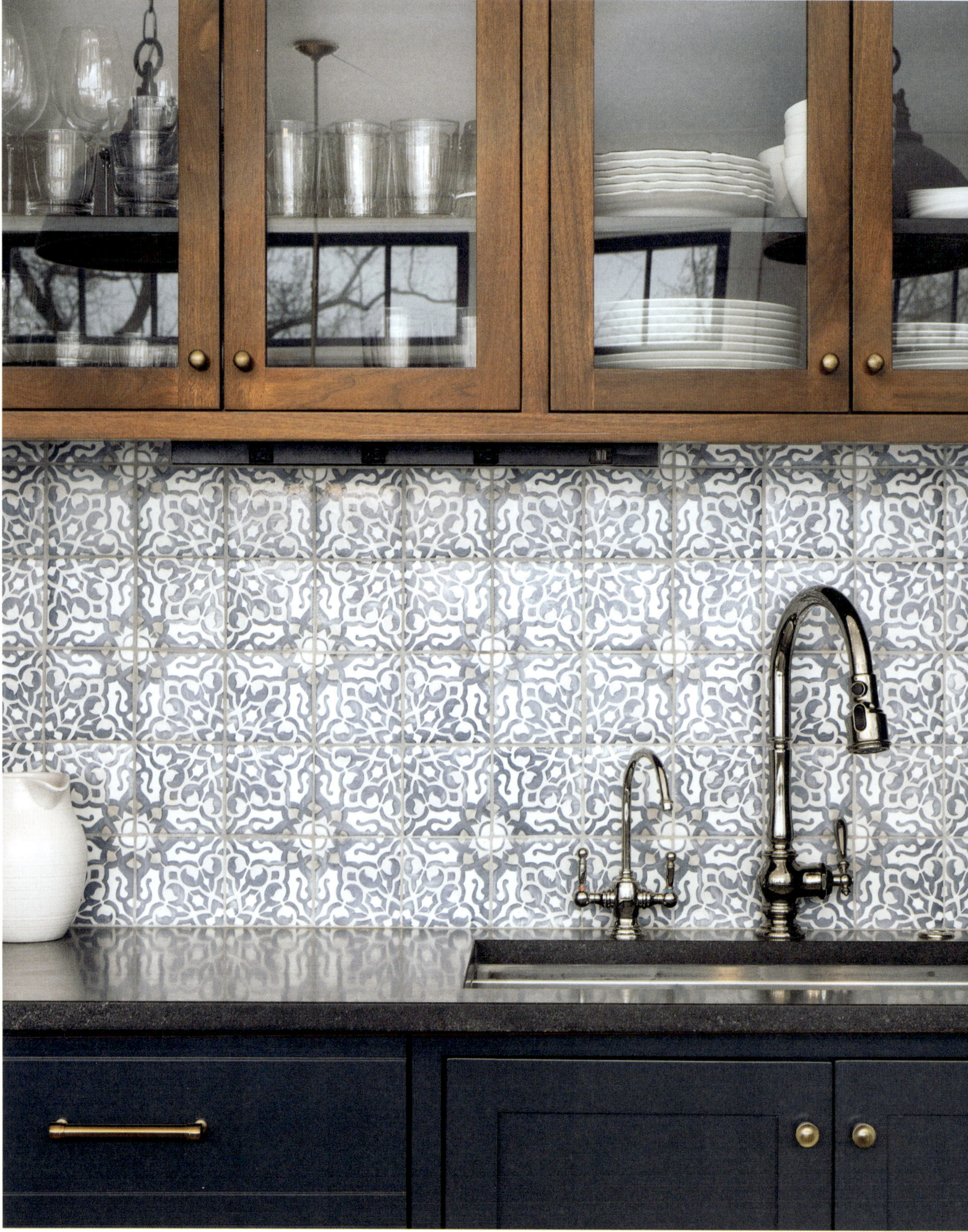

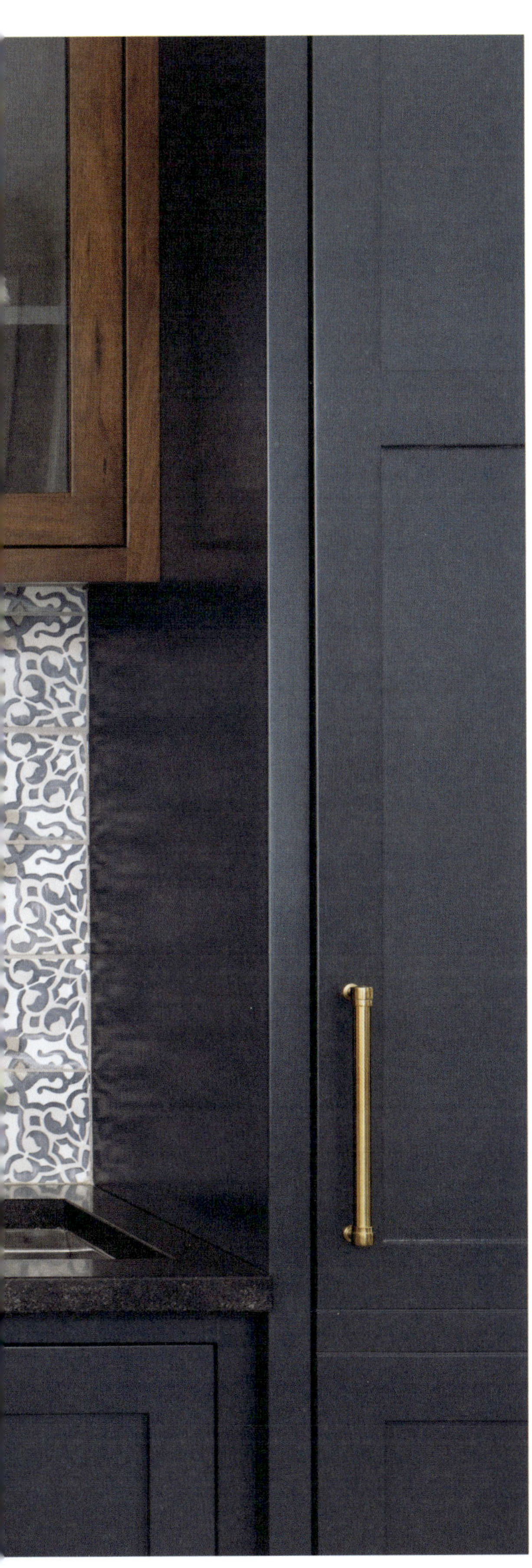

This kitchen features key elements of modern country style, including a rich colour palette inspired by nature and a balance of finishes in wood, steel and brass, with a marble-effect benchtop. The tiled splashback creates a 'farmhouse-of-old' look.

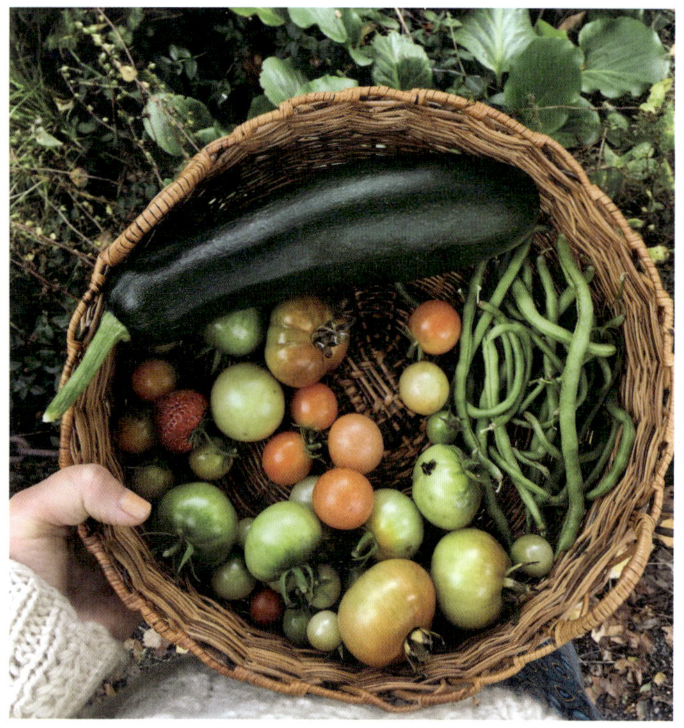

Carefully-chosen vintage items, such as the florist scissors pictured right, lend a lovely authentic touch to the modern country home.

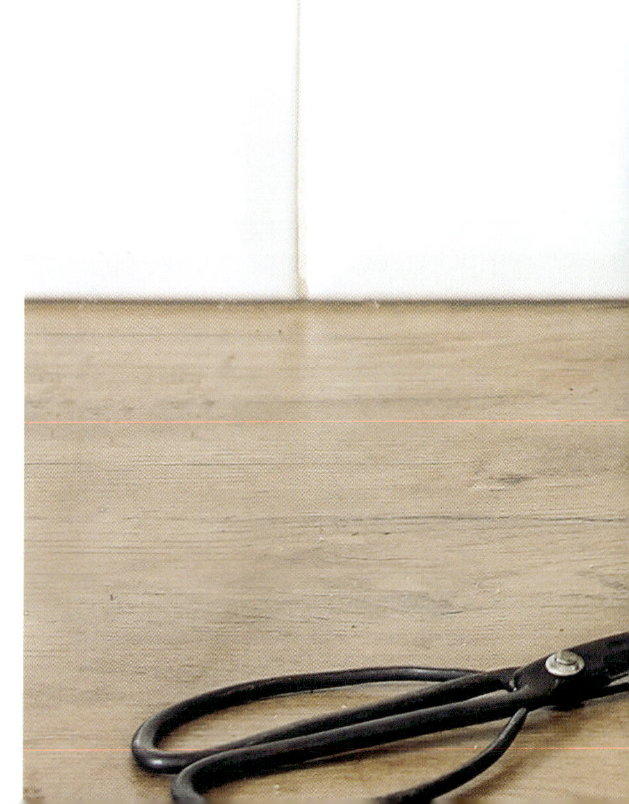

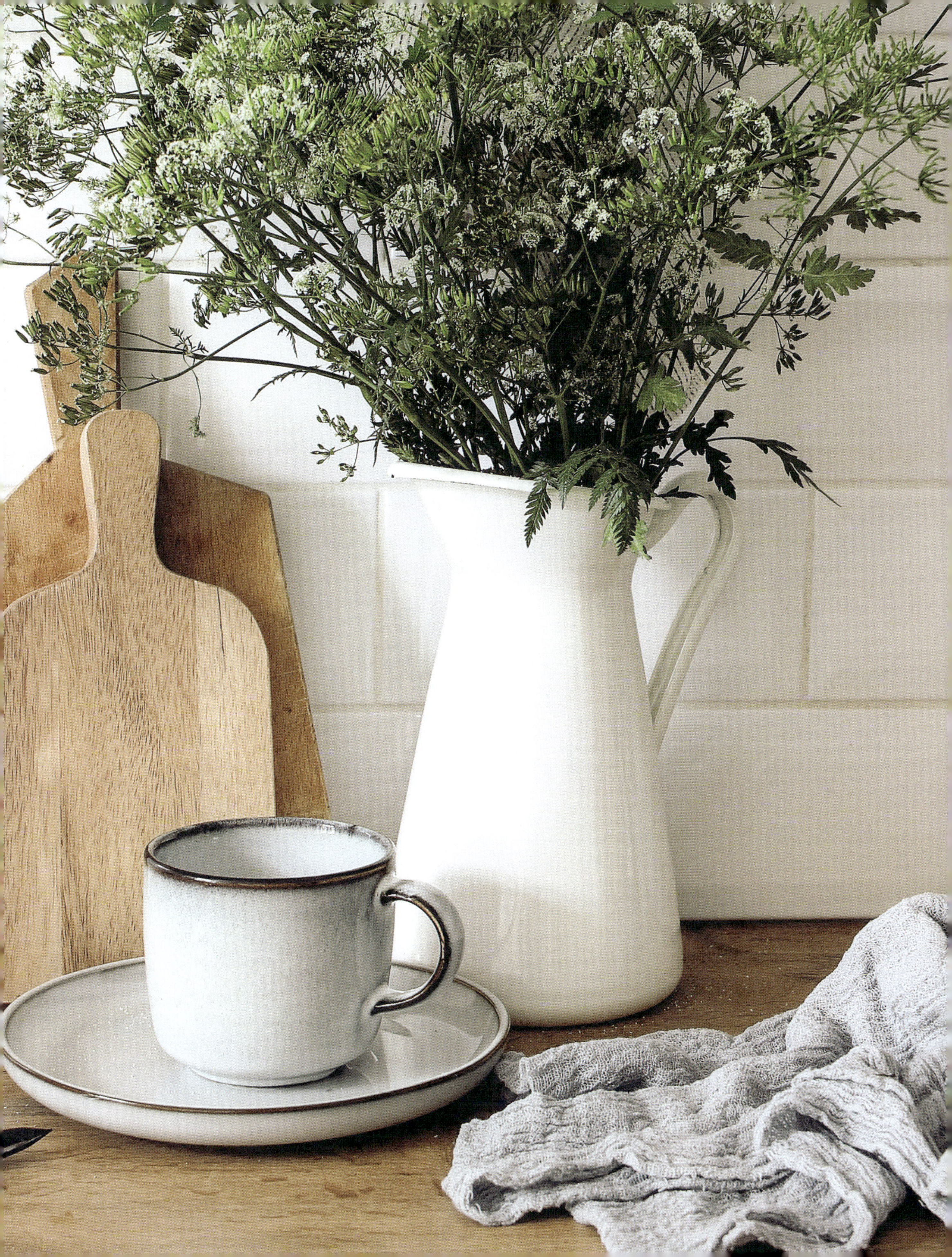

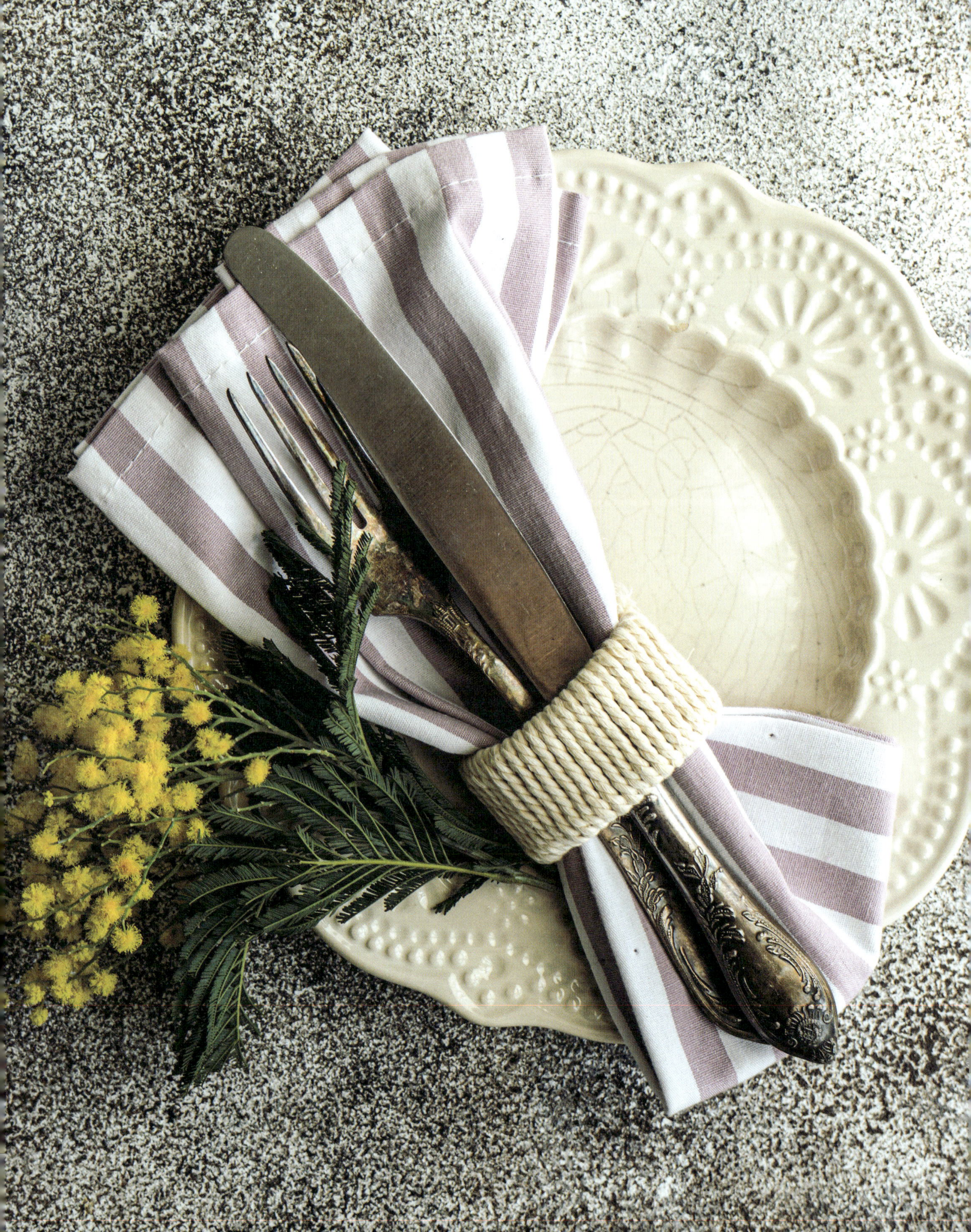

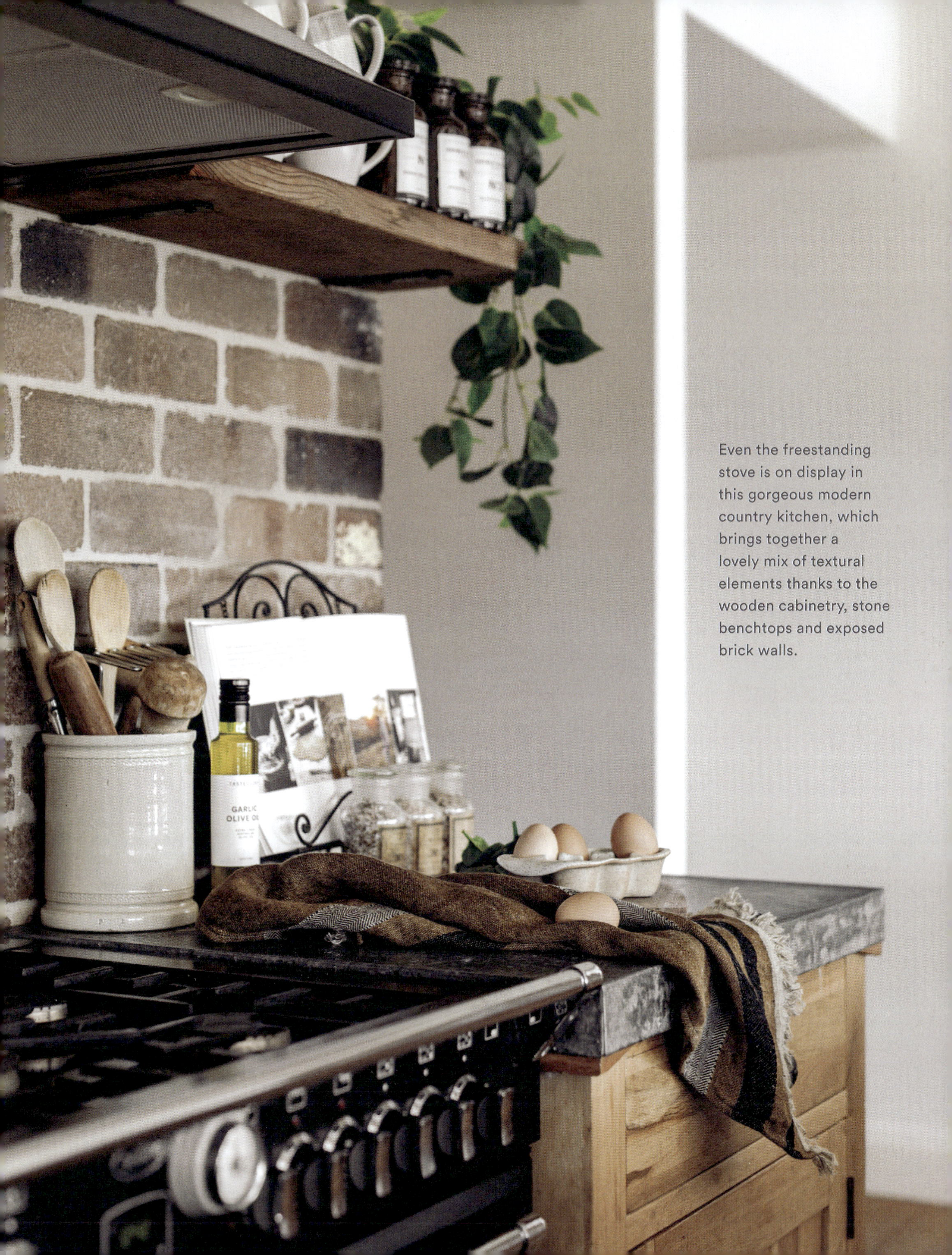

Even the freestanding stove is on display in this gorgeous modern country kitchen, which brings together a lovely mix of textural elements thanks to the wooden cabinetry, stone benchtops and exposed brick walls.

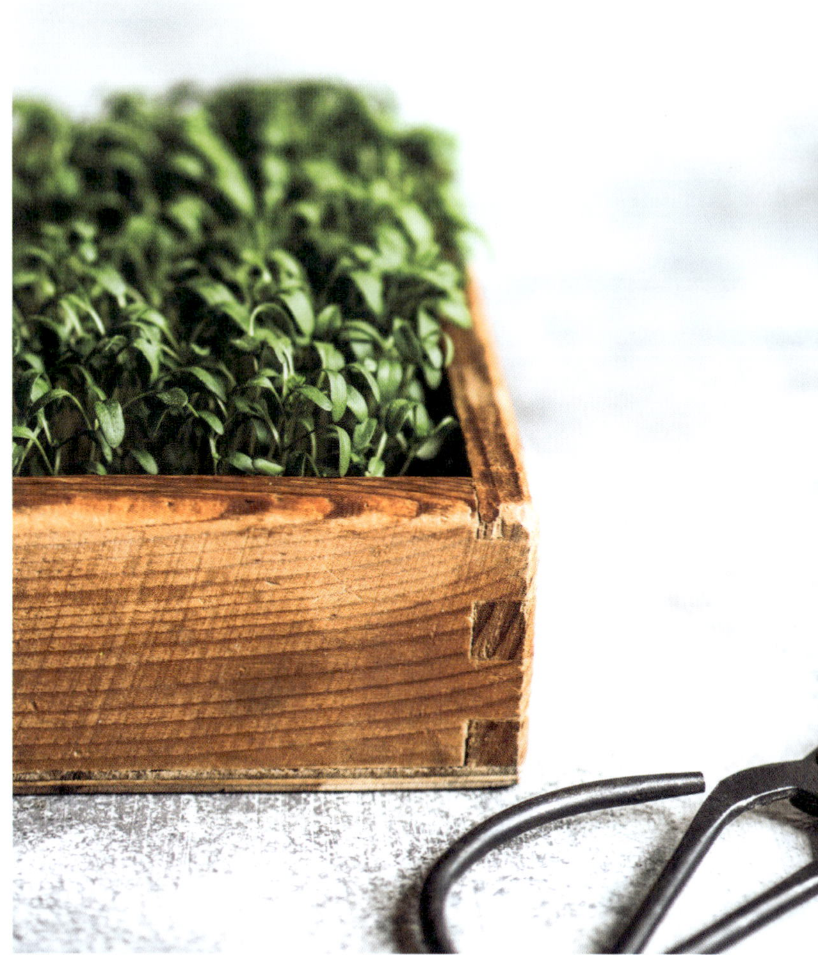

Nature's bounty on display – in the form of fresh herbs and eggs, fruit from the garden or freshly-baked bread, creates a mood of timeless pleasure and easy hospitality.

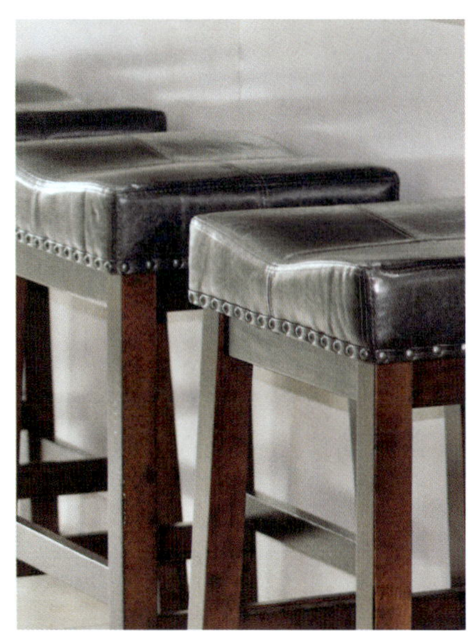

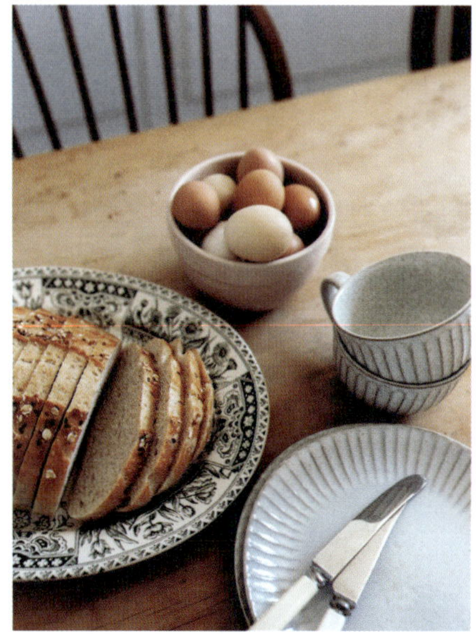

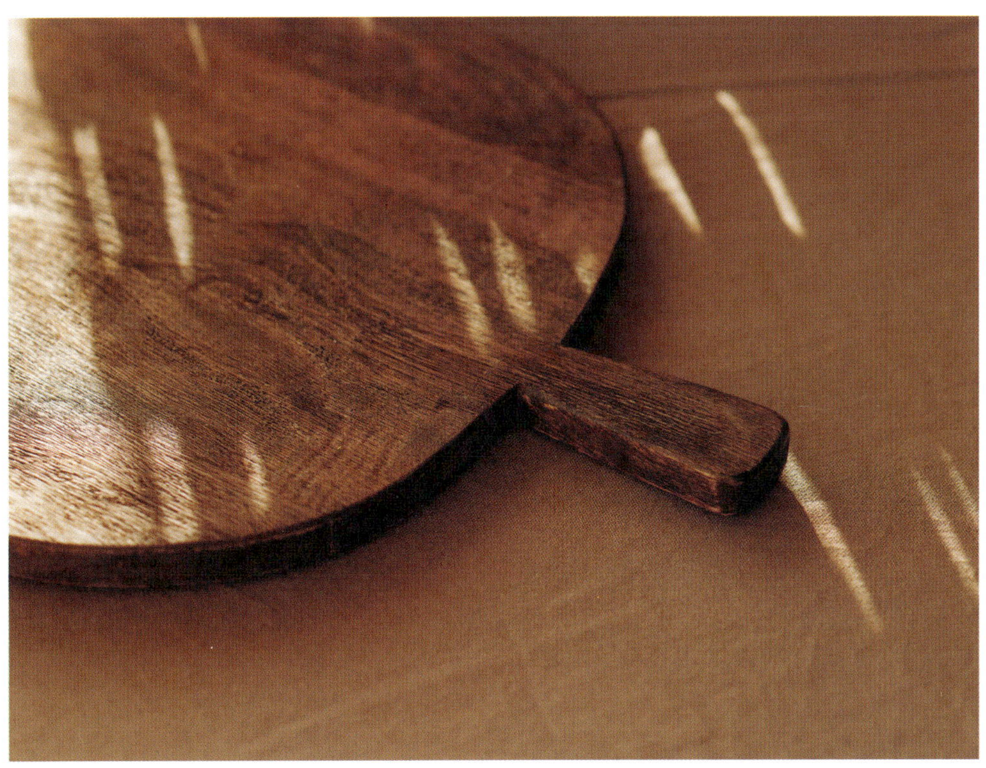

Rough-hewn wooden chopping boards provide the perfect blend of form and function in a modern country kitchen.

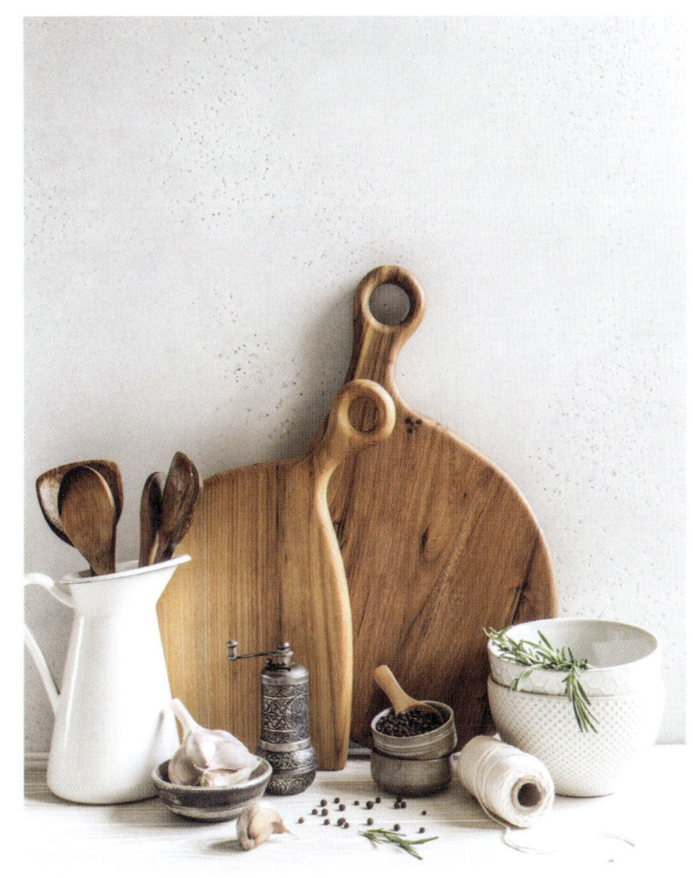

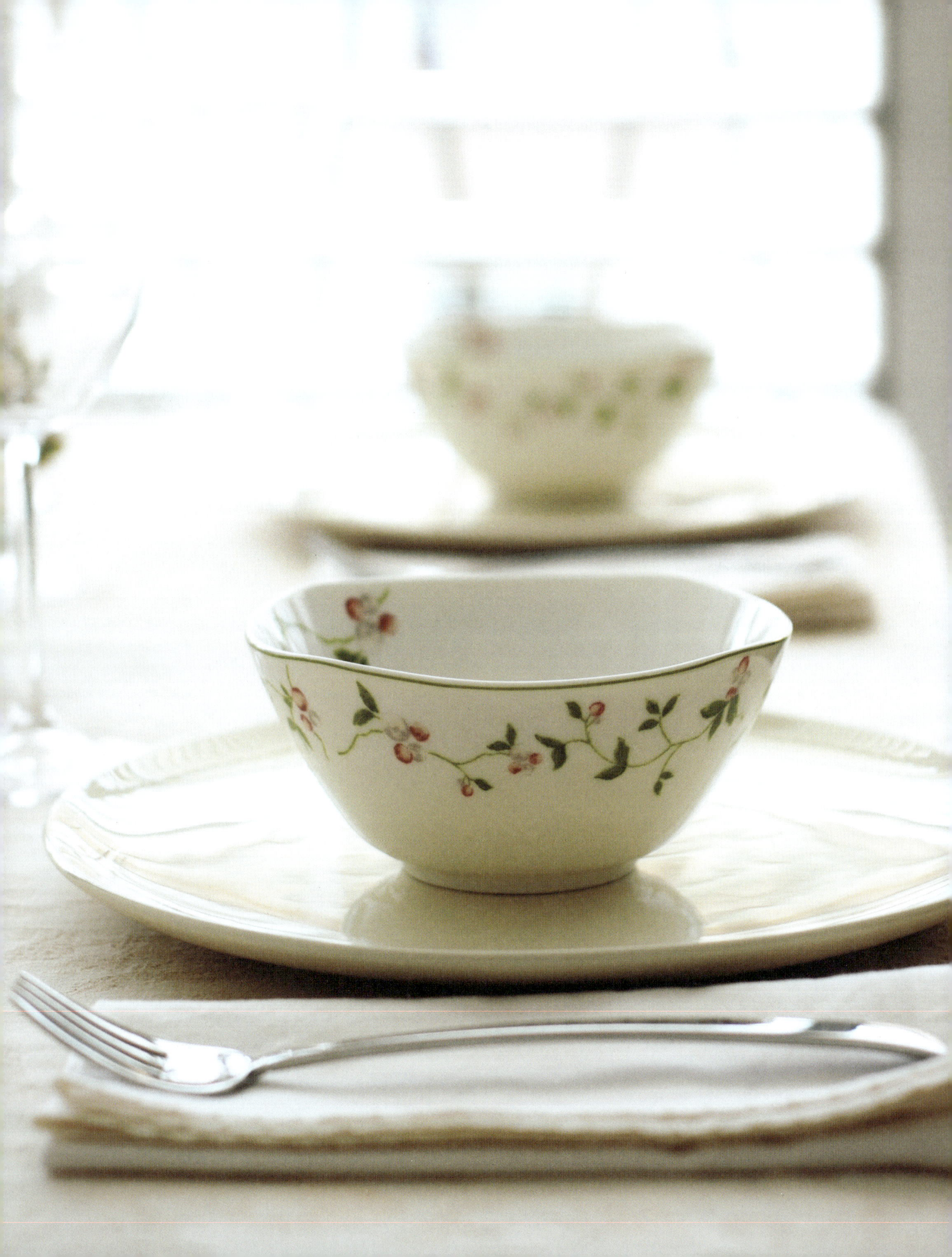

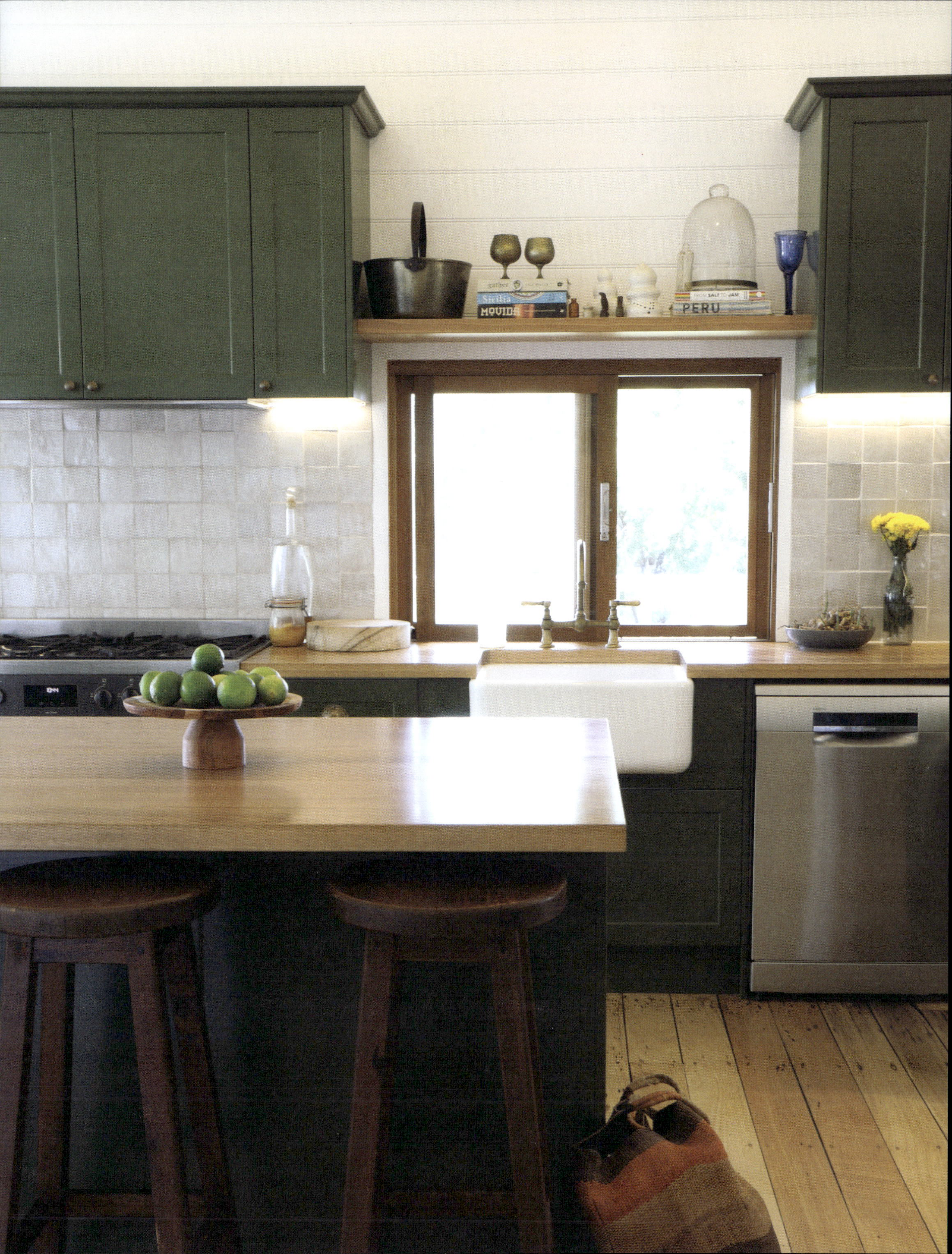
gather
Sicilia
MOVIDA
FROM SALT TO JAM
PERU

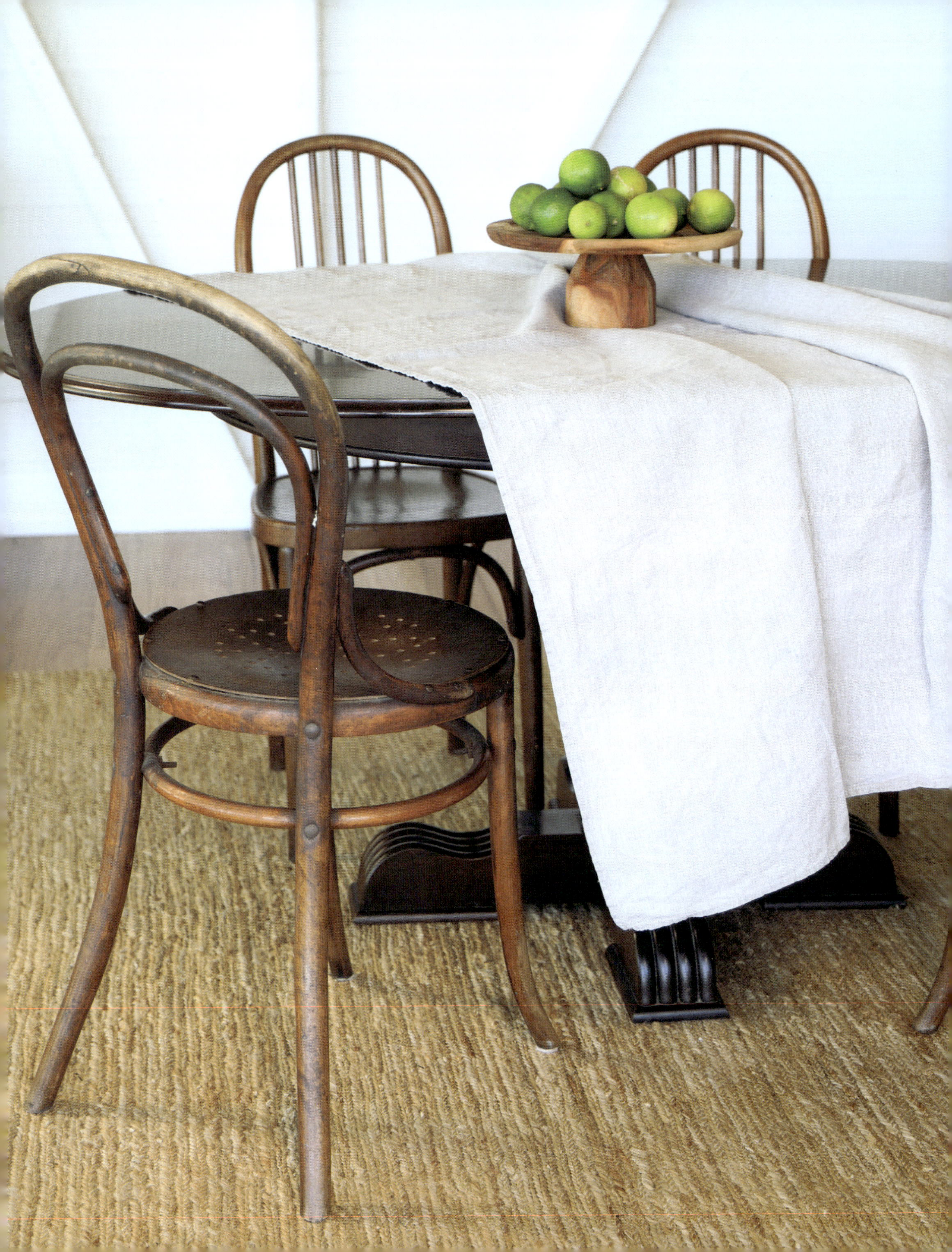

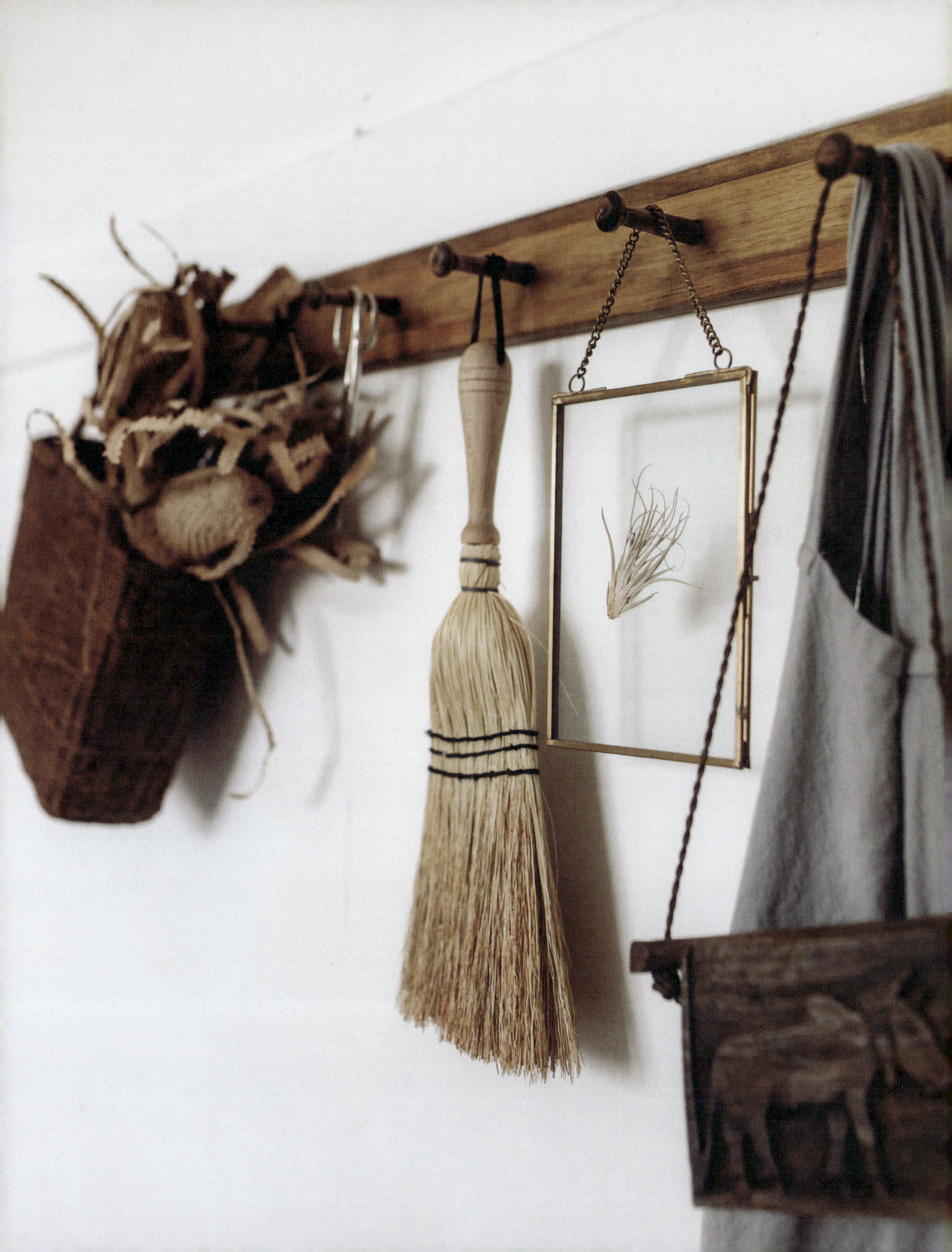

The Quick List

Open shelving to display crockery and glassware

Under-bench open shelving for pots and pans

Concrete benchtops

Farmhouse dining tables

Cabinetry in colours inspired by nature, from soft grey to sage greens

Eclectic or mismatched tableware

High-quality linen napkins and tablecloths

Pendant lighting for workspaces and dining areas

Quirky collections of less frequently used objects on high shelves

Loved glasses for summer evening drinks

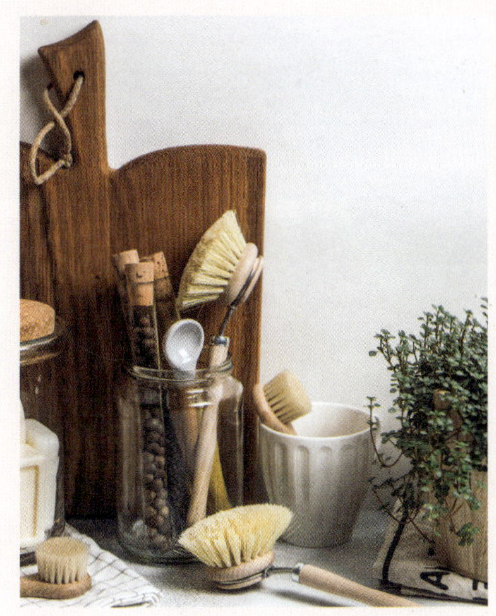

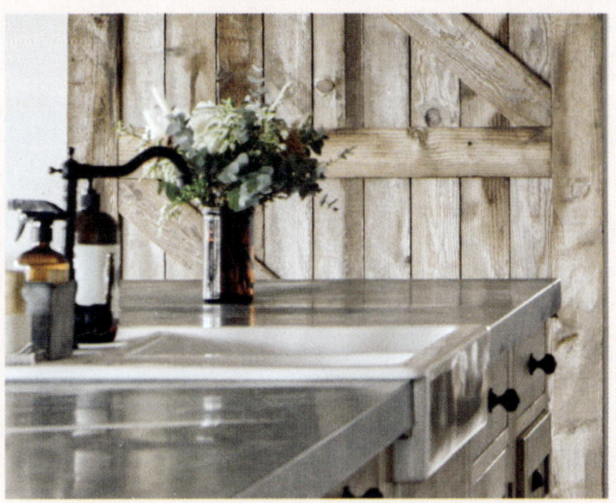

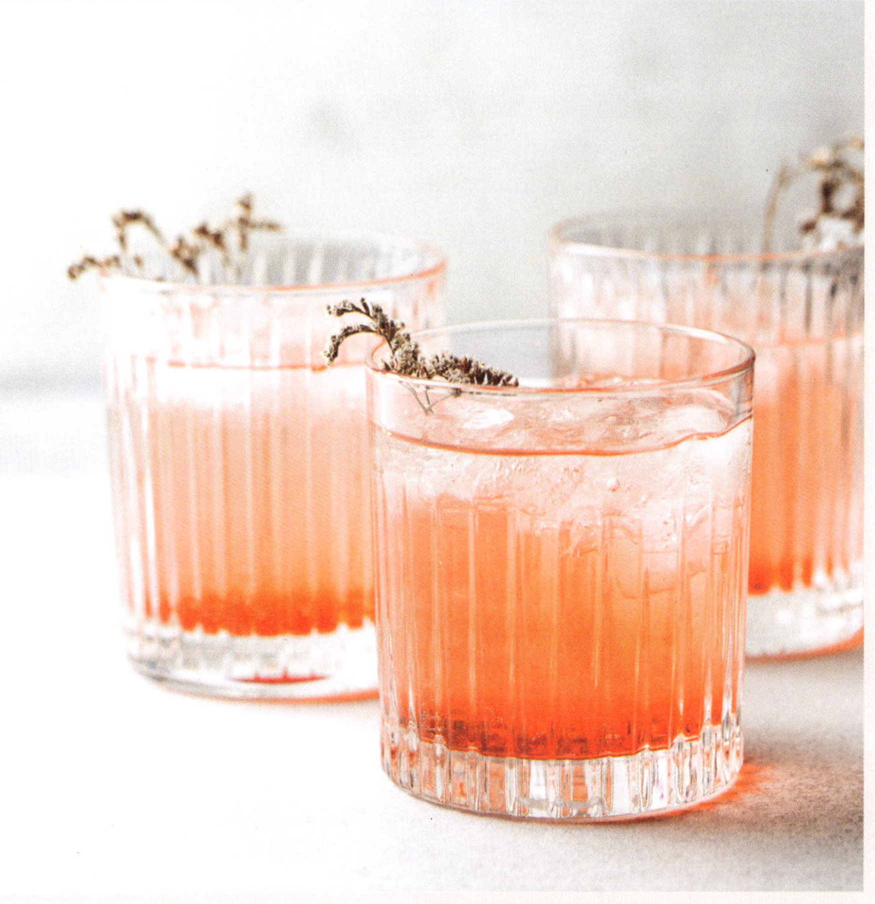

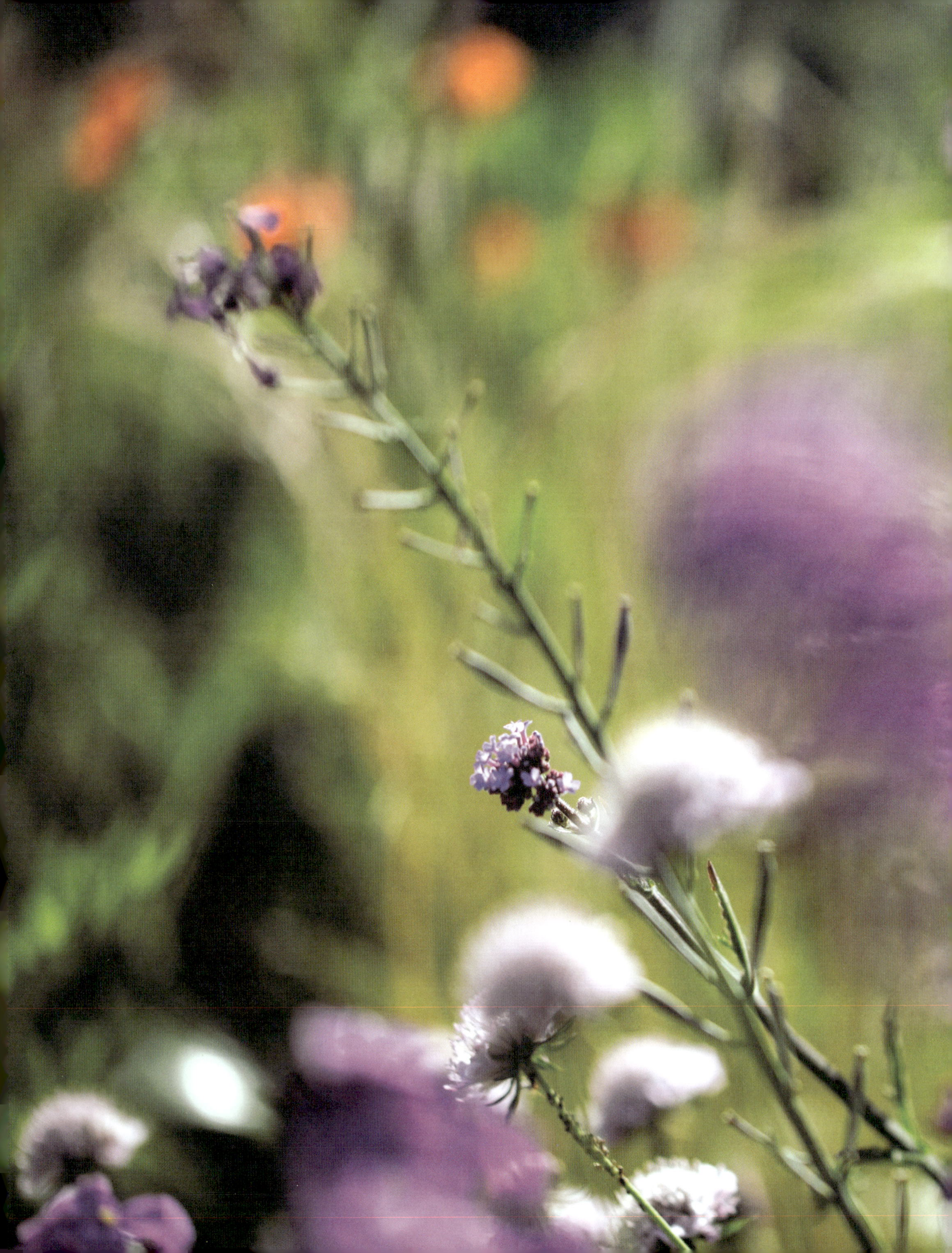

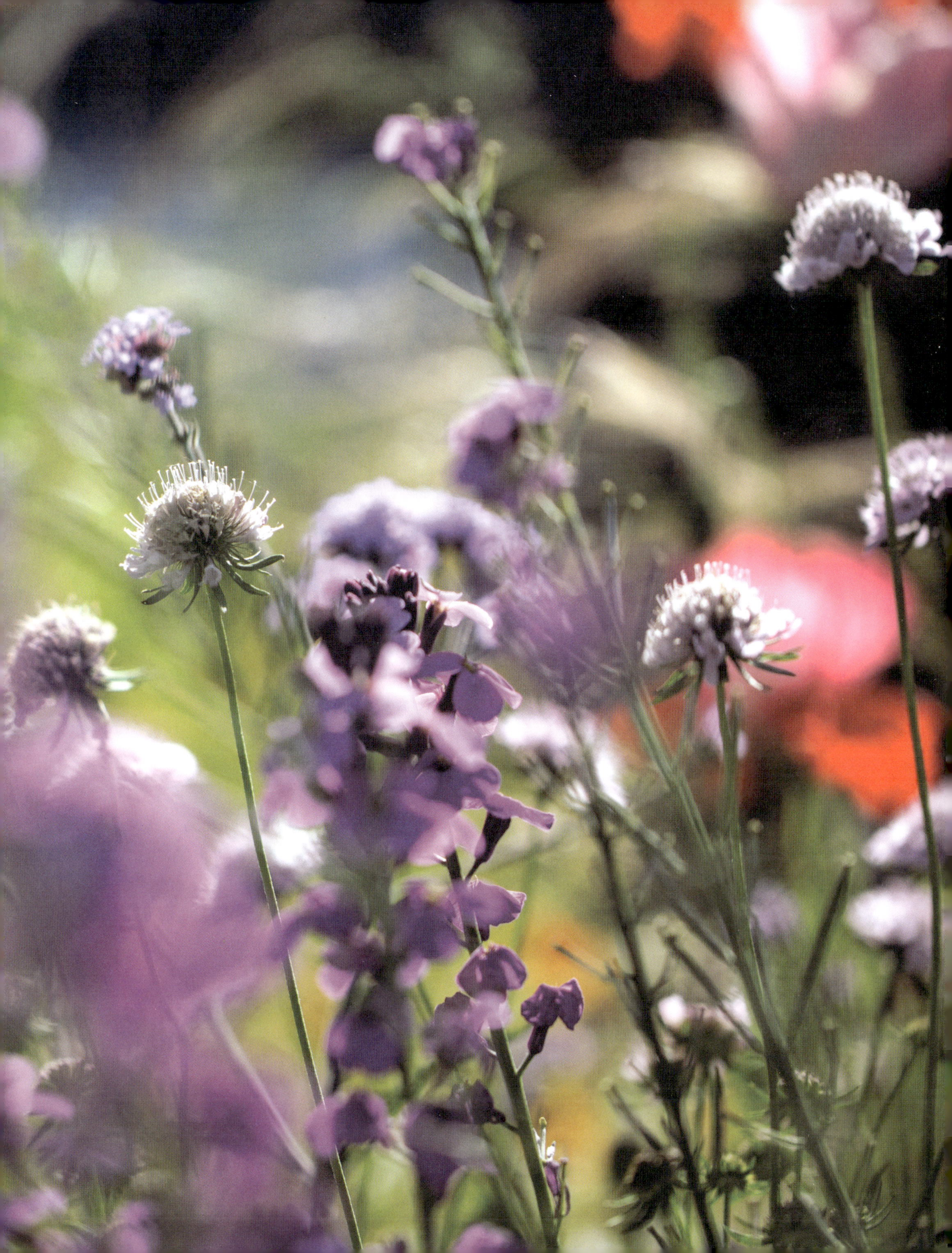

chapter six

bathing

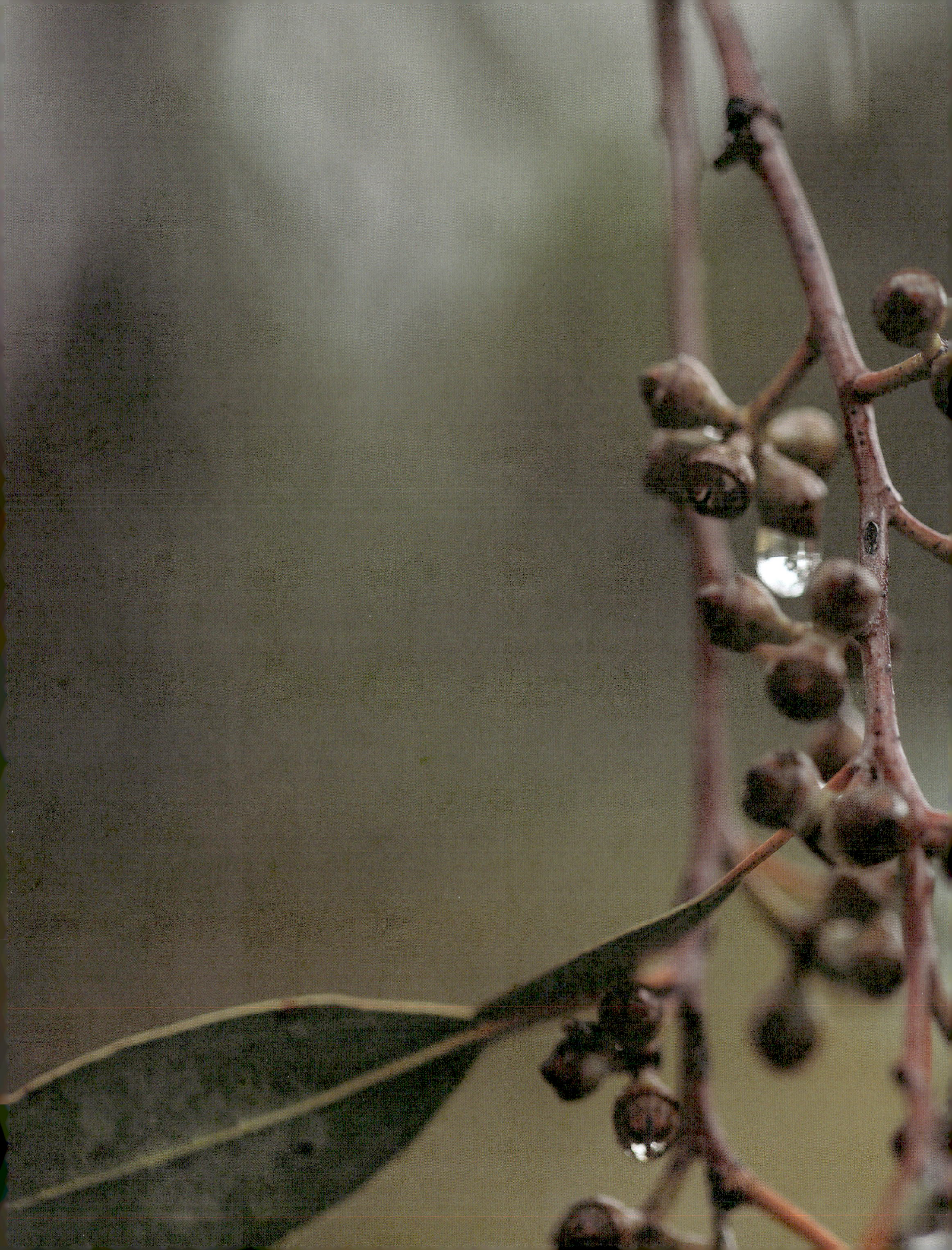

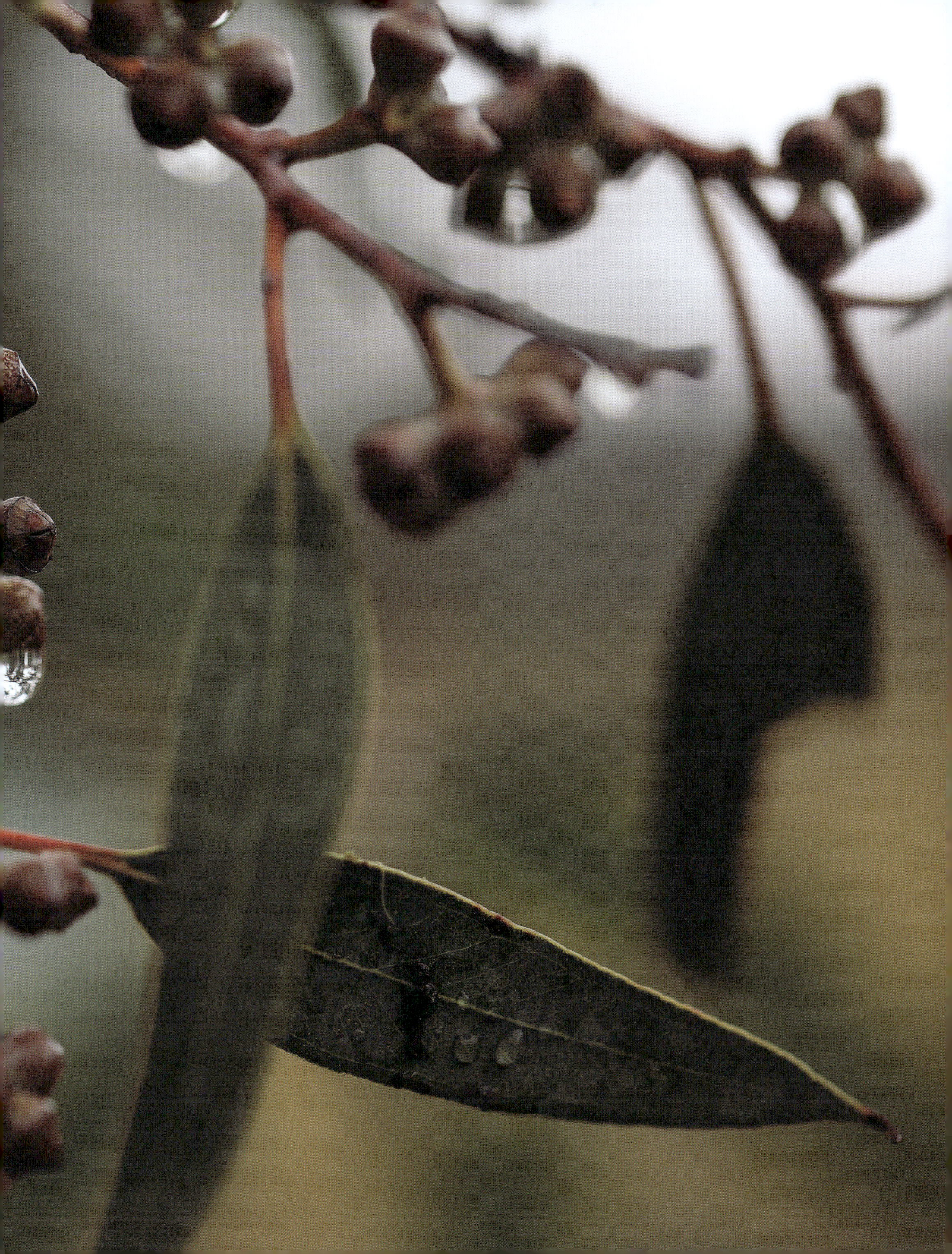

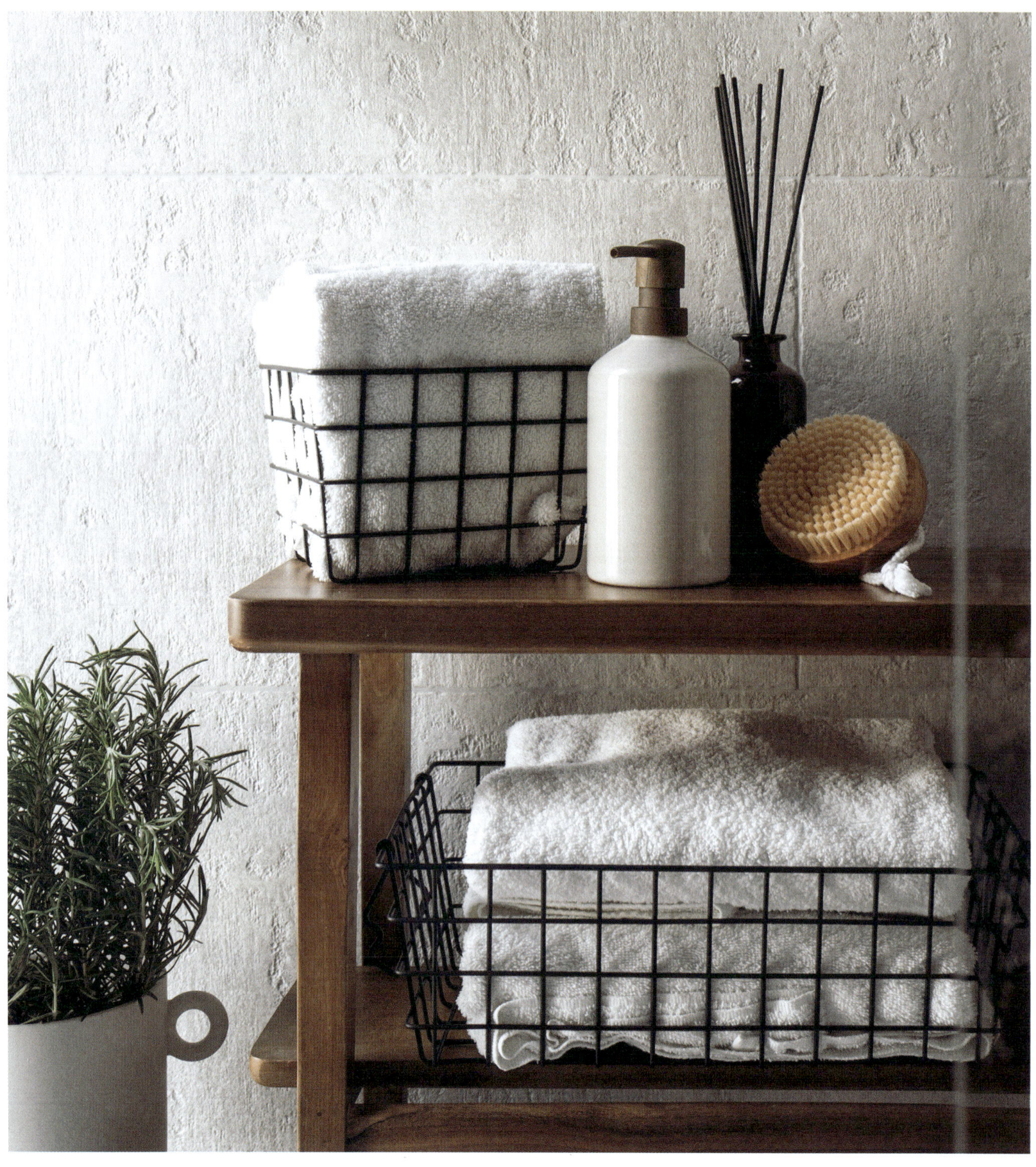

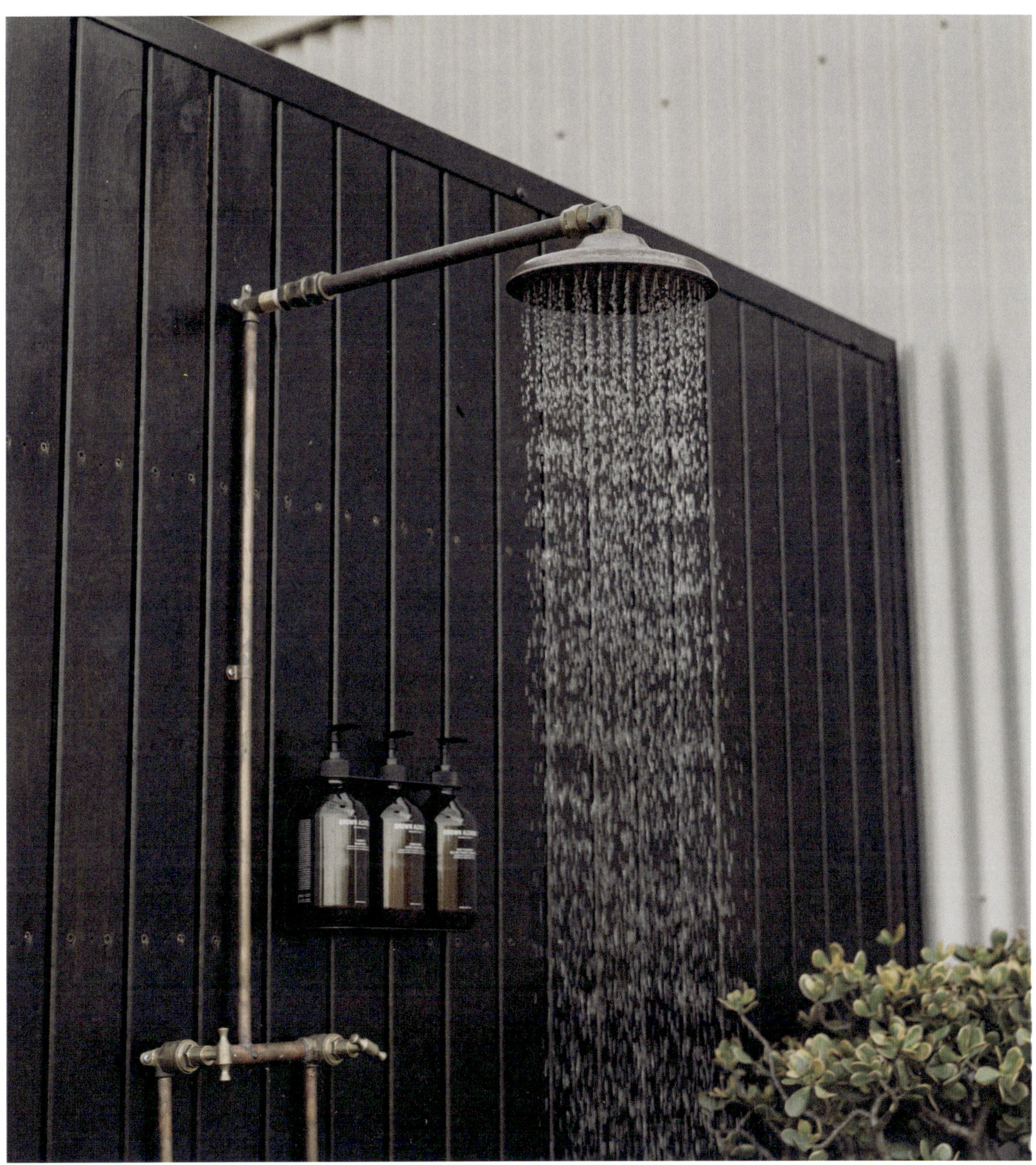

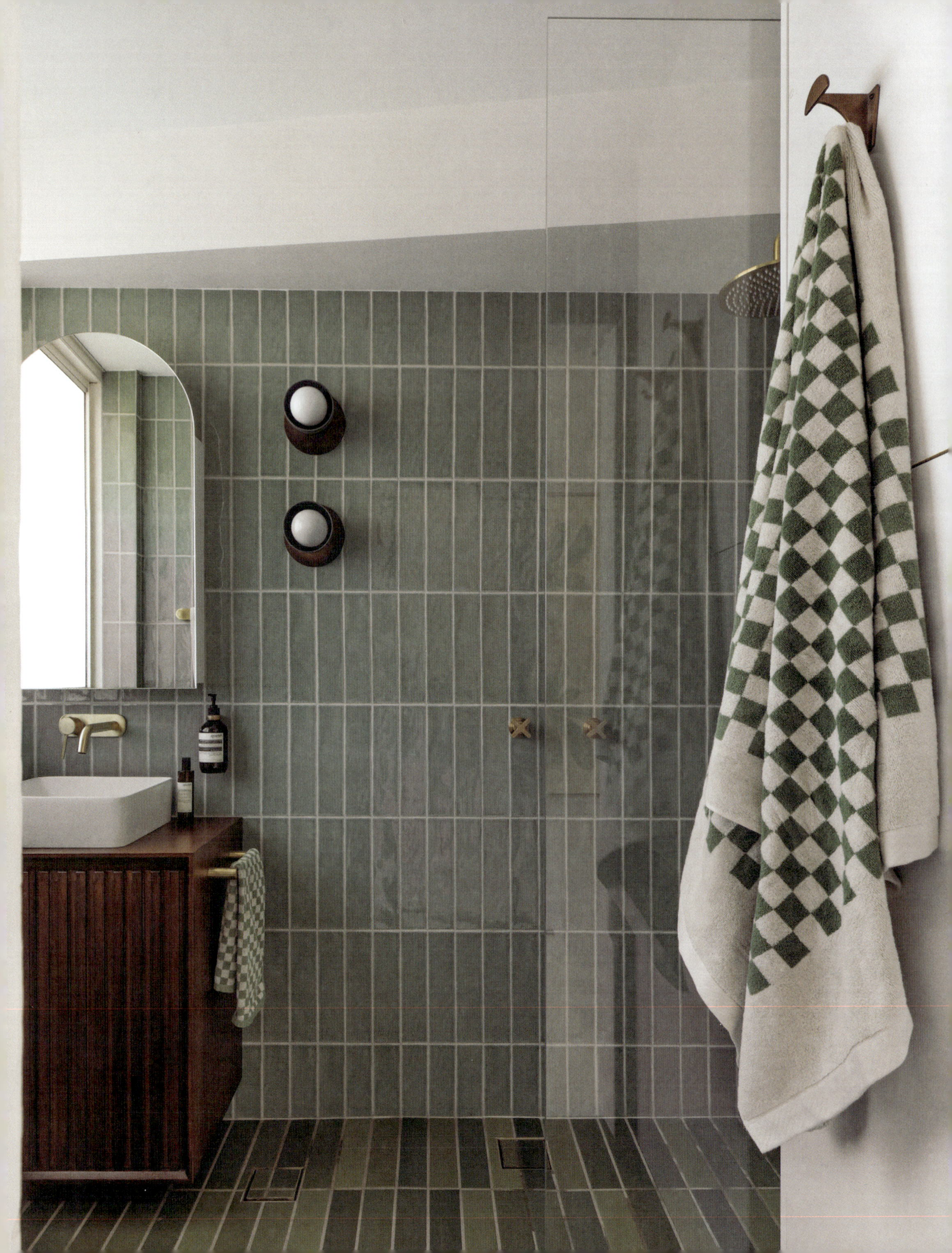

Country-style bathrooms traditionally feature hard-wearing surfaces like weathered timber and finishes like brass, setting them up to withstand the tough demands of country living.

Times have changed and bathroom design in general has gone in the direction of functional, simple and slick, but modern country bucks this trend to a certain degree.

Nothing says farmstead or rural country idyll more than a claw-foot bath in front of a large window opening over rolling hills and a vintage timber milking stool to park your book or wine – the ultimate in relaxation after a hard day in the fields. But you don't need to follow the script. Whatever bath you have is just fine. The joy in styling a bathroom in the modern country look is that it's achievable without too much effort or expense.

A useful tip to keep in mind is to style the bathroom as you would any other room. Freestanding furniture, such as stools, chairs or a dresser, works well, as does greenery – plants and plenty of them bring energy and life into the bathroom. You could even consider a nice rug – why not upgrade from that old bathmat to something more luxurious to enjoy?

If you are renovating or looking to replace fixtures and fittings in your bathroom, keep in mind that timber (think shiplap or VJ panelling for walls, or timber dressers) is an essential material in the country bathroom. It pairs well with aged brass or copper. You can get the shiny new versions of these materials or go old-style and consider exposed copper pipes or bricks as a deliberate styling choice if available to you.

Timeless elegance is the look to go for in the modern country bathroom, with a mix of purpose-built or freestanding furniture, beautiful linen and towels, united by a soft, natural colour palette and enlivened by plants, natural soaps and oils, and perhaps the odd vintage display item or two.

TOP FIVE

1\.

Freestanding furniture

2\.

Personal or vintage touches

3\.

Natural soaps, oils and cleaning products

4\.

Tiles paired in different styles

5\.

Classic materials such as timber and brass

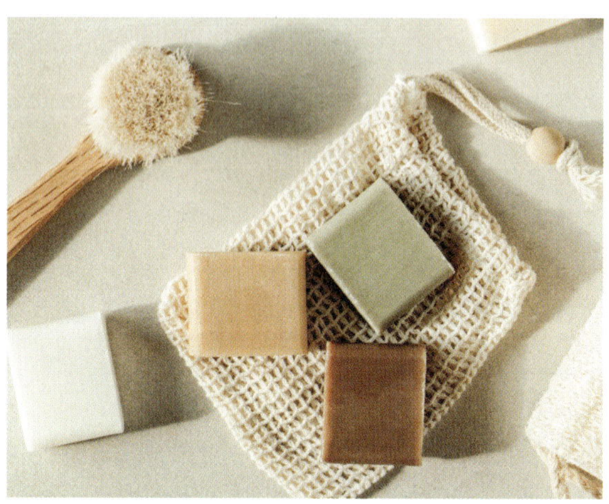

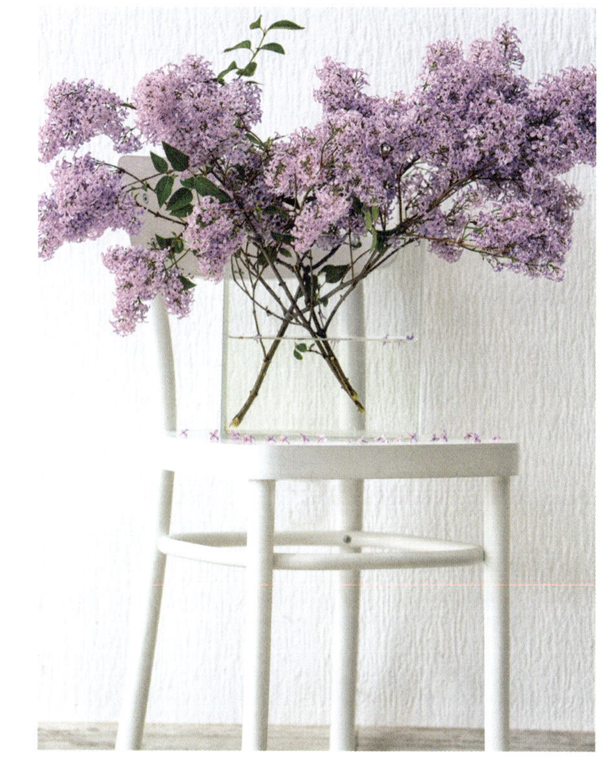

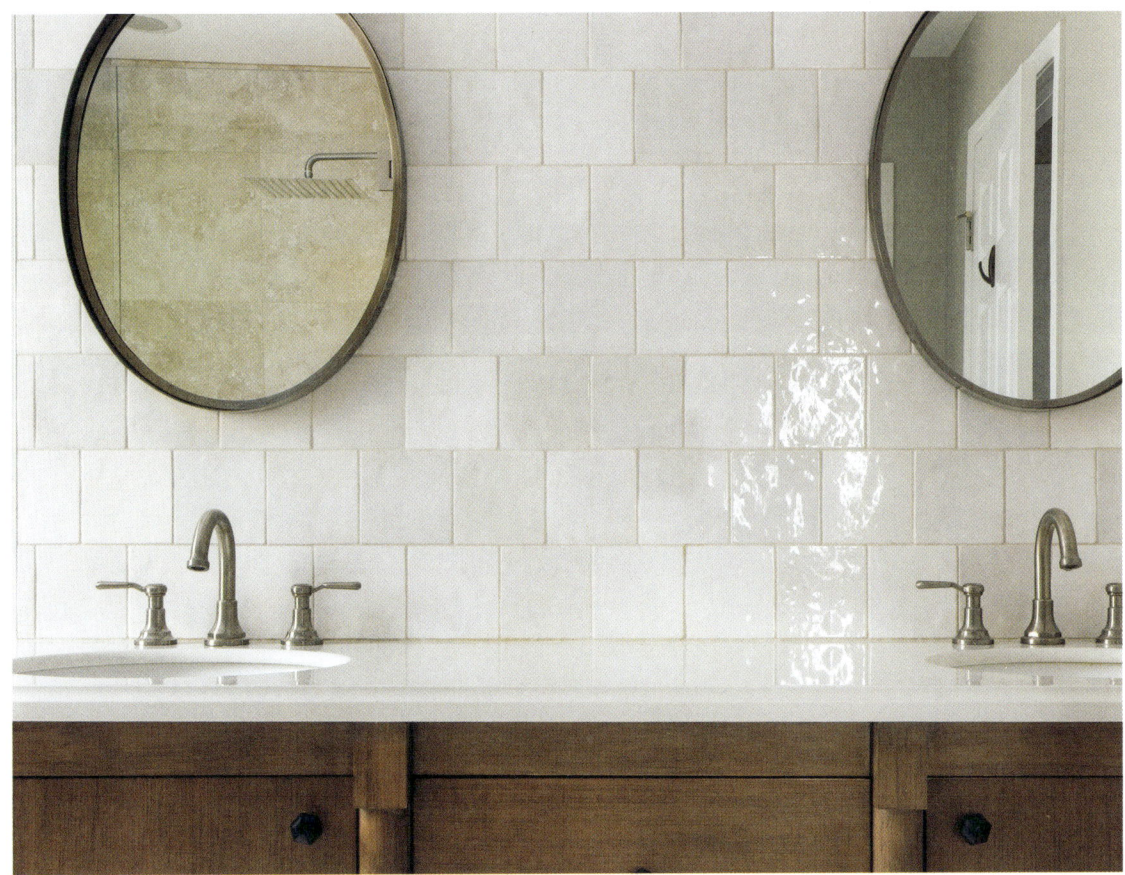

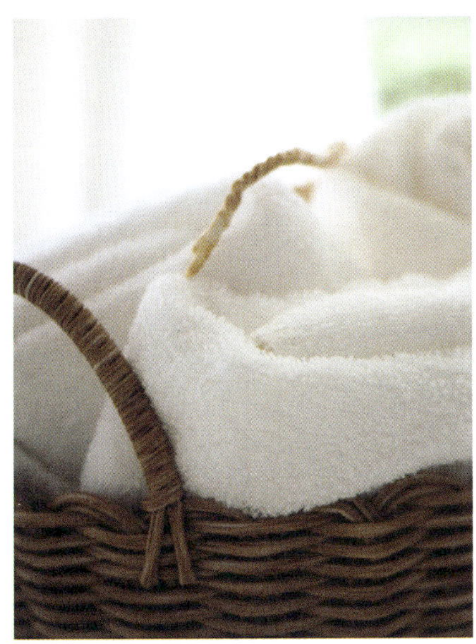

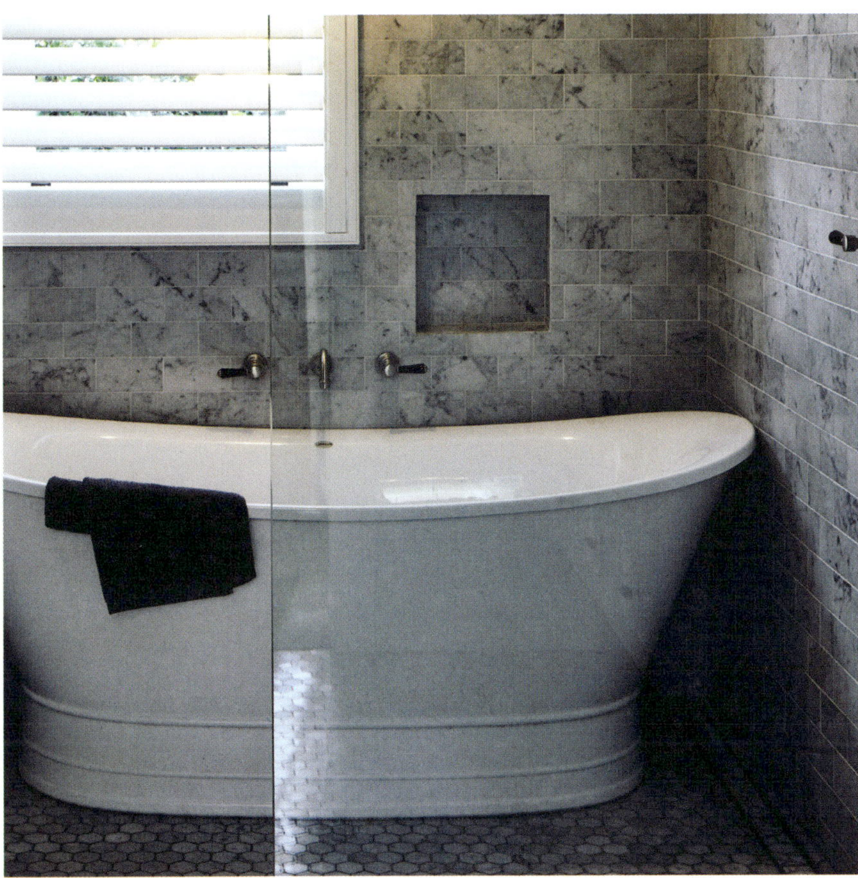

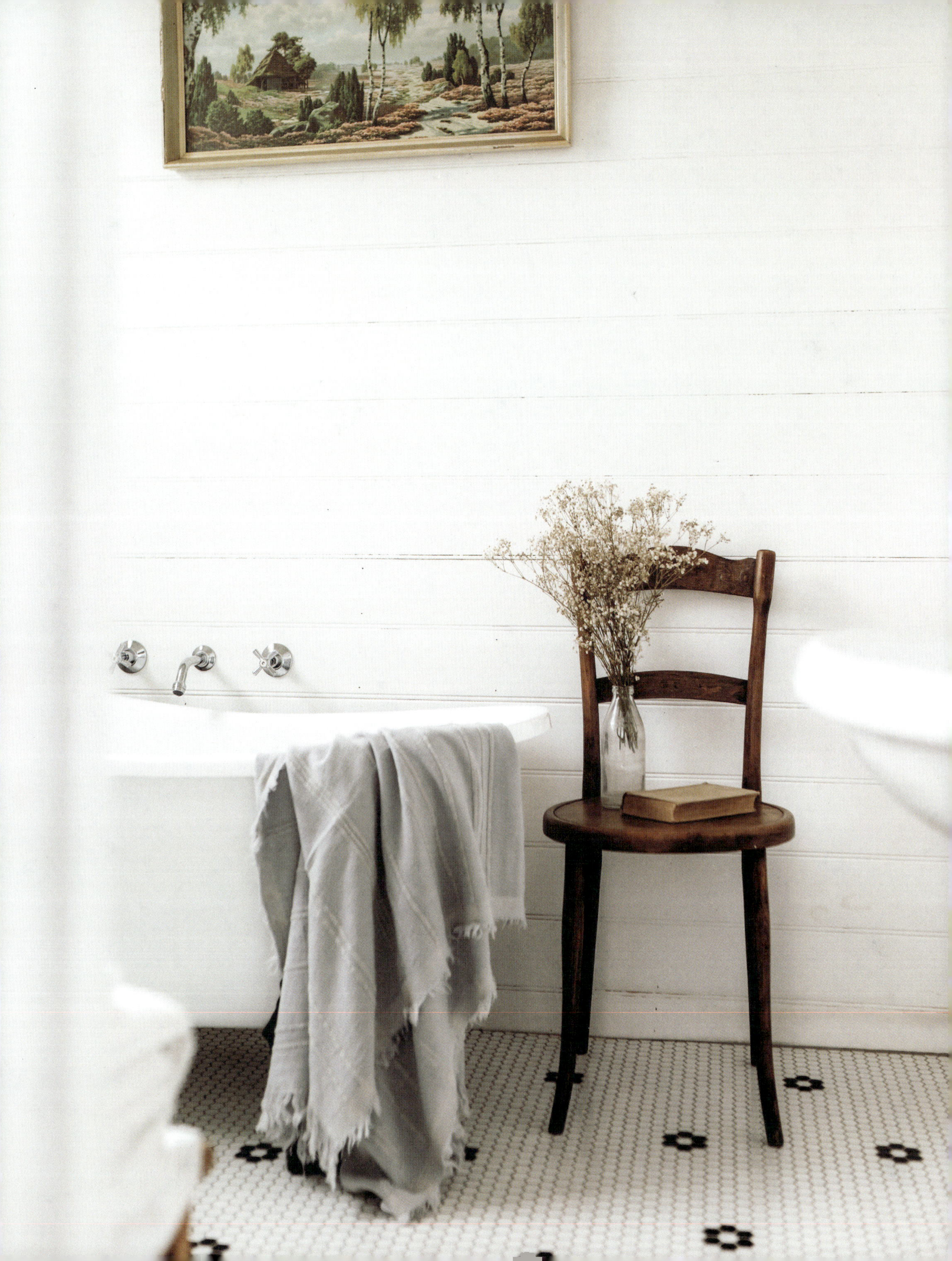

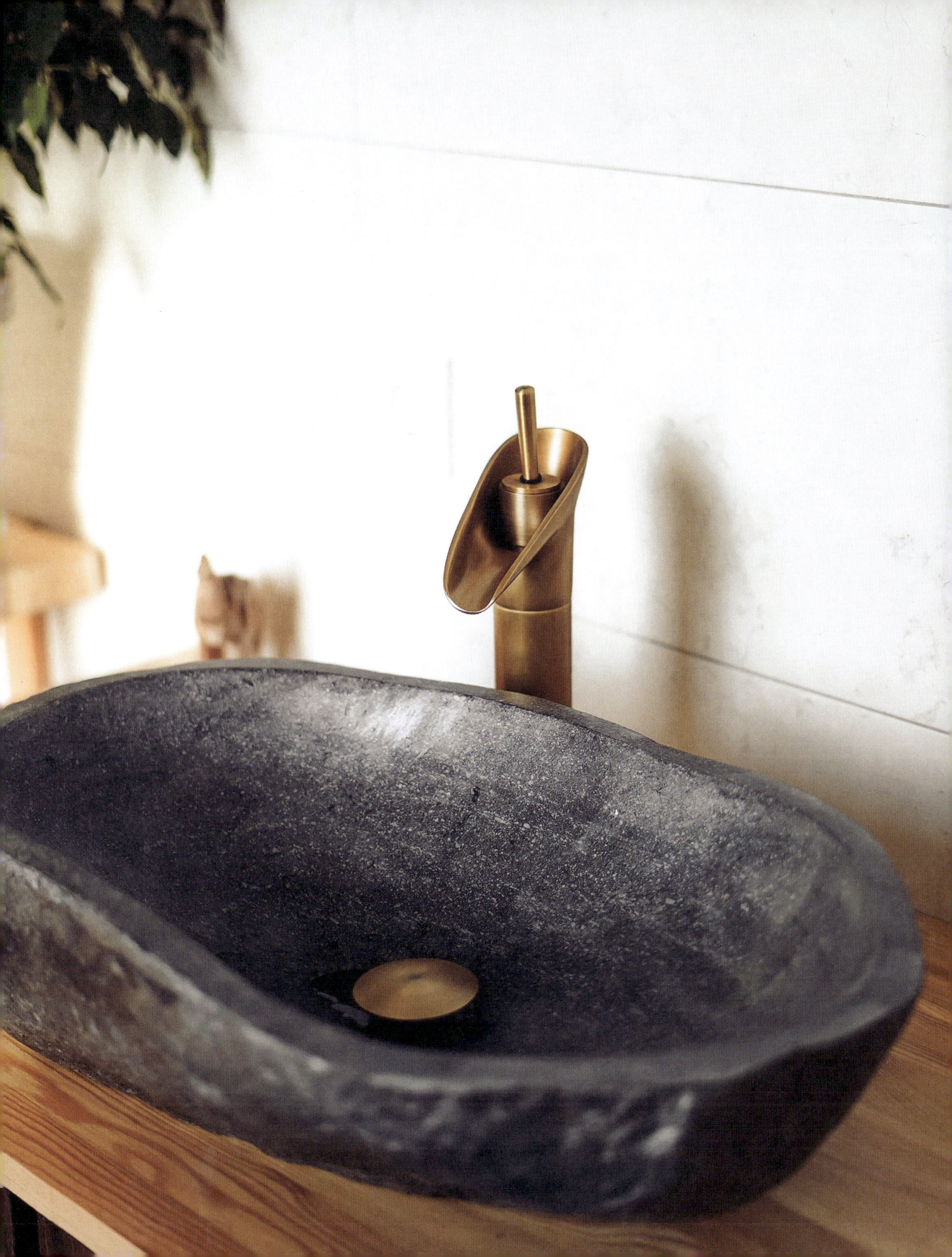

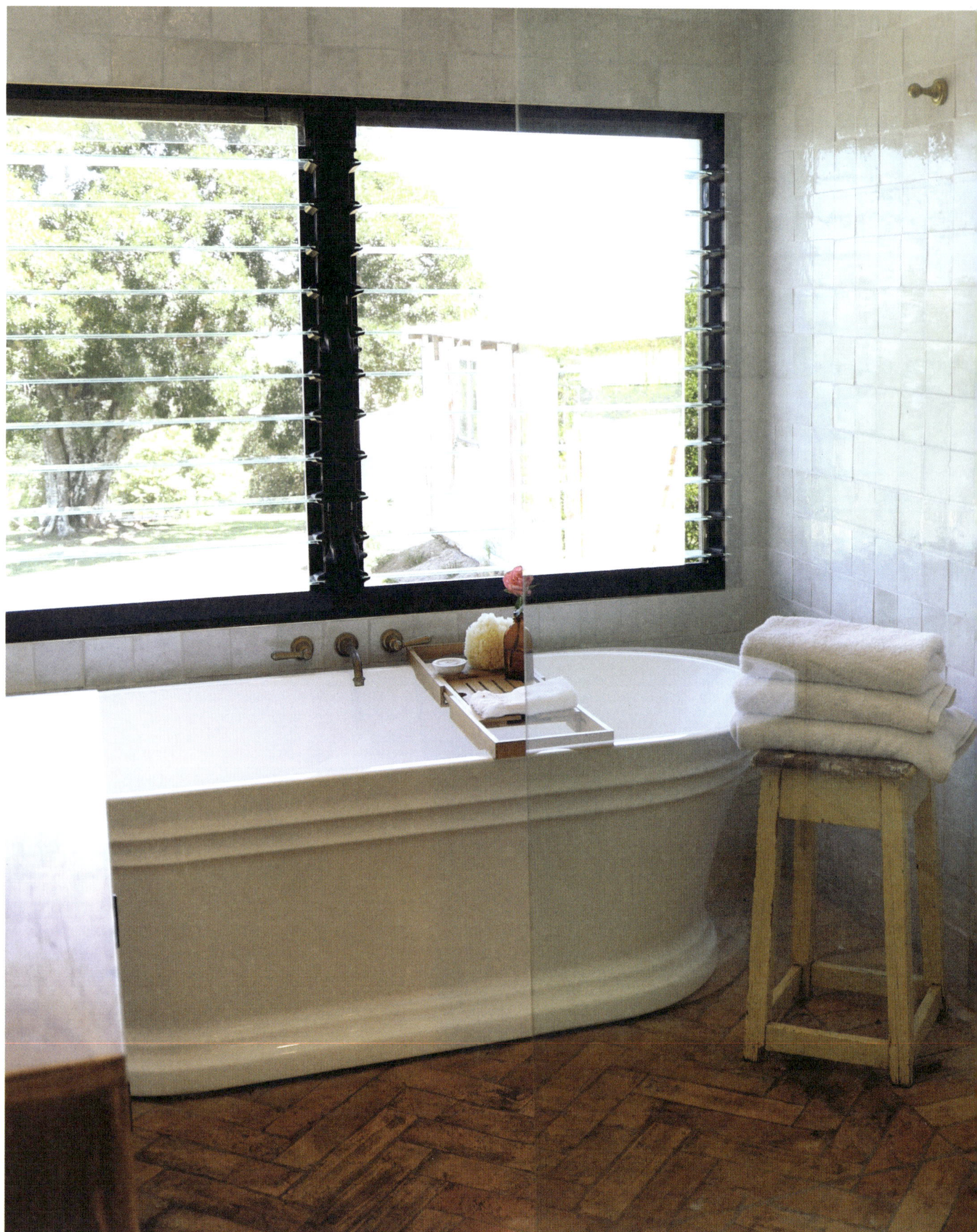

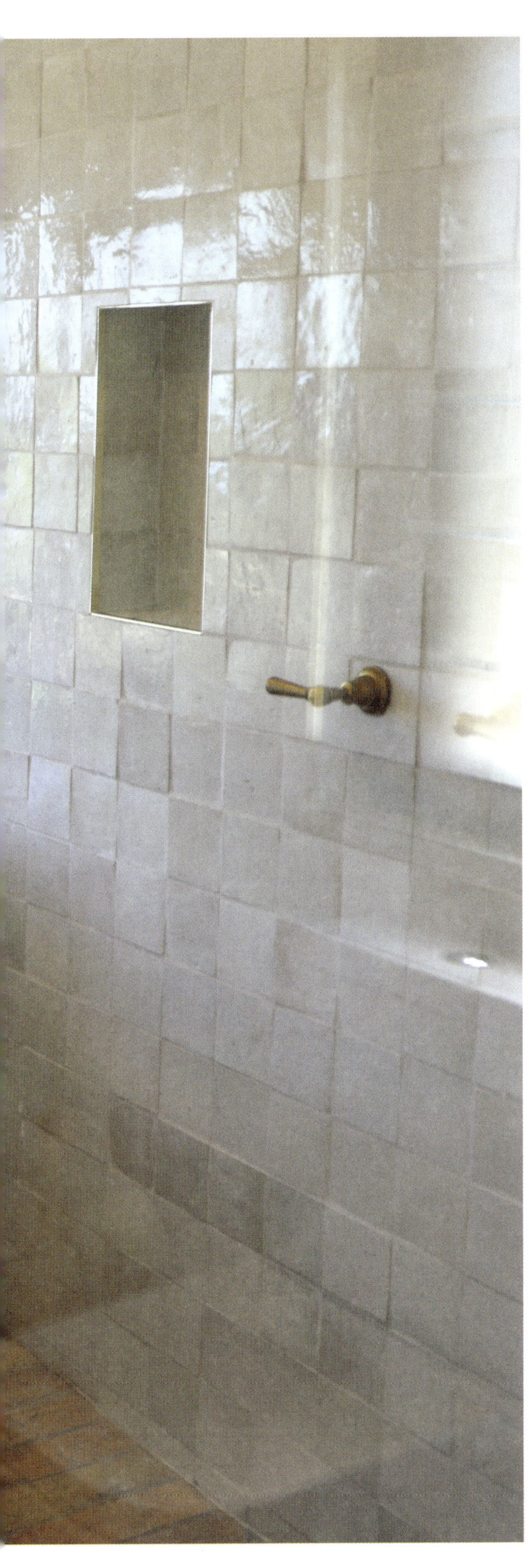

A perfect execution of modern country style, this simple family bathroom confidently pairs herringbone and square tiles, features brass tapware, a freestanding bath and vanity and a vintage stool topped with plump and inviting fresh towels. Bliss.

Carefully-curated displays are as important in the bathroom as any other room in the house. The warm, honeyed tones of the wood and natural fibres on display here lend an air of calm and tranquility to the space.

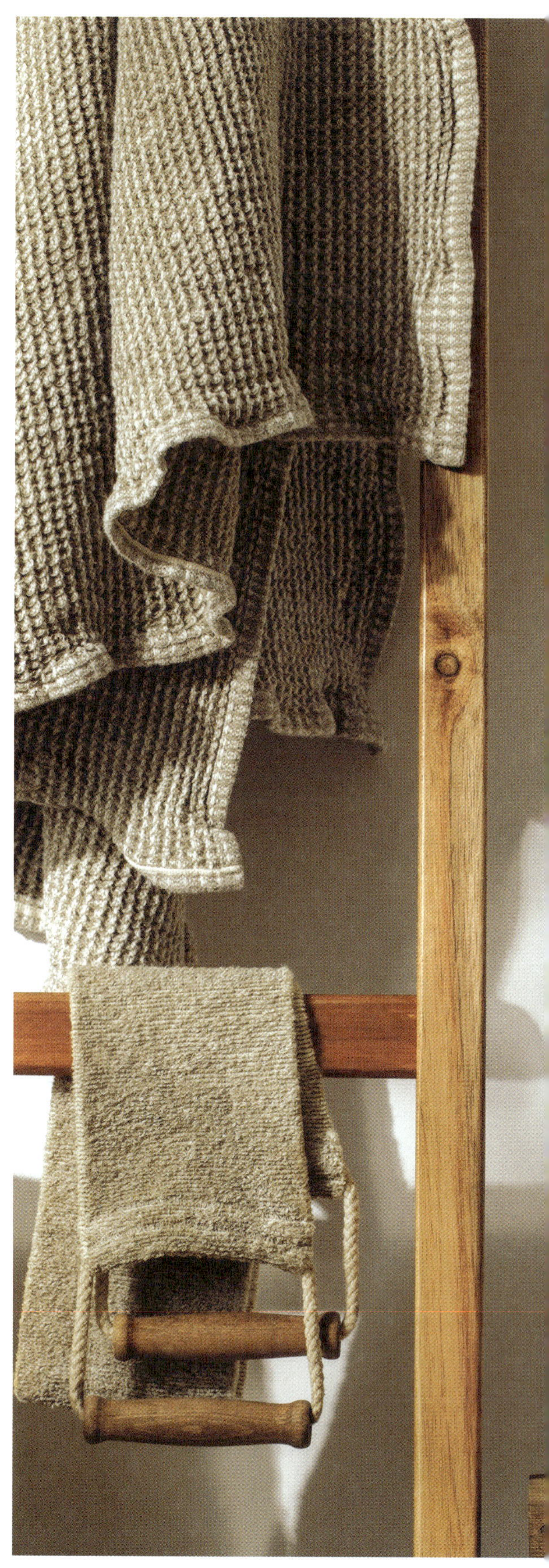

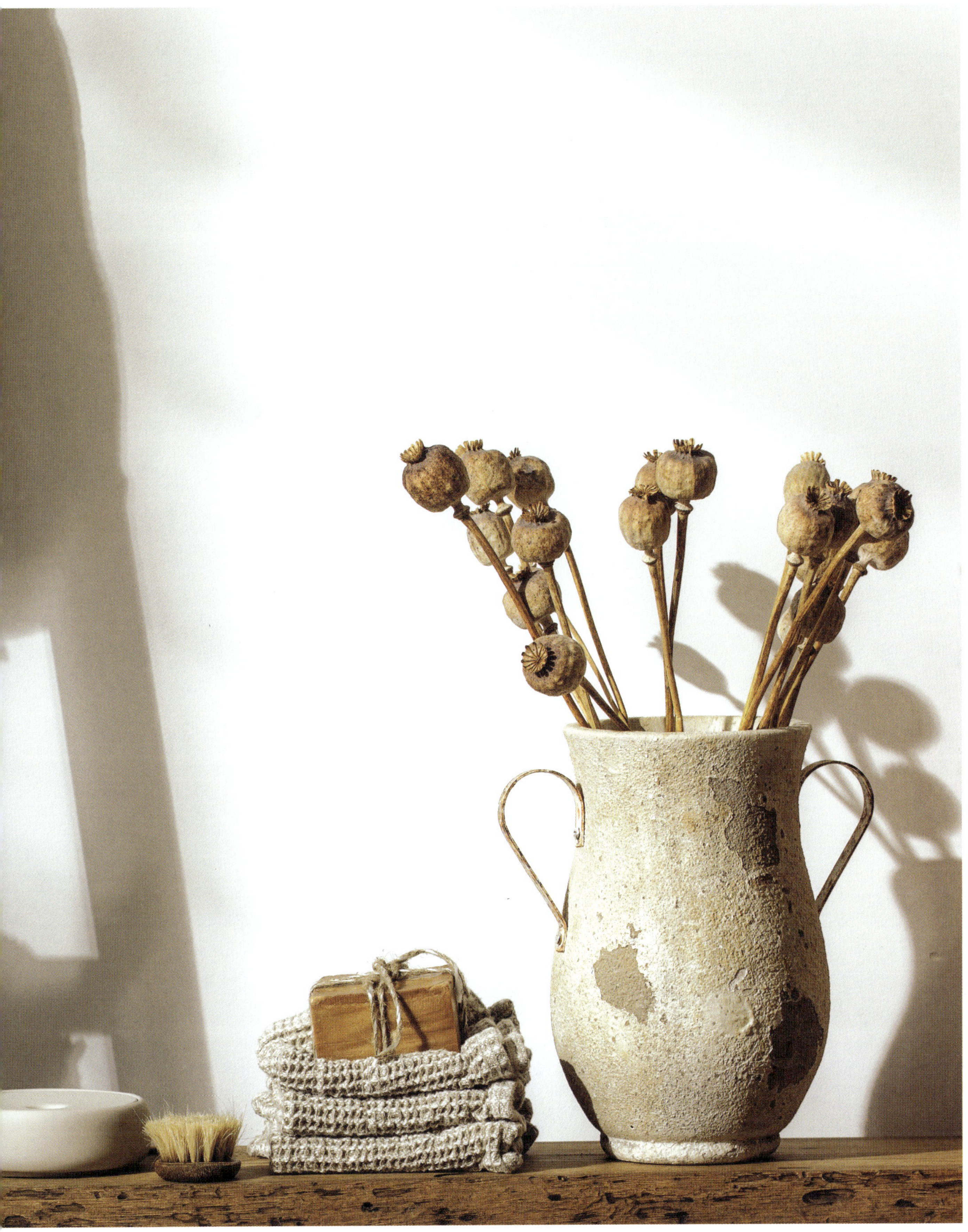

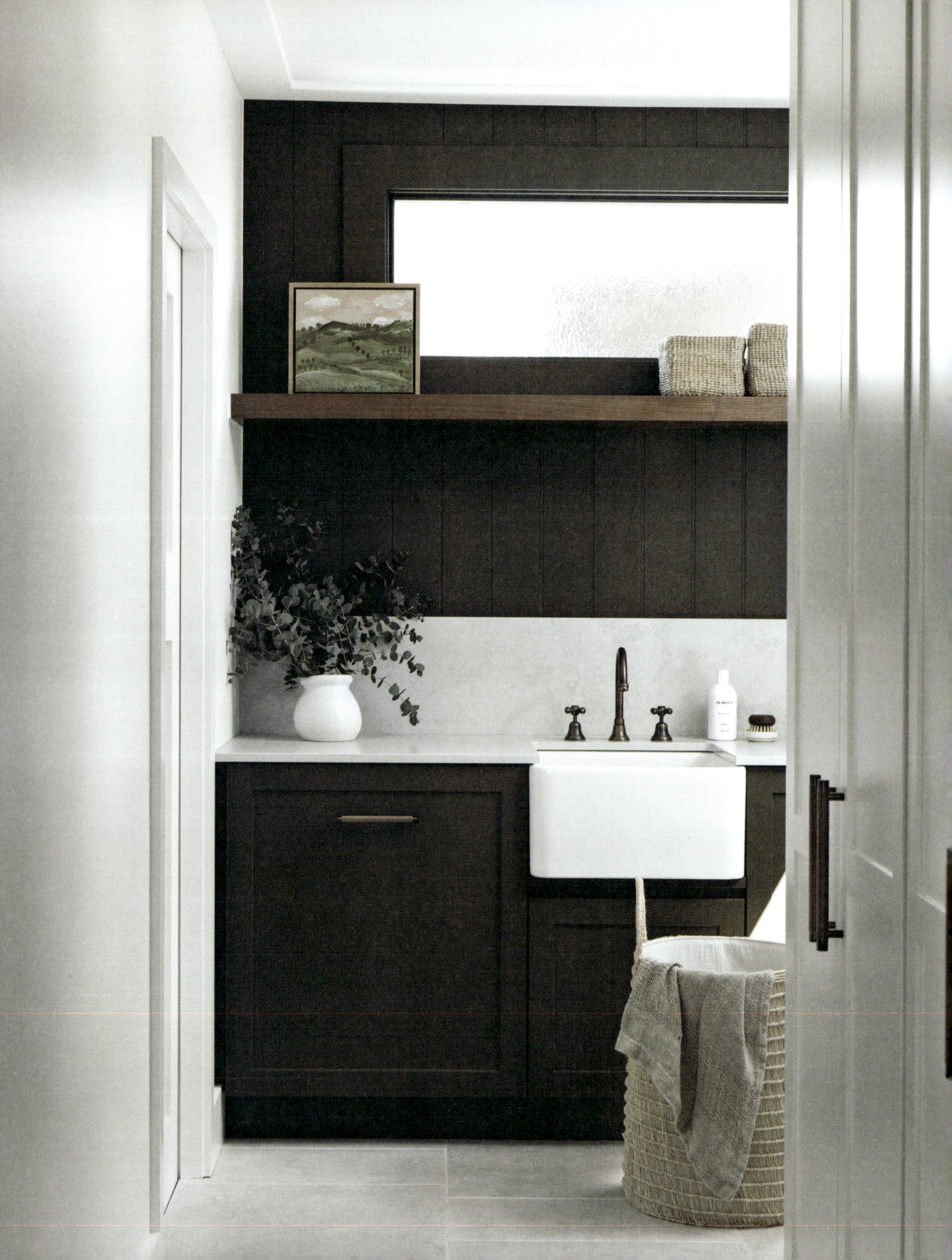

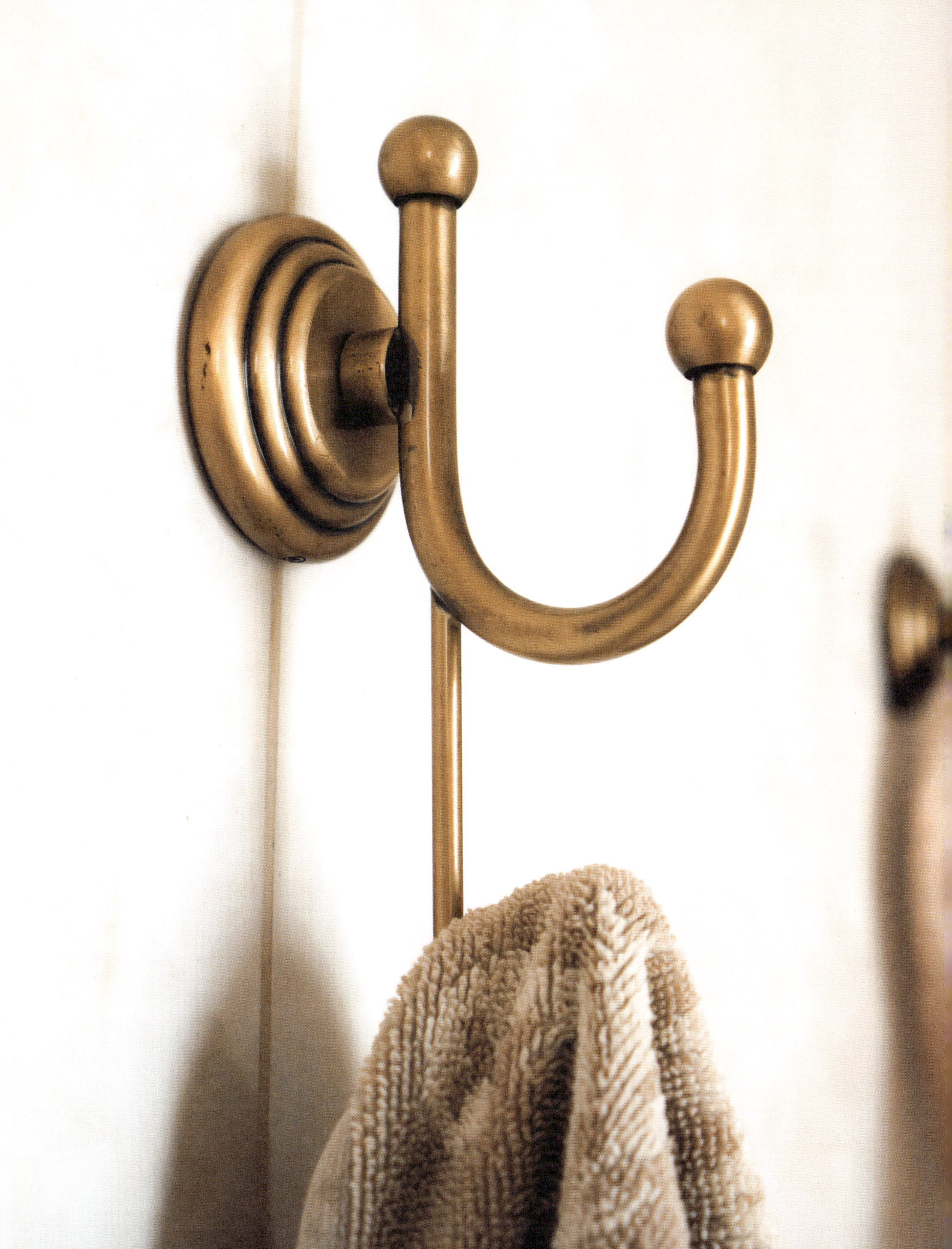

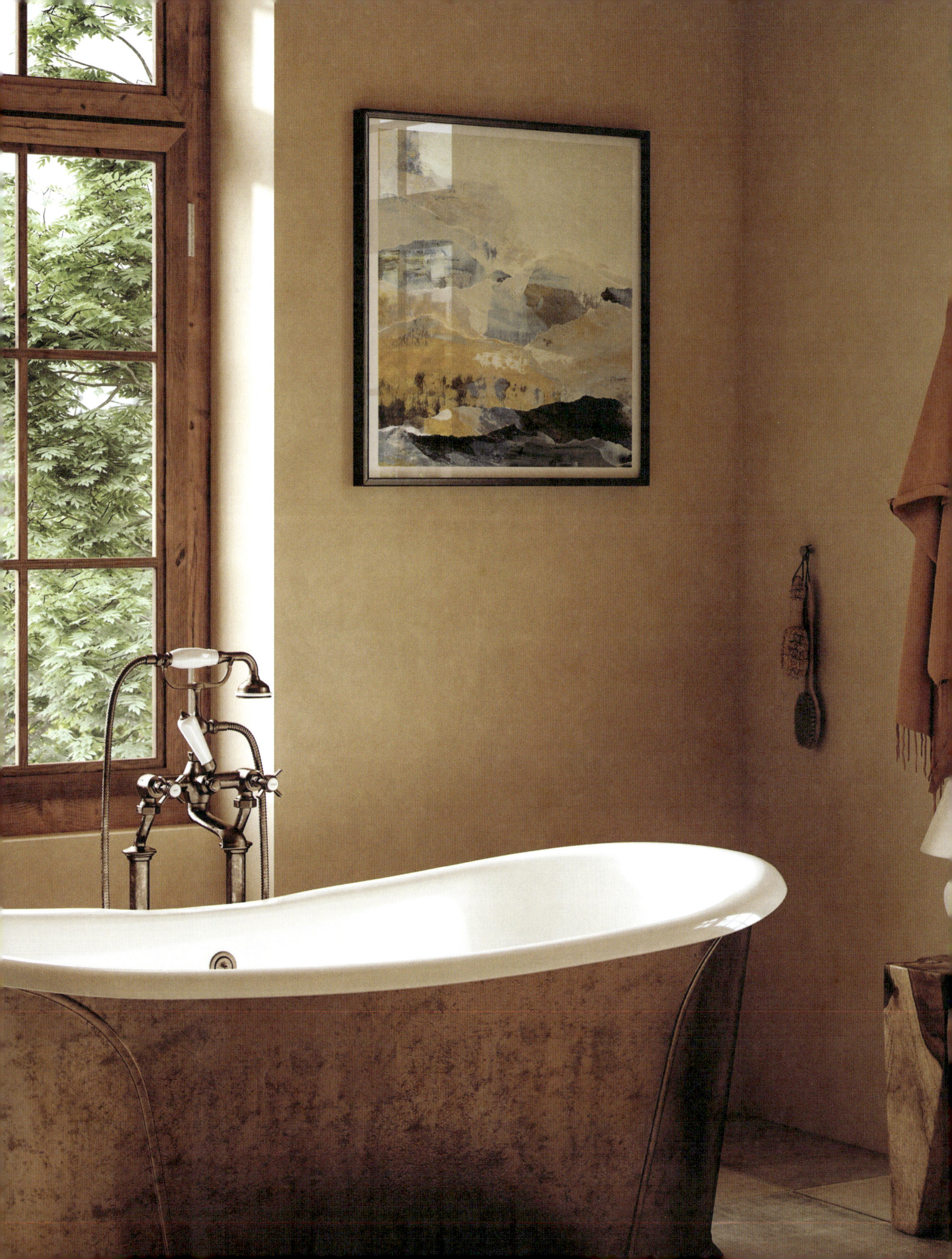

'Ah! There is nothing like staying at home for real comfort.'

JANE AUSTEN

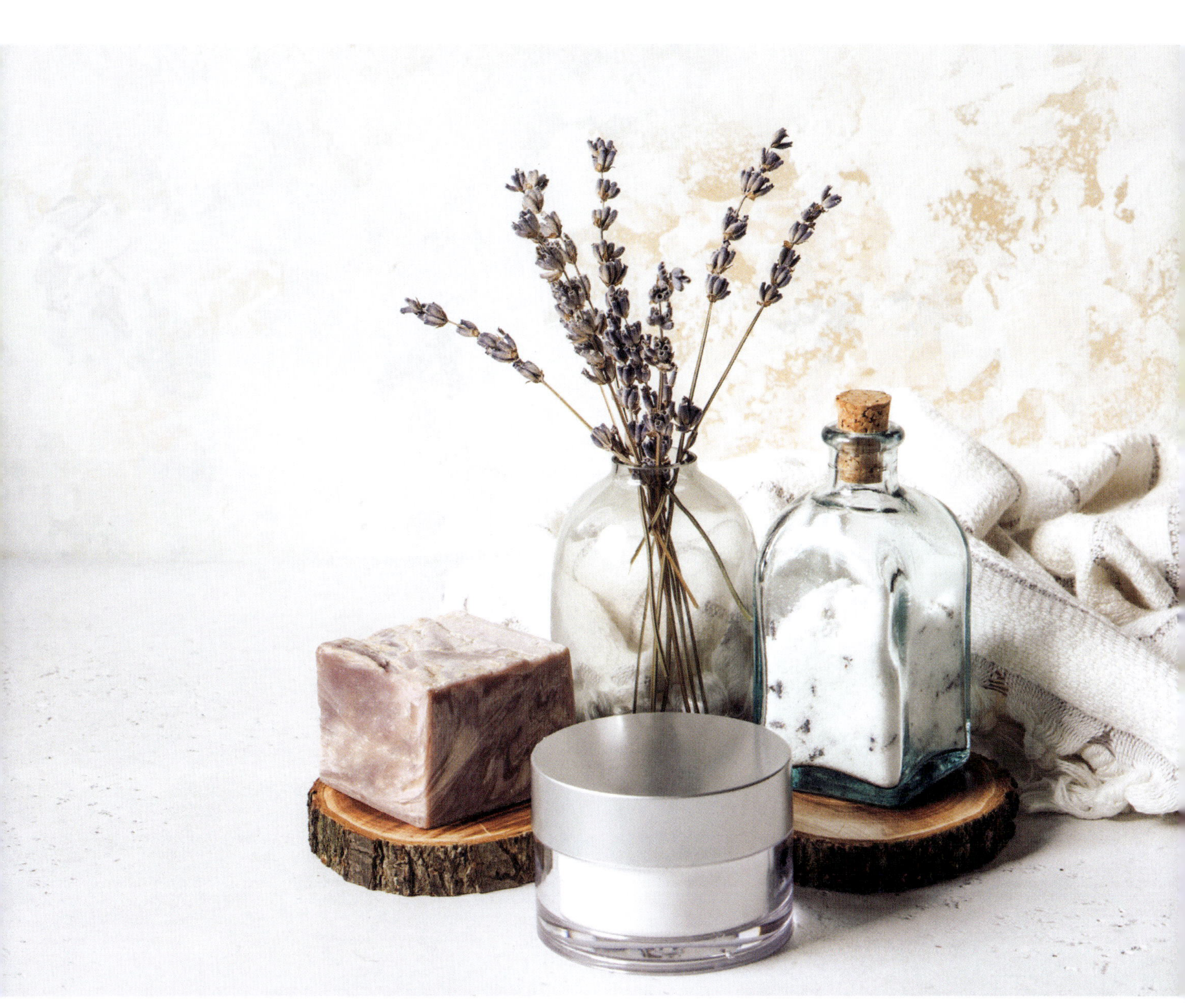

The Quick List

Freestanding furniture that creates a link to the past

Milking stools – the perfect side table

Artworks, vases of flowers, even rugs to enhance the style

Soft, white towels, a failsafe way to add a luxury element

Hooks and shelving that make the functional beautiful

Lighting to help create a mood of tranquillity

Touches of green – plants, herbs or accent colour

Beautiful natural soaps, oils and handmade candles on display

STANDARD SUPPLY
LOT NO. 1009-A

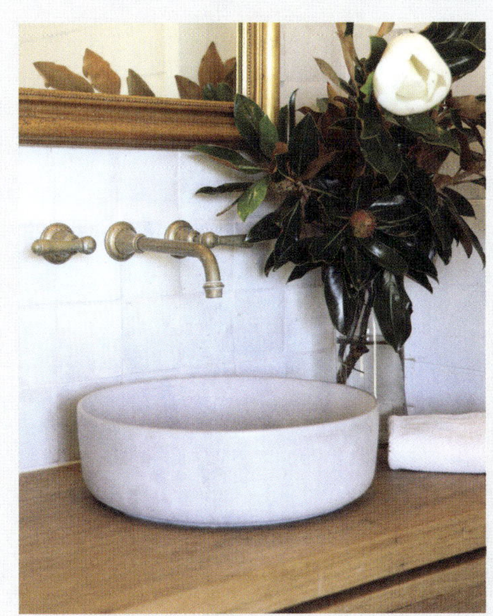

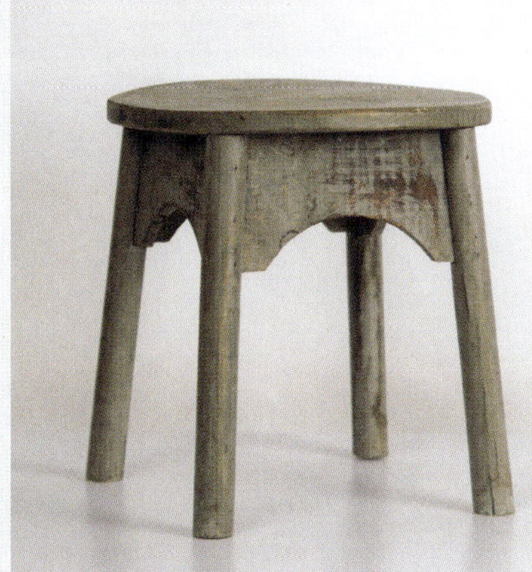

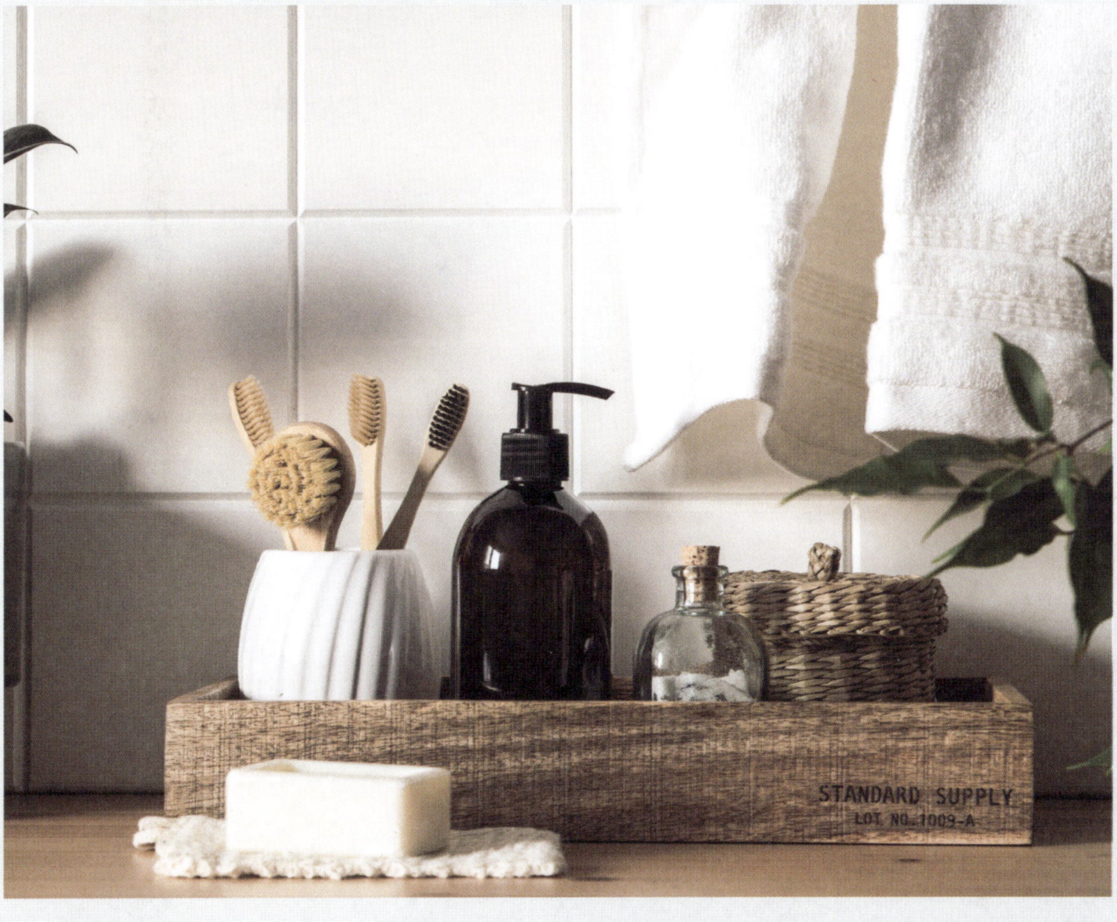

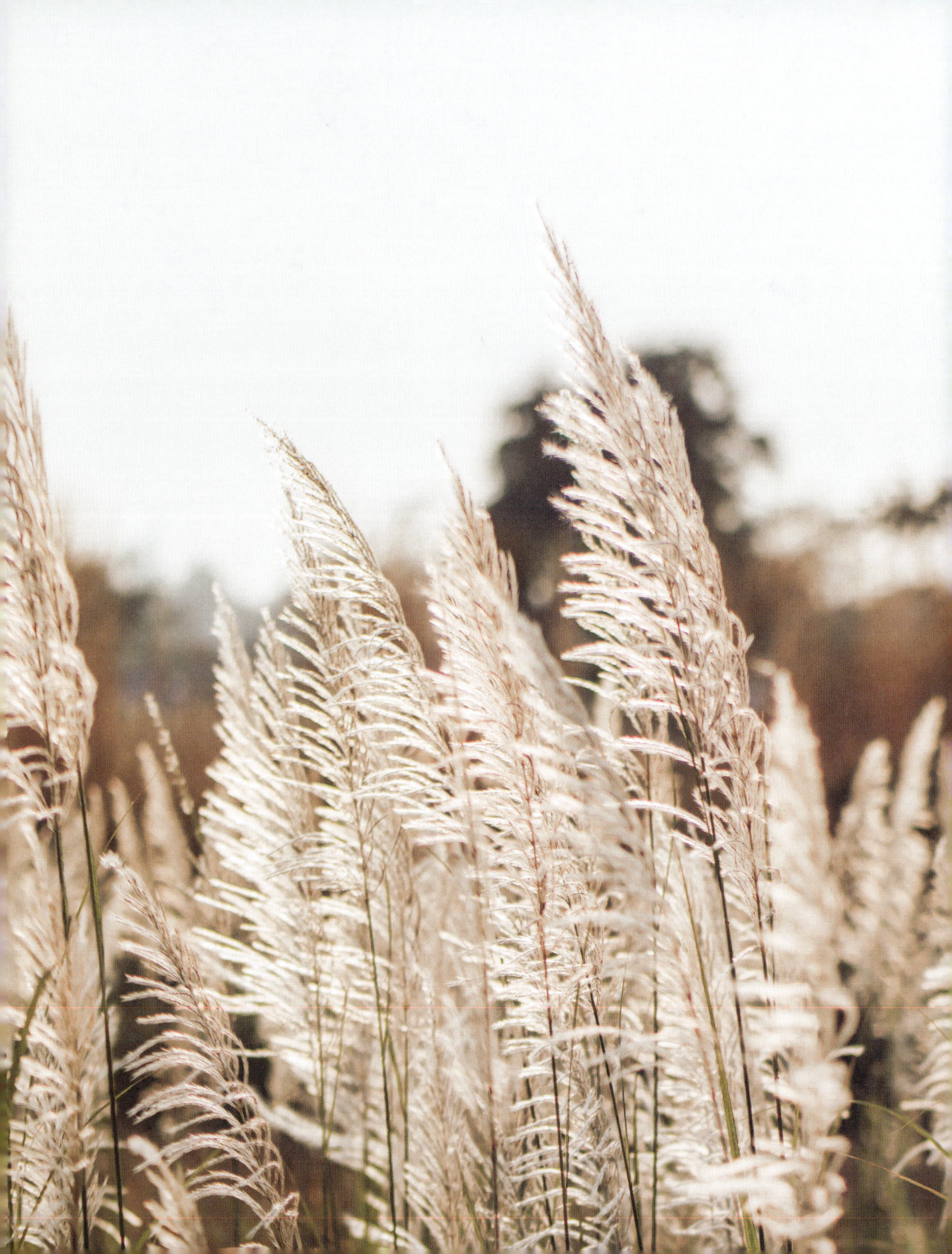

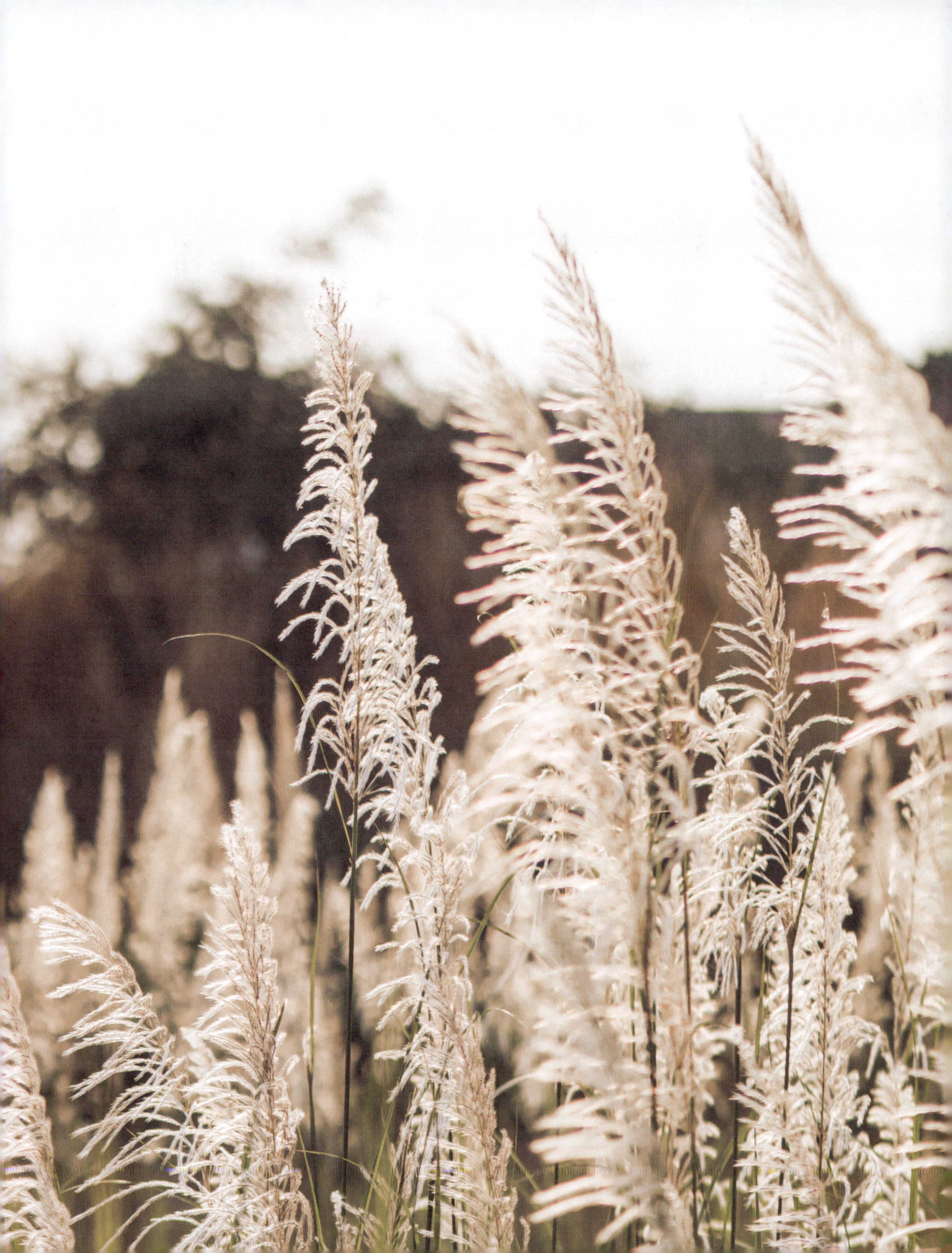

chapter seven

outside

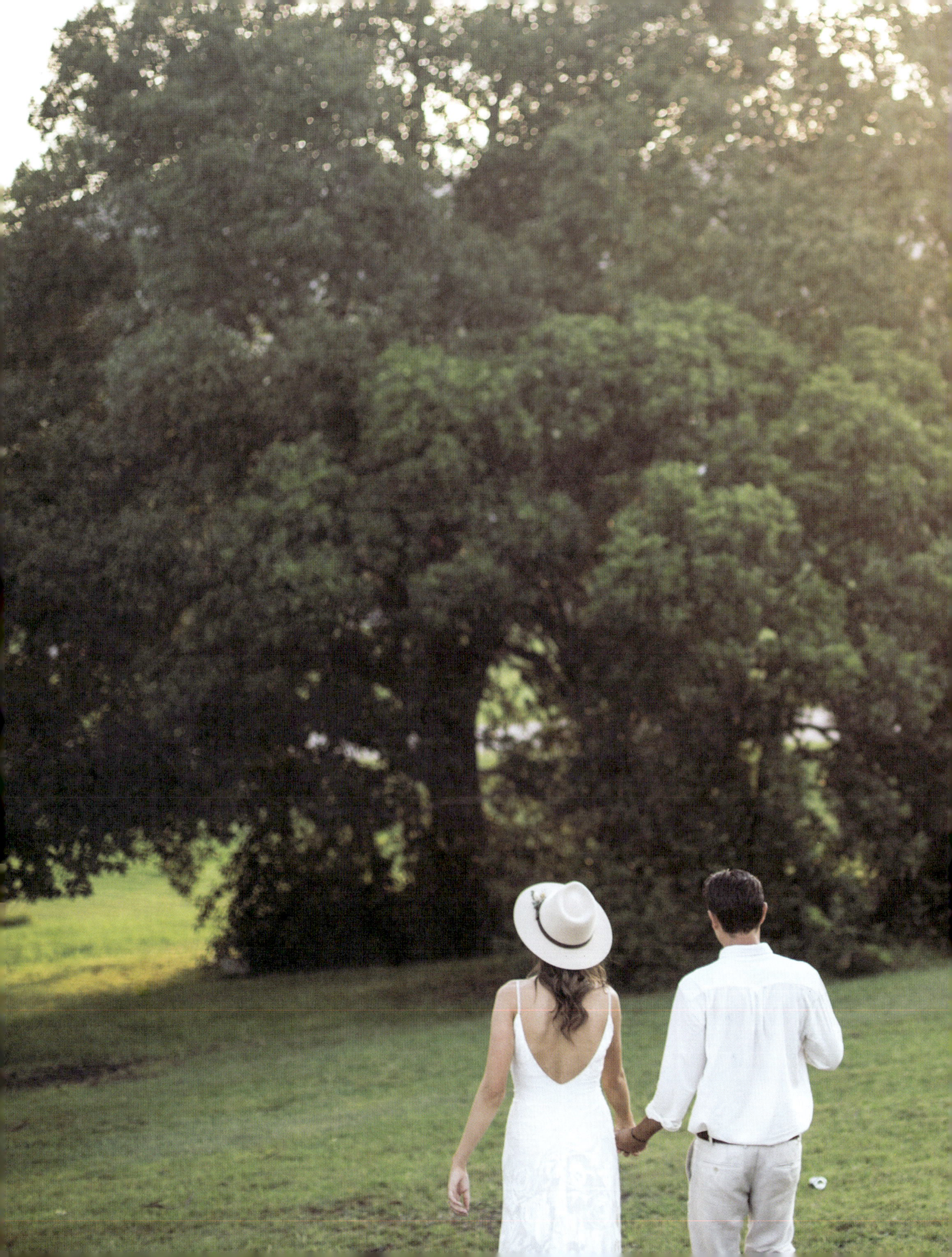

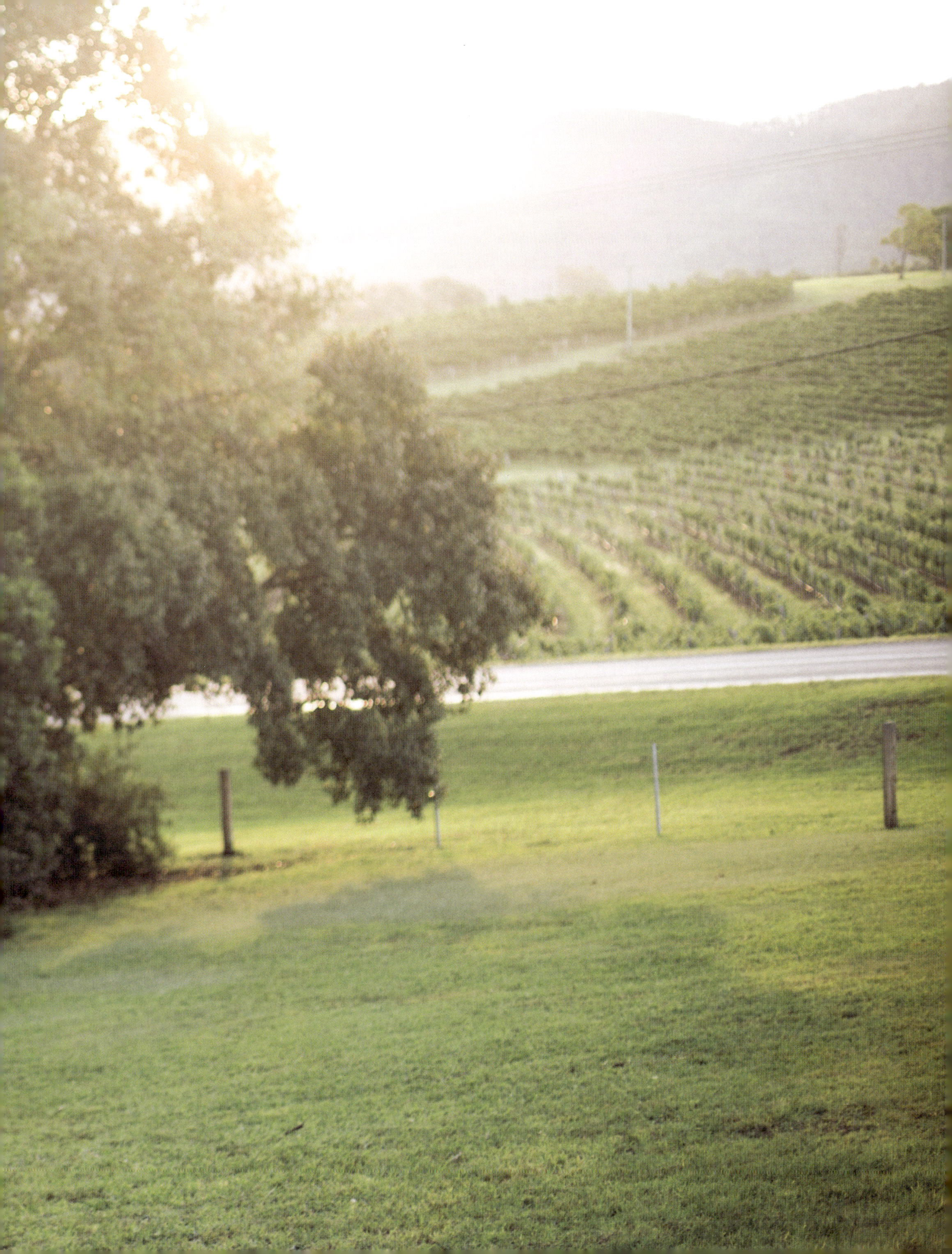

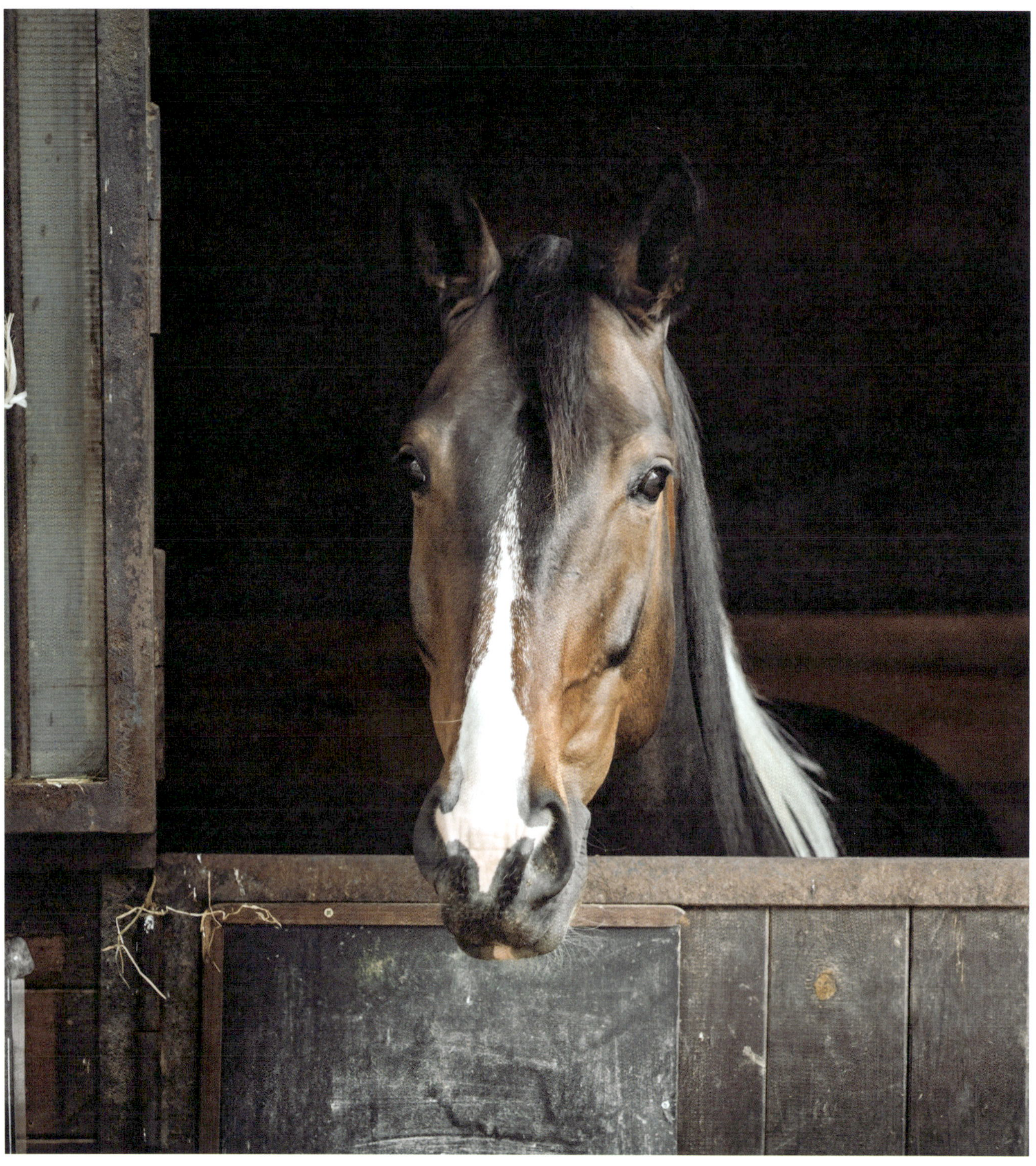

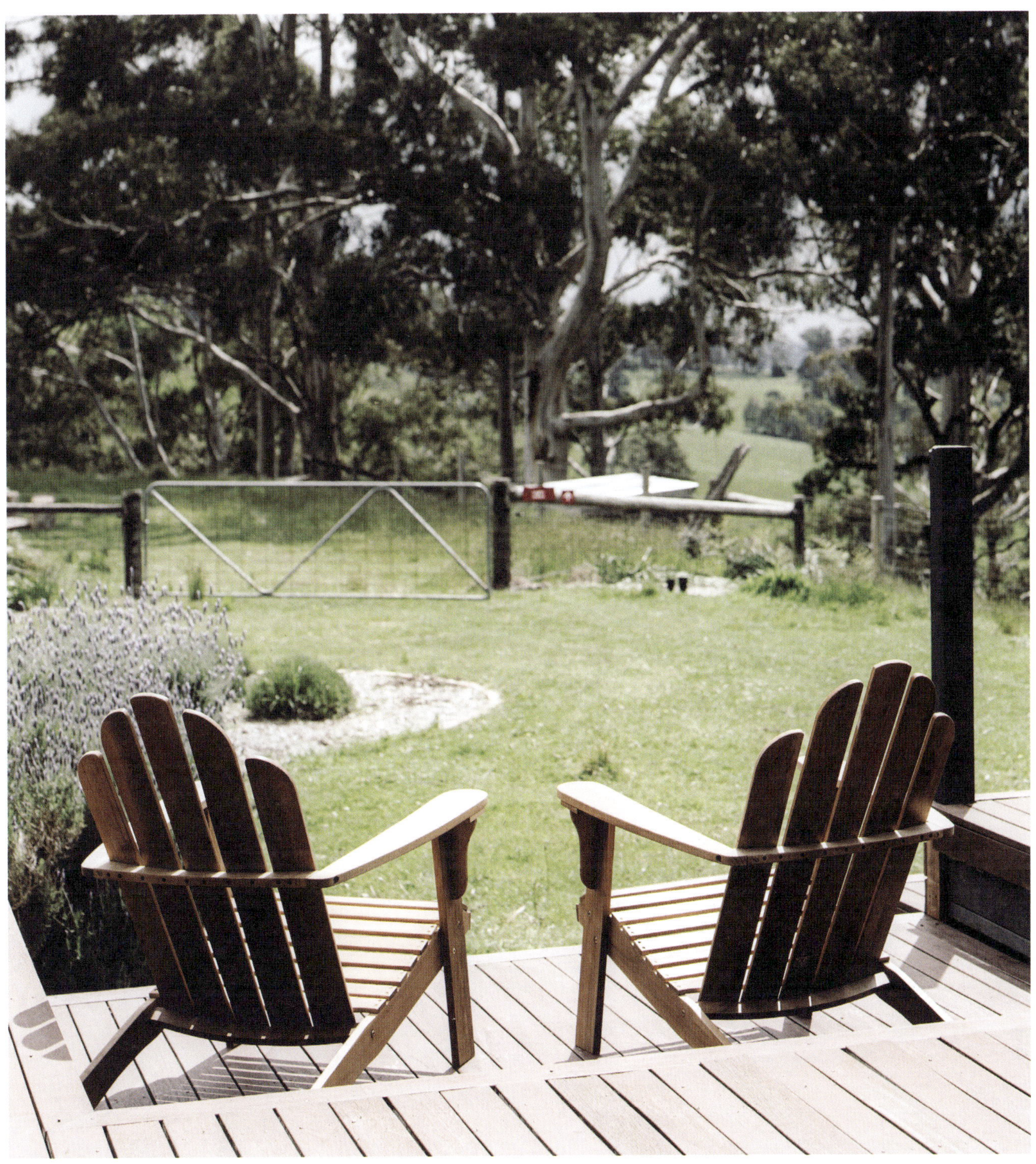

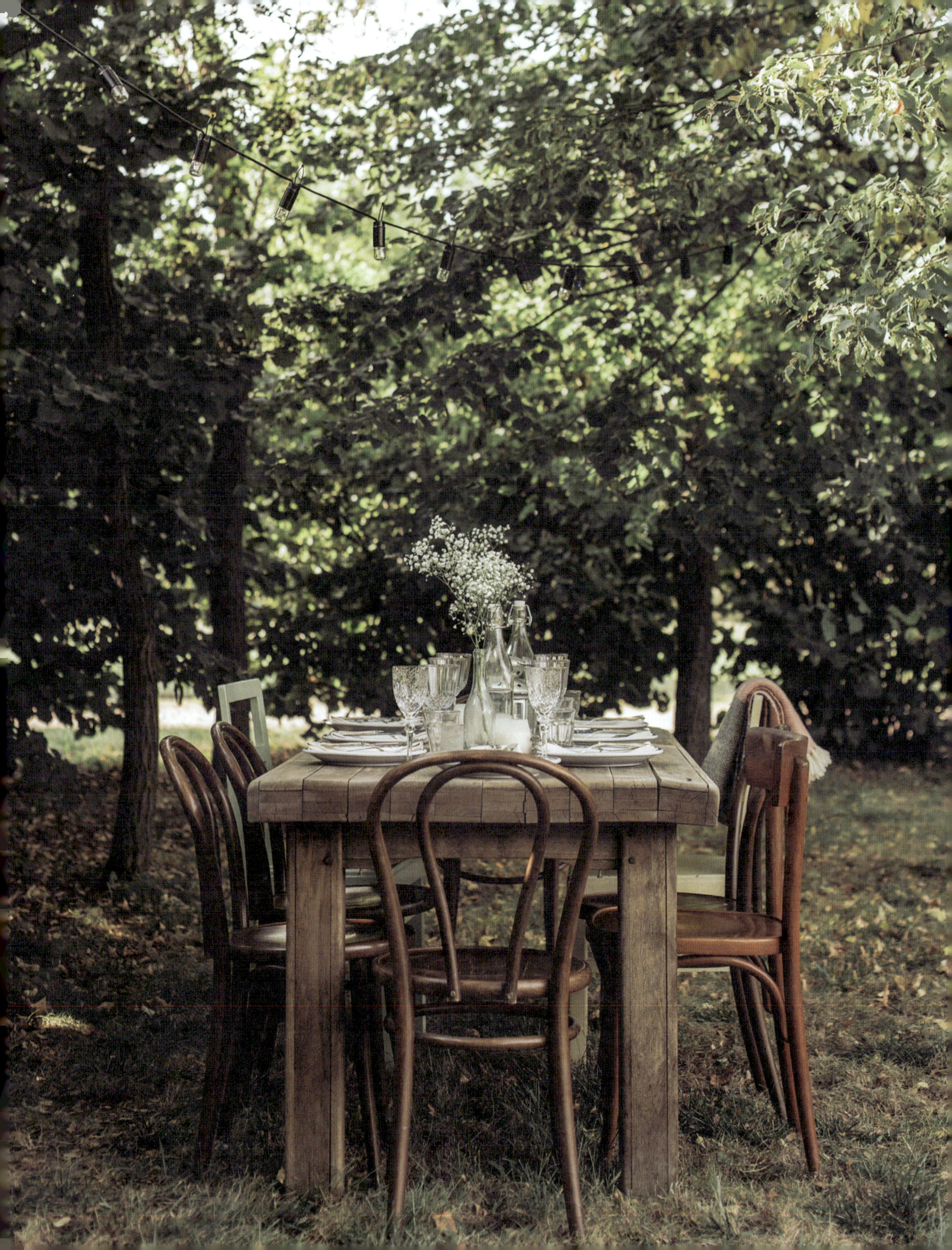

Modern country home style is a homage to nature. Everything about the style is natural, organic and beautiful, inspired by nature and inspiring us to be in nature. So, it goes without saying that outdoor spaces are integral to this style of home.

A seamless indoor-outdoor flow (think sliding doors from dining area to patio) is highly desirable, enabling an easy transition into outdoor living. To maximise the flow, make deliberate choices to extend the same fixtures (such as flooring) inside and out. And mirror the furnishing elements (colour palette, choice of textiles and even furniture) in both spaces to create a strong visual link.

Where possible, from your indoor rooms create direct lines of sight to greenery or other highlighted features of your garden. If a window faces a wall, introduce climbing plants such as wisteria or star jasmine to transform the outlook.

At the end of the day (when the sun dips beneath the horizon and the glasses are empty), it's all about the love you have for your outdoor space, and a big part of that love, for most of us, is a place where we can enjoy the company of friends and family in the blissful surrounds of nature.

When creating your outdoor haven, set yourself up with spaces that cater to the elements (think shade and shelter), introduce purposeful relaxation zones (for eating, taking a nap, reading a book or chatting with friends). Pay attention to the details such as lighting, sound, comfort and the aesthetic of your spaces. Wicker baskets, flowers and pot plants, rugs, throws and even artworks all have a place and add comfort to the outdoor room.

If space and budget allow, don't forget to focus on three hallmarks of Australian outdoor living: a fire pit, an eating area (with barbecue) and an outdoor shower or bathroom.

TOP FIVE

1.

Somewhere to sit and look at the garden

2.

Herbs for country cooking

3.

A place to eat together

4.

A fire pit for cold nights and long stories

5.

Outdoor bath or shower

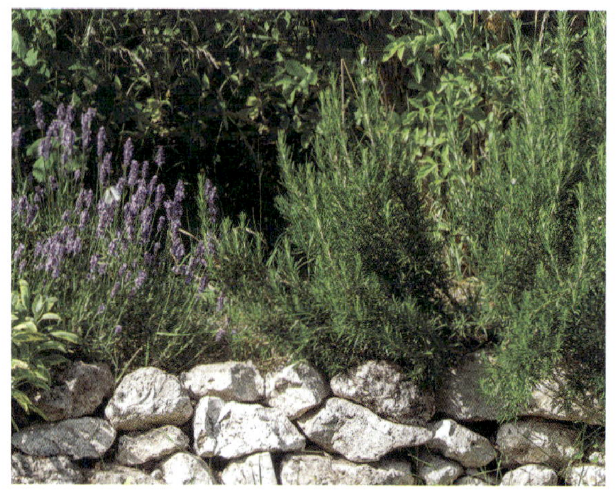

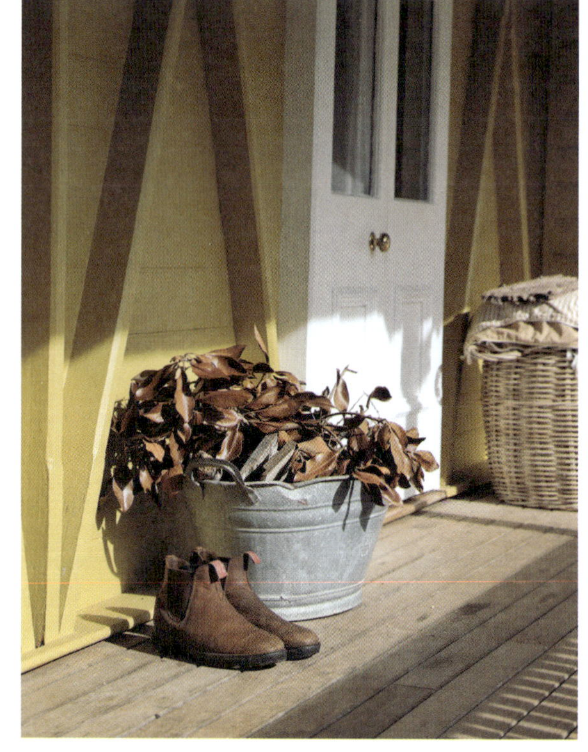

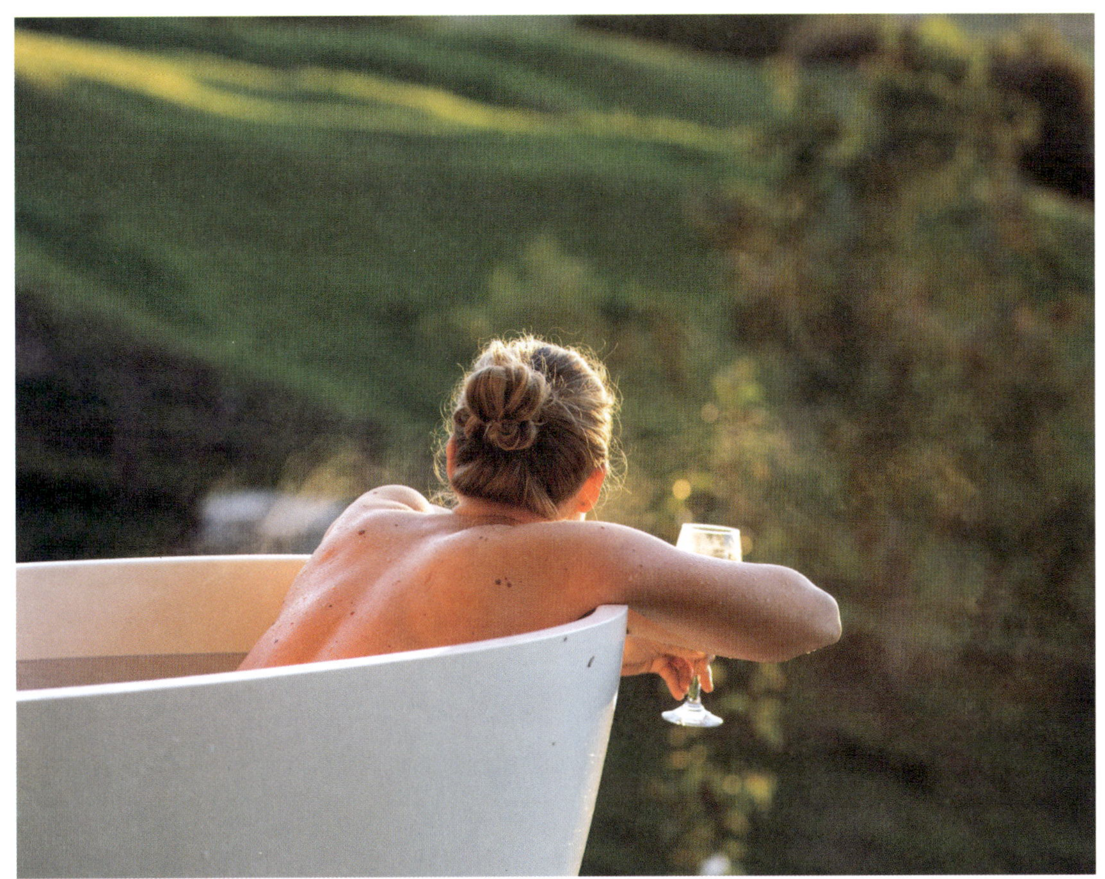

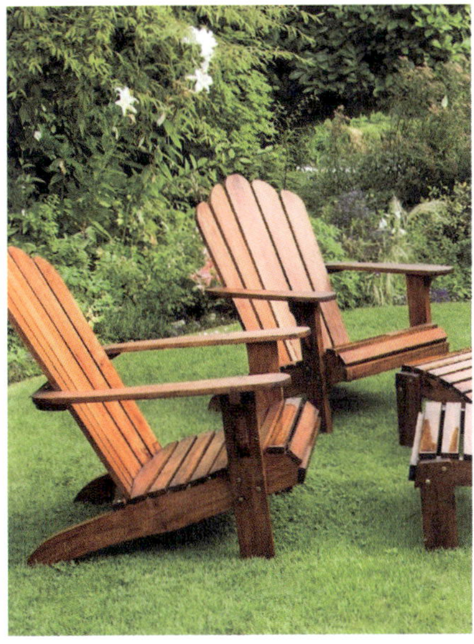

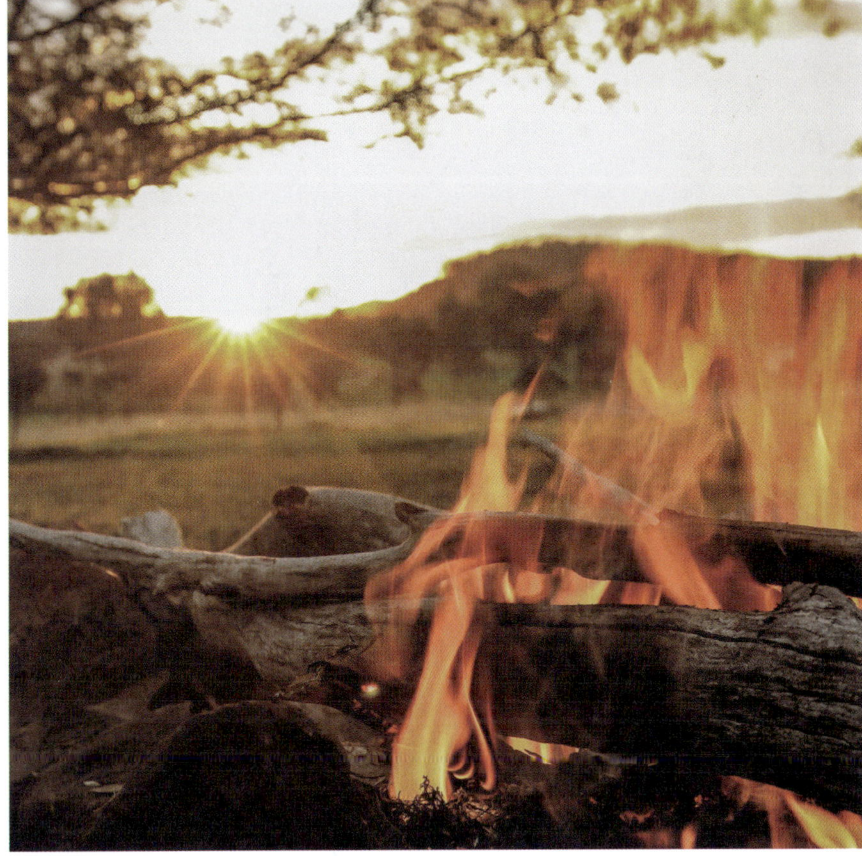

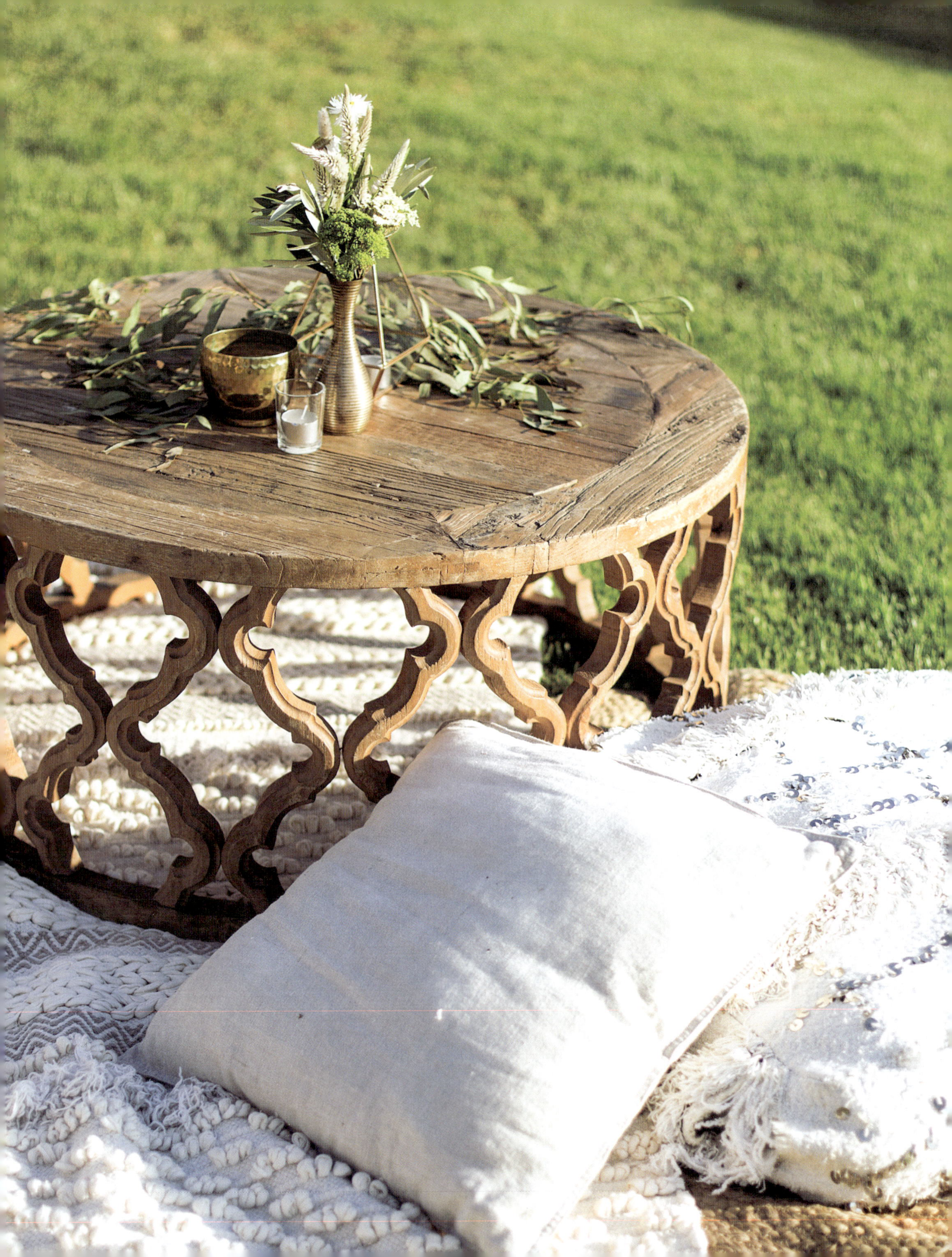

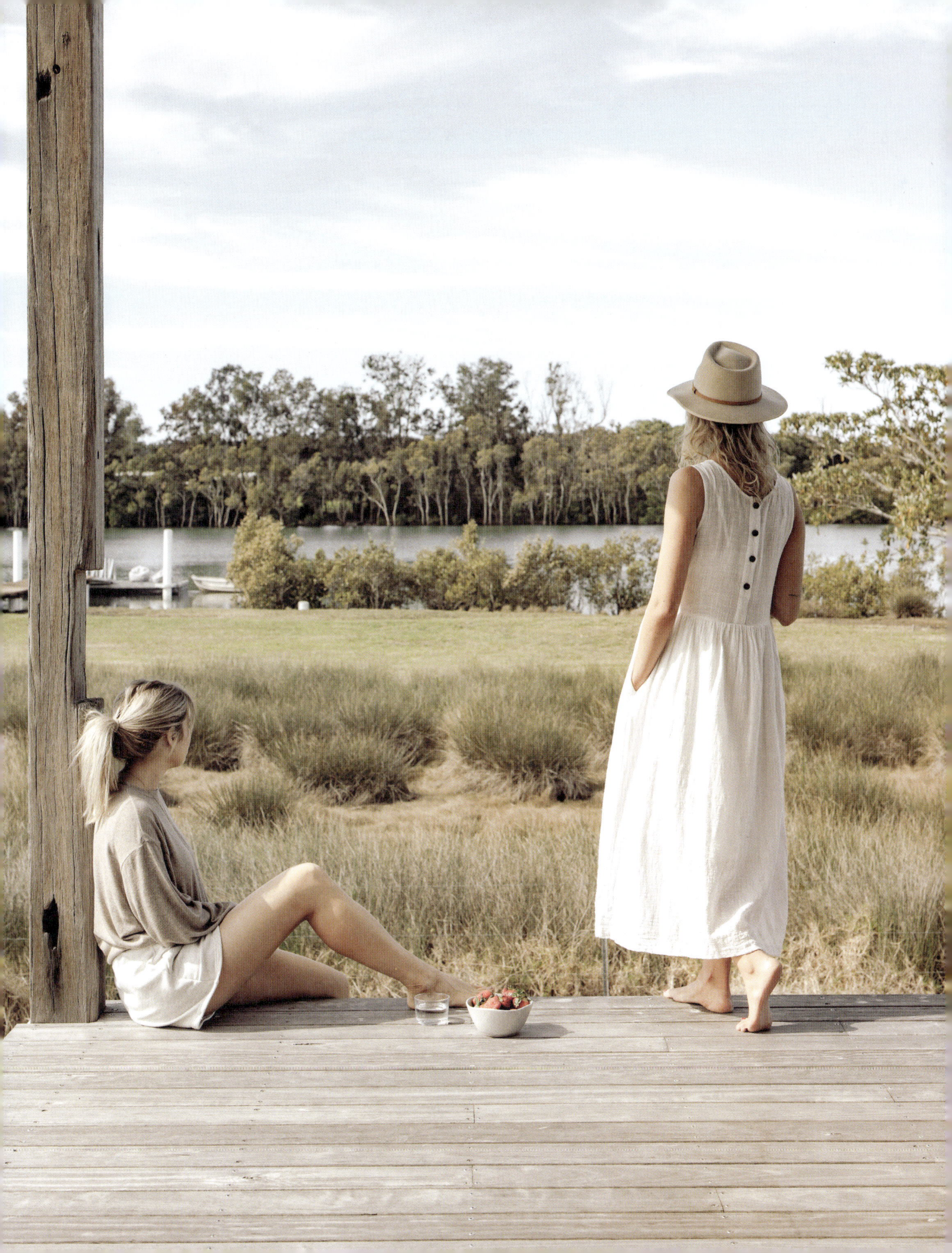

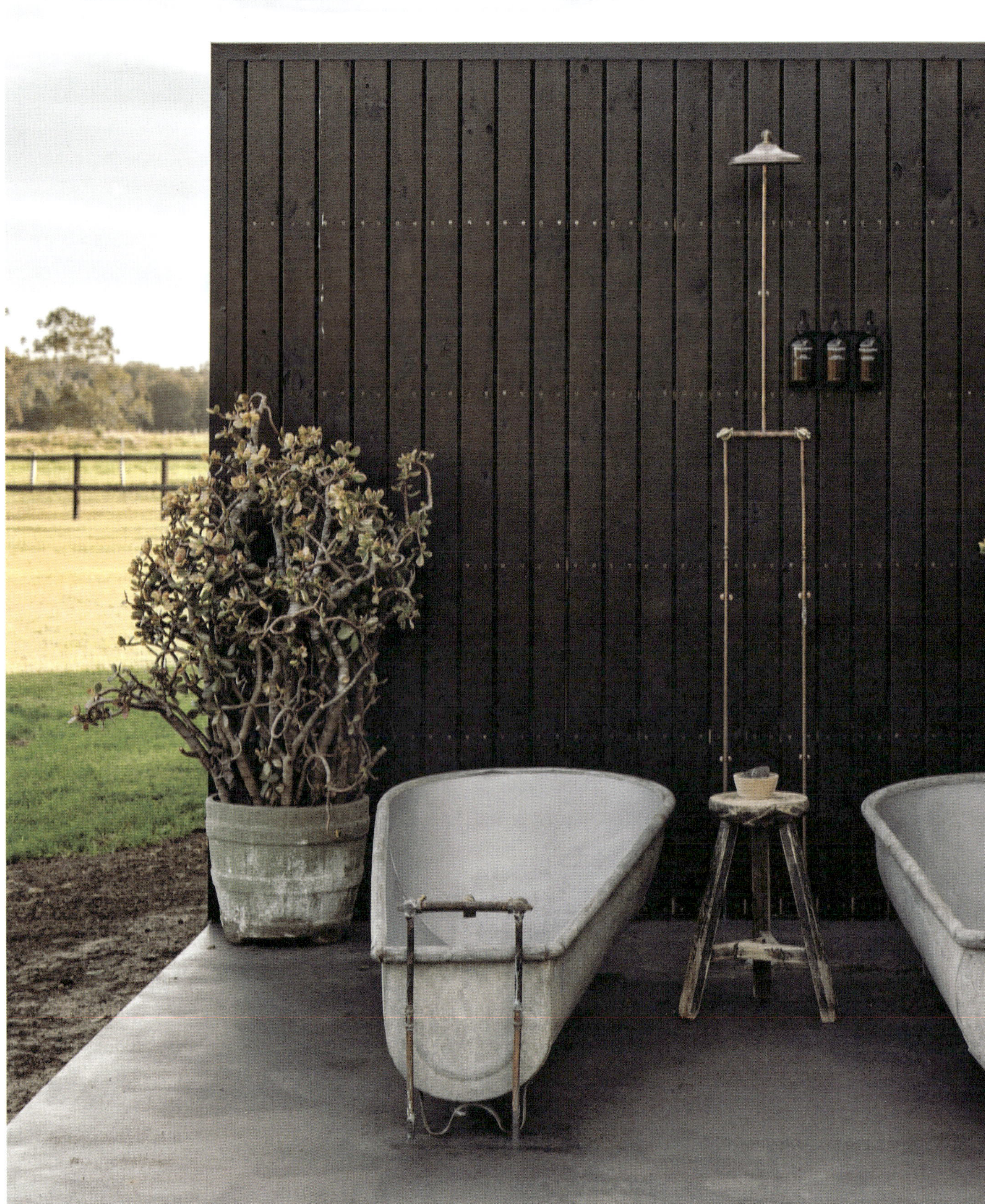

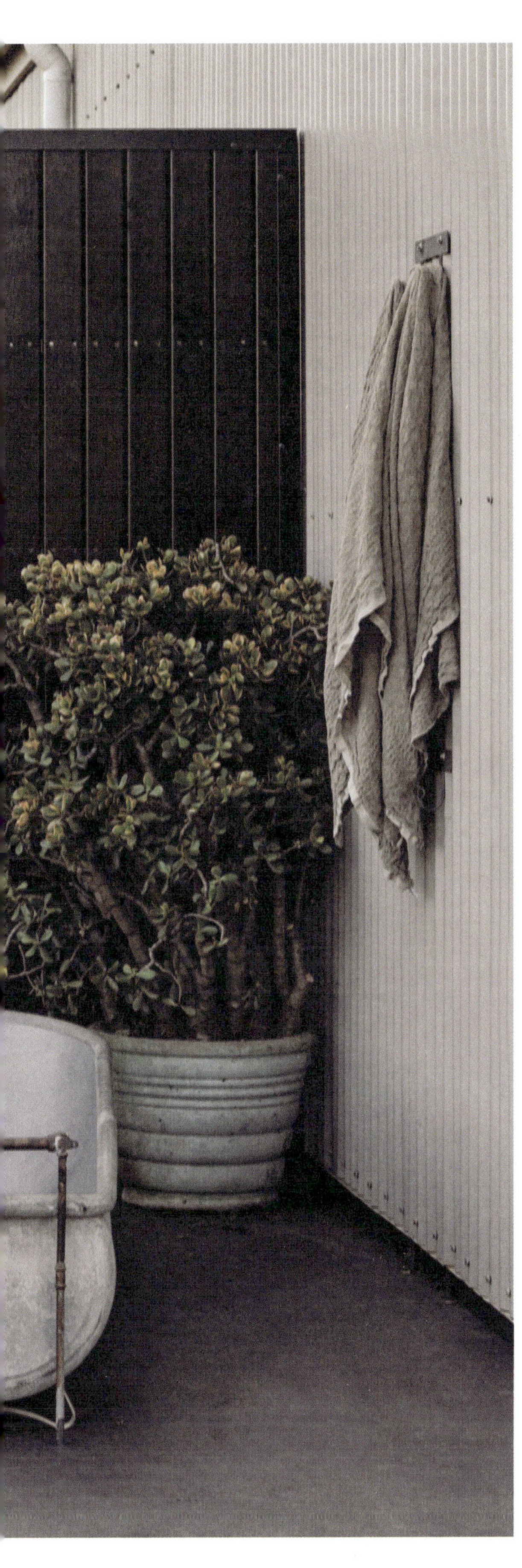

Whether it's a bare tap with which to rinse off muddy feet, a copper pipe that doubles as a shower, or a full-blown outdoor bathroom, having a wet room set-up of sorts is an important element of outdoor living in the Australian climate and way of life.

These feathered friends have become something of a style accessory (an emblem of country life regardless of where you live), as well as a productive members of the family.

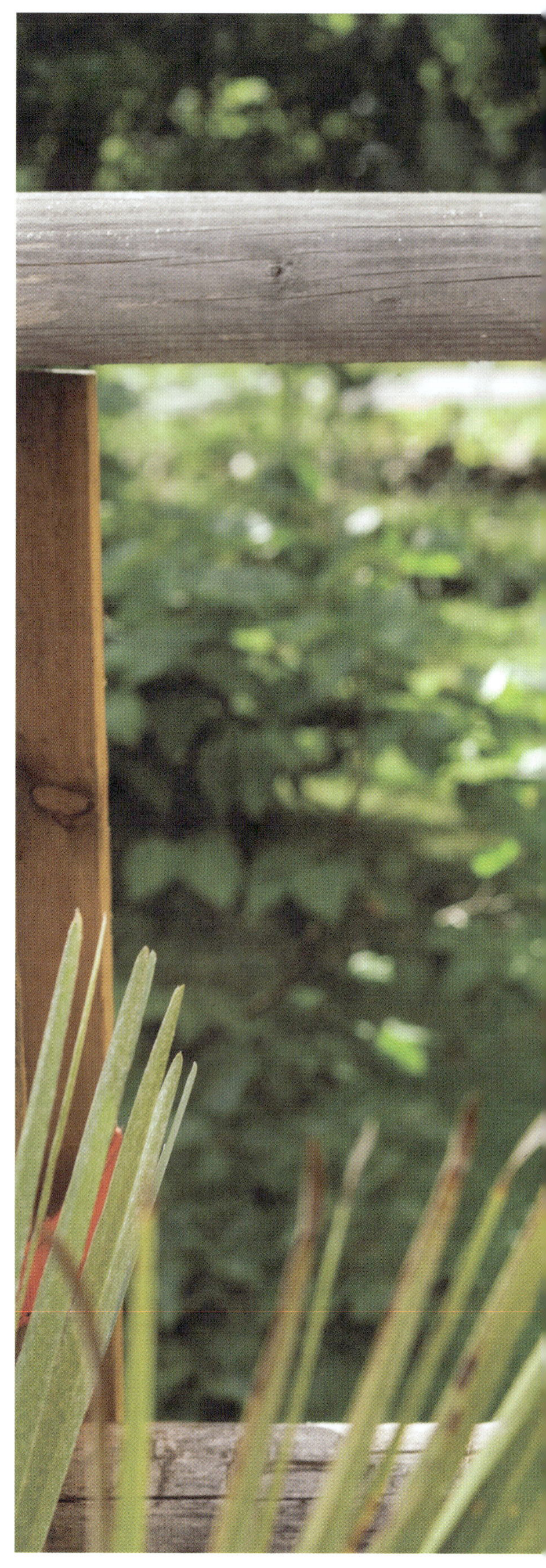

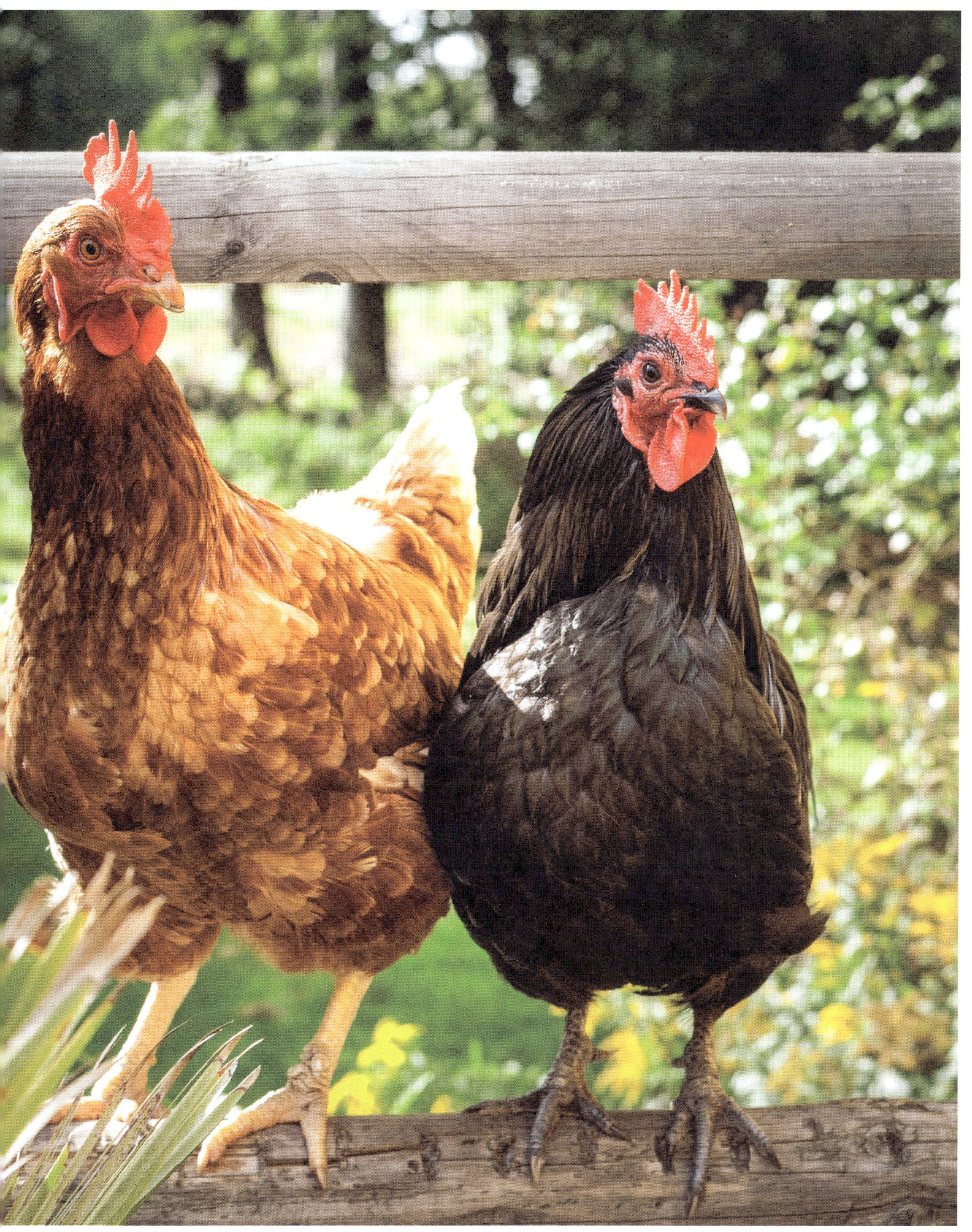

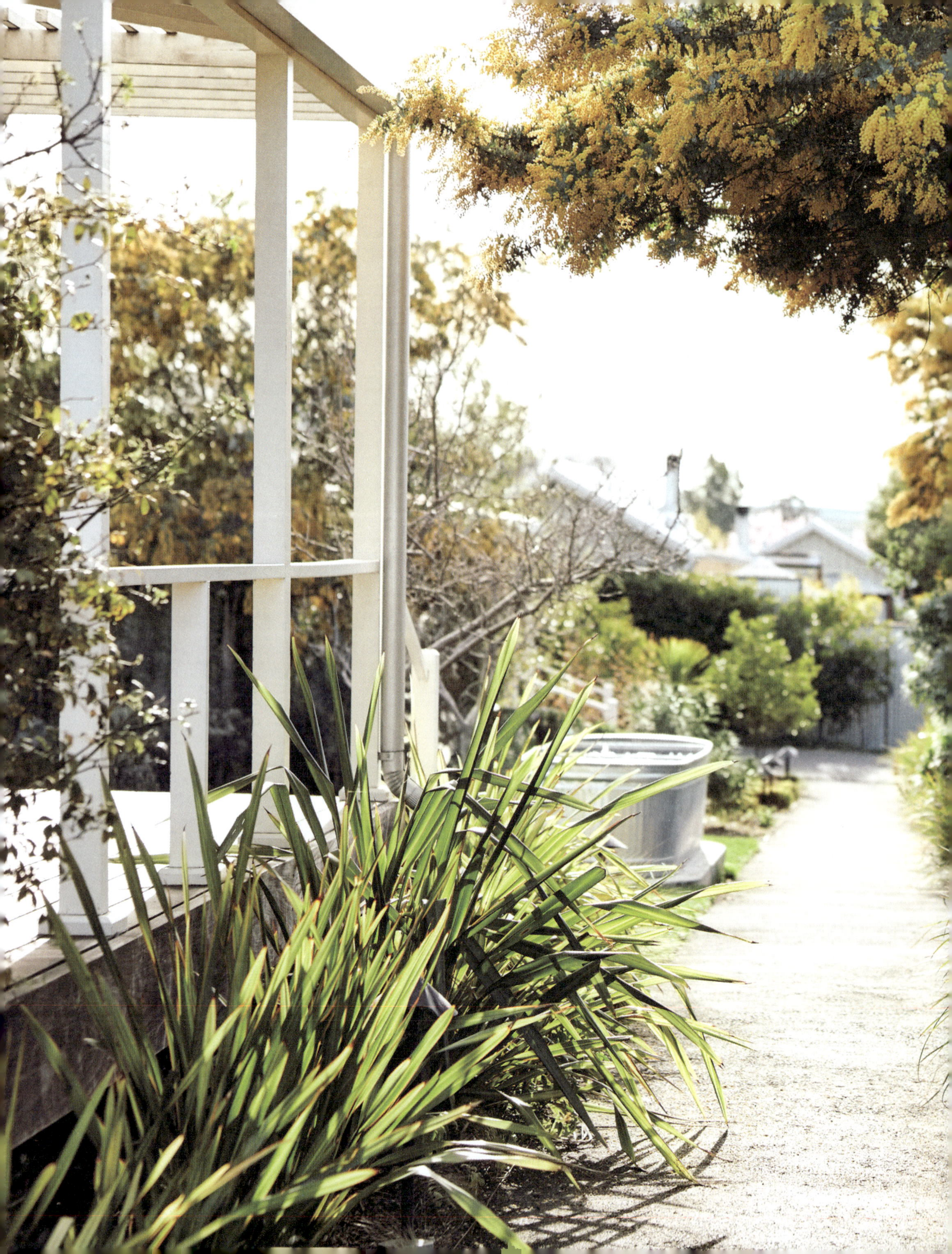

'The garden suggests there might be a place where we can meet nature halfway.'

MICHAEL POLLAN

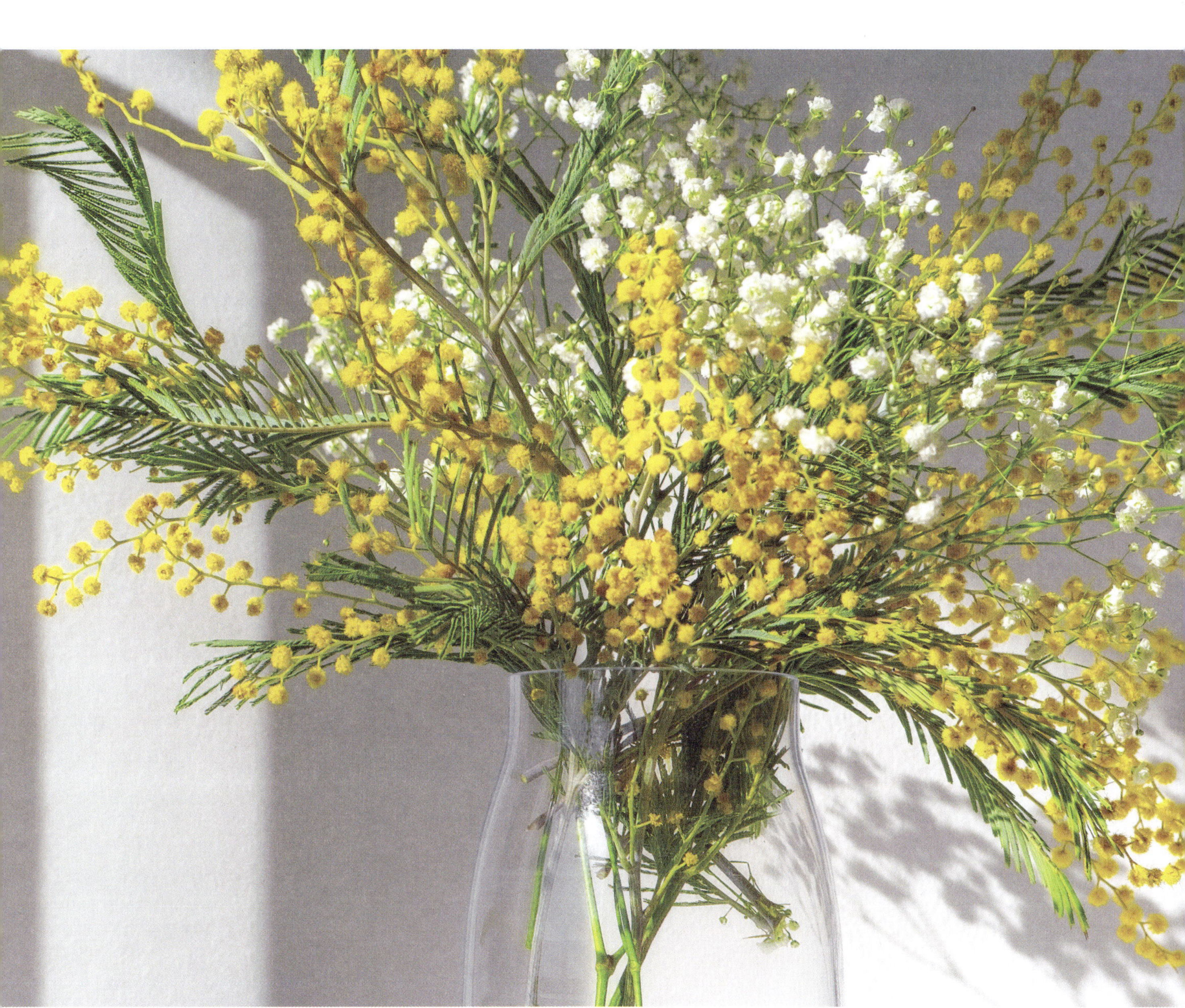

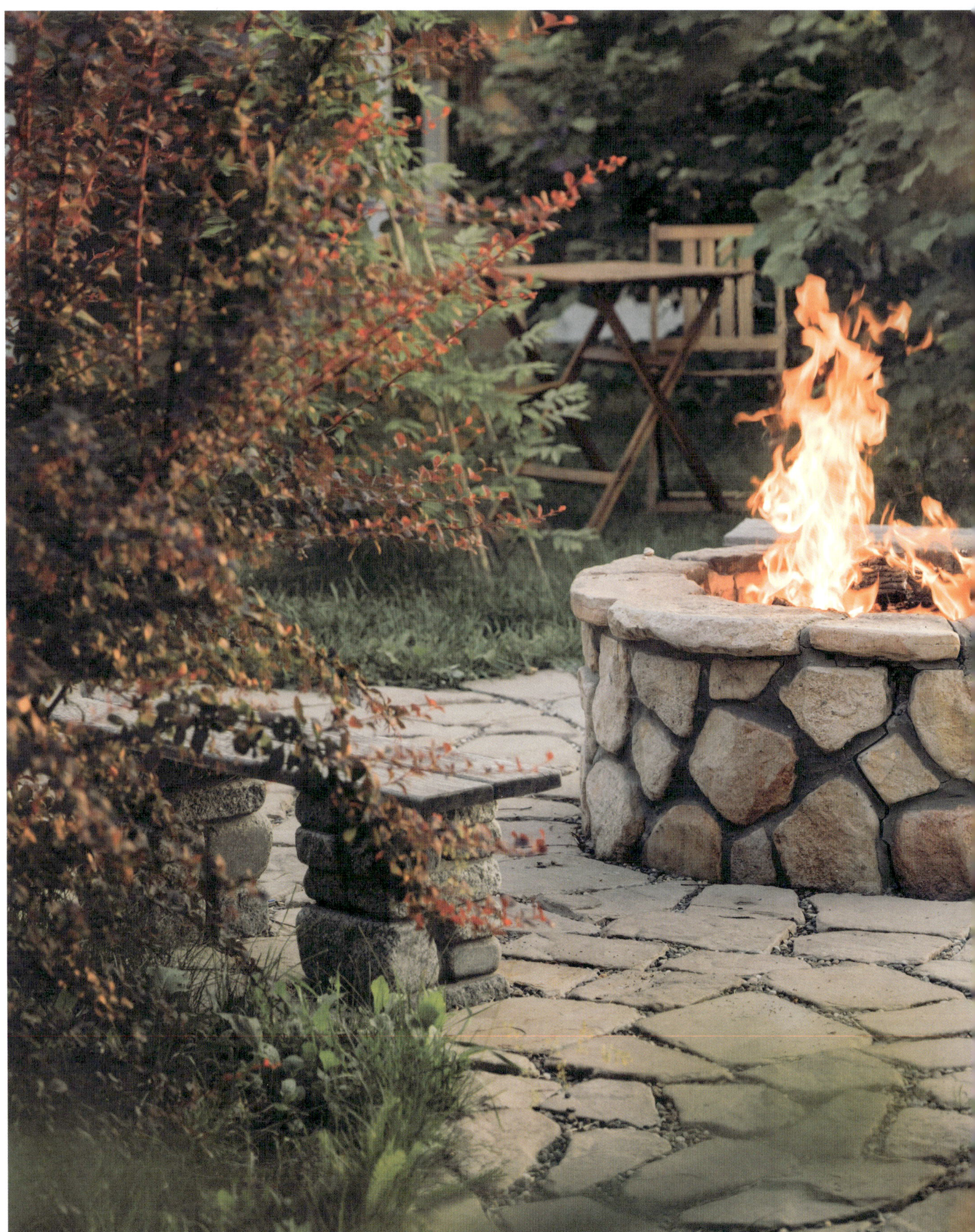

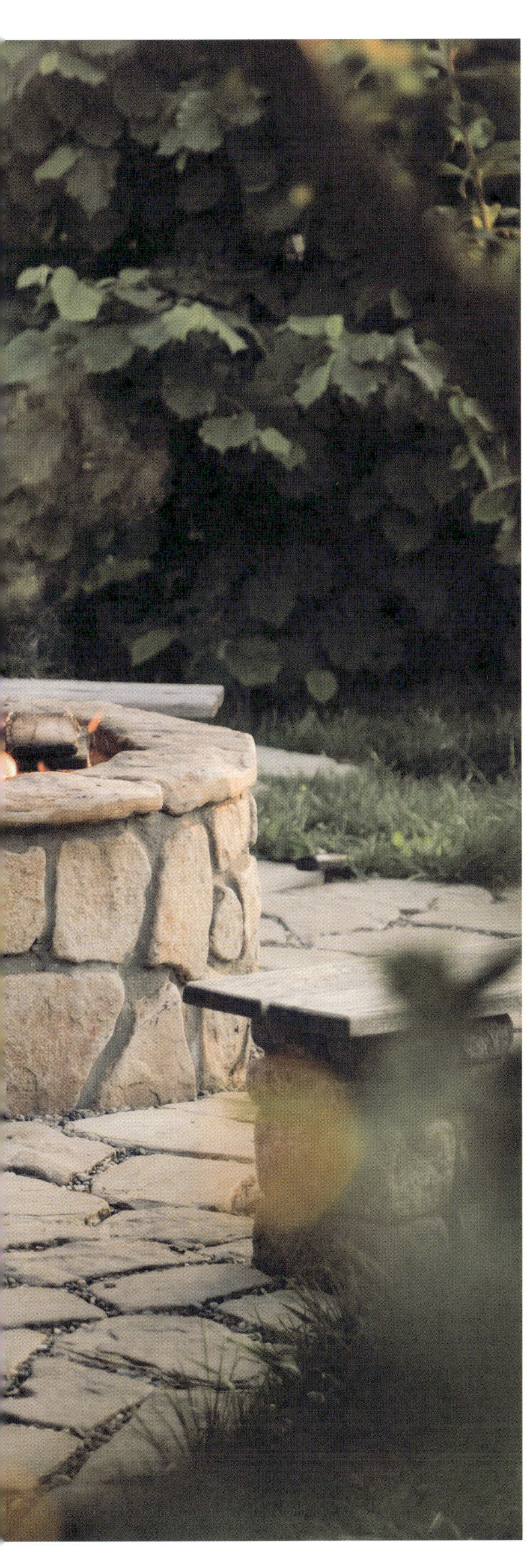

Toasting marshmallows around an open fire, or sitting up late star-gazing and spinning yarns, are time-honoured traditions of country life. A fire pit is where the action happens, and is bound to be a much-loved element of any modern country home's outdoor landscape.

Regardless of location, it's likely that your modern-country-style home will include Australian natives in the garden. These hardy plants are heat- and drought-resistant, and they look perfect in the place where they belong, adding bold colour and scent to attract birdlife and filtering the harsh, bright sun. Include a birdbath to attract native birds to your outdoor space.

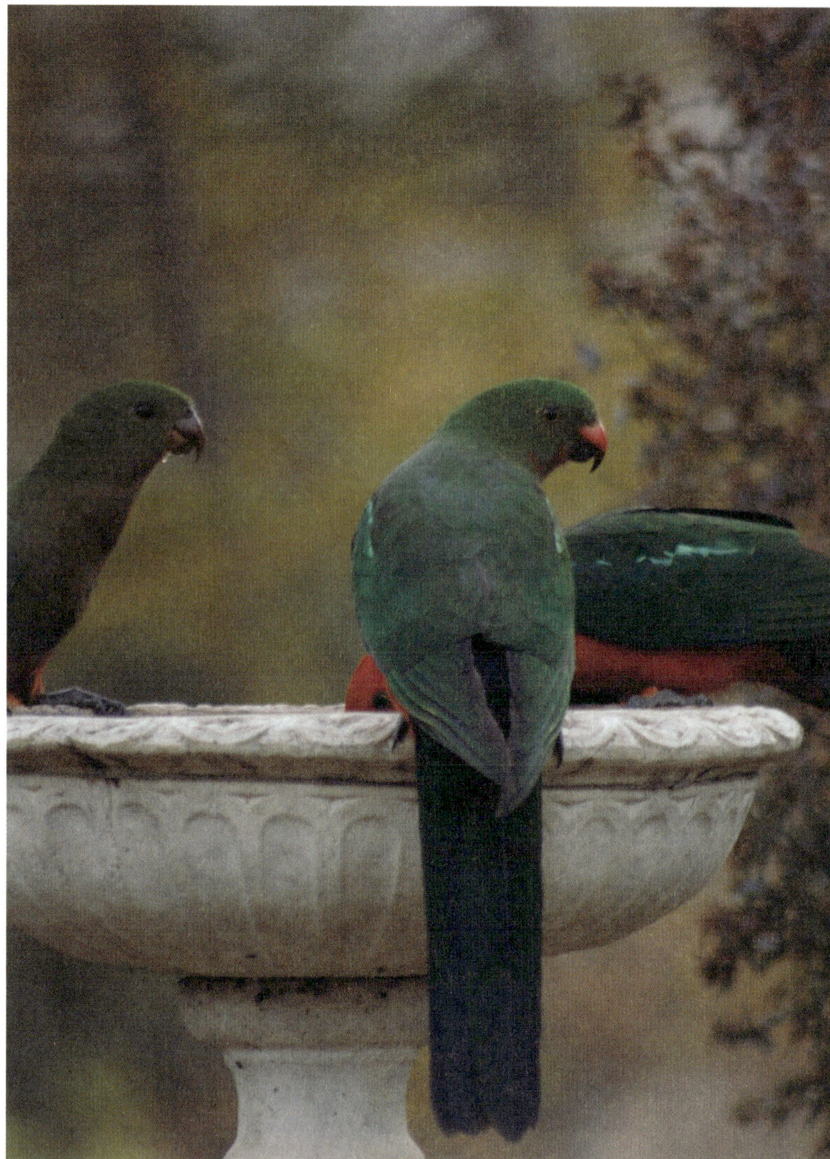

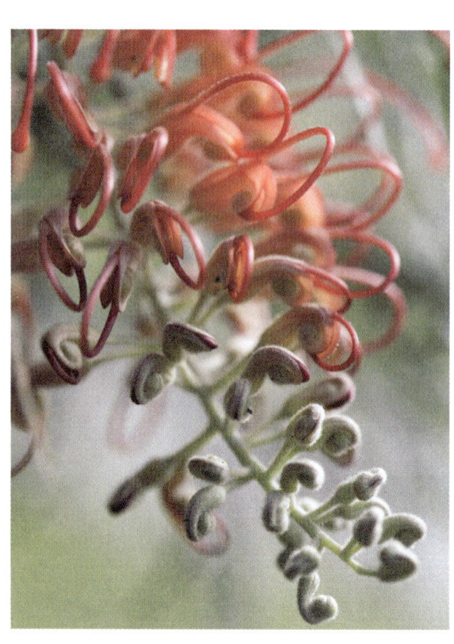

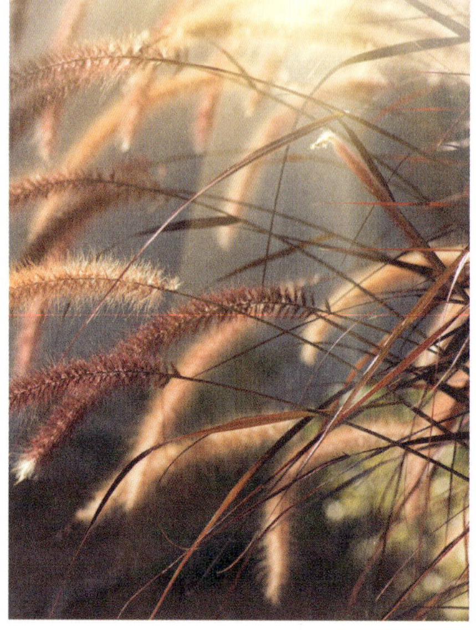

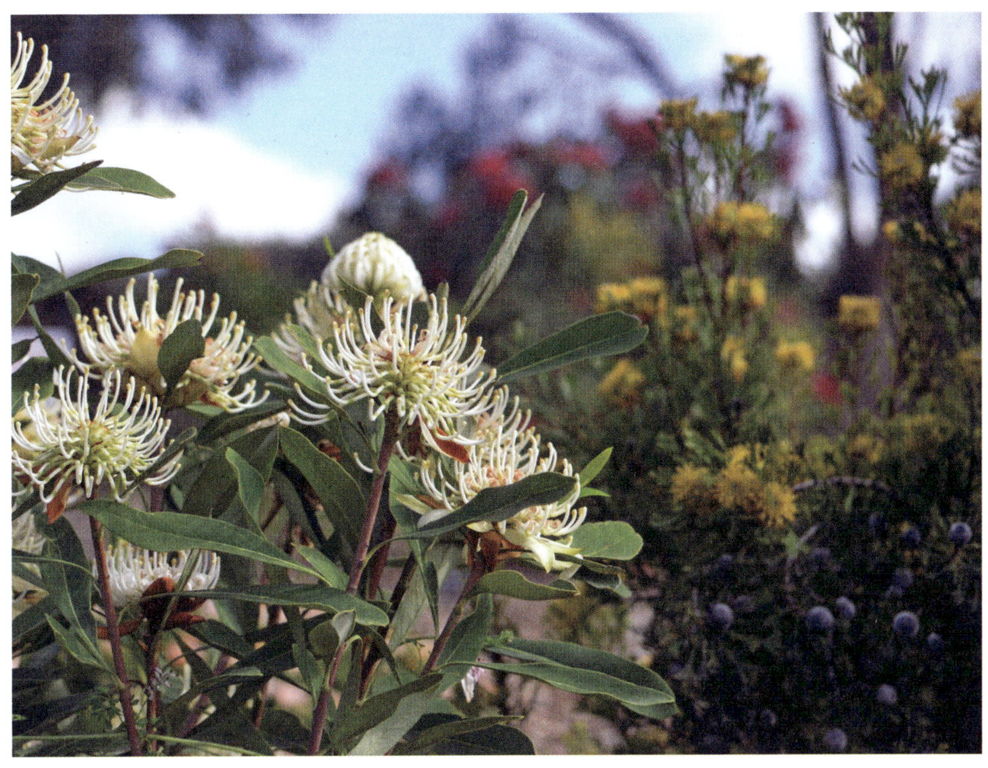

Lavender is also a drought-resistant and hardy plant, with a fragrant aroma, which adds an on-trend Mediterranean vibe to the garden.

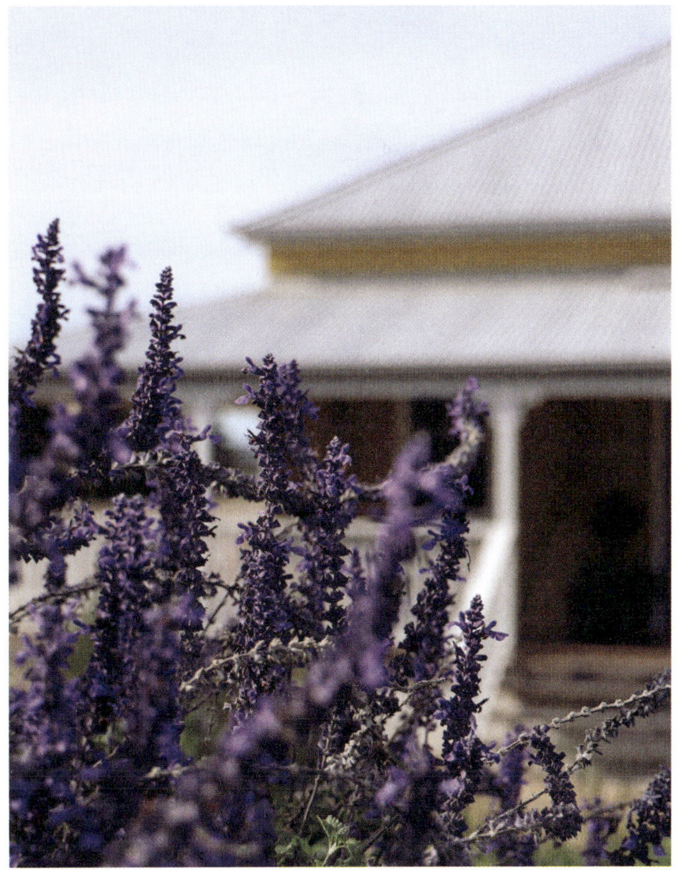

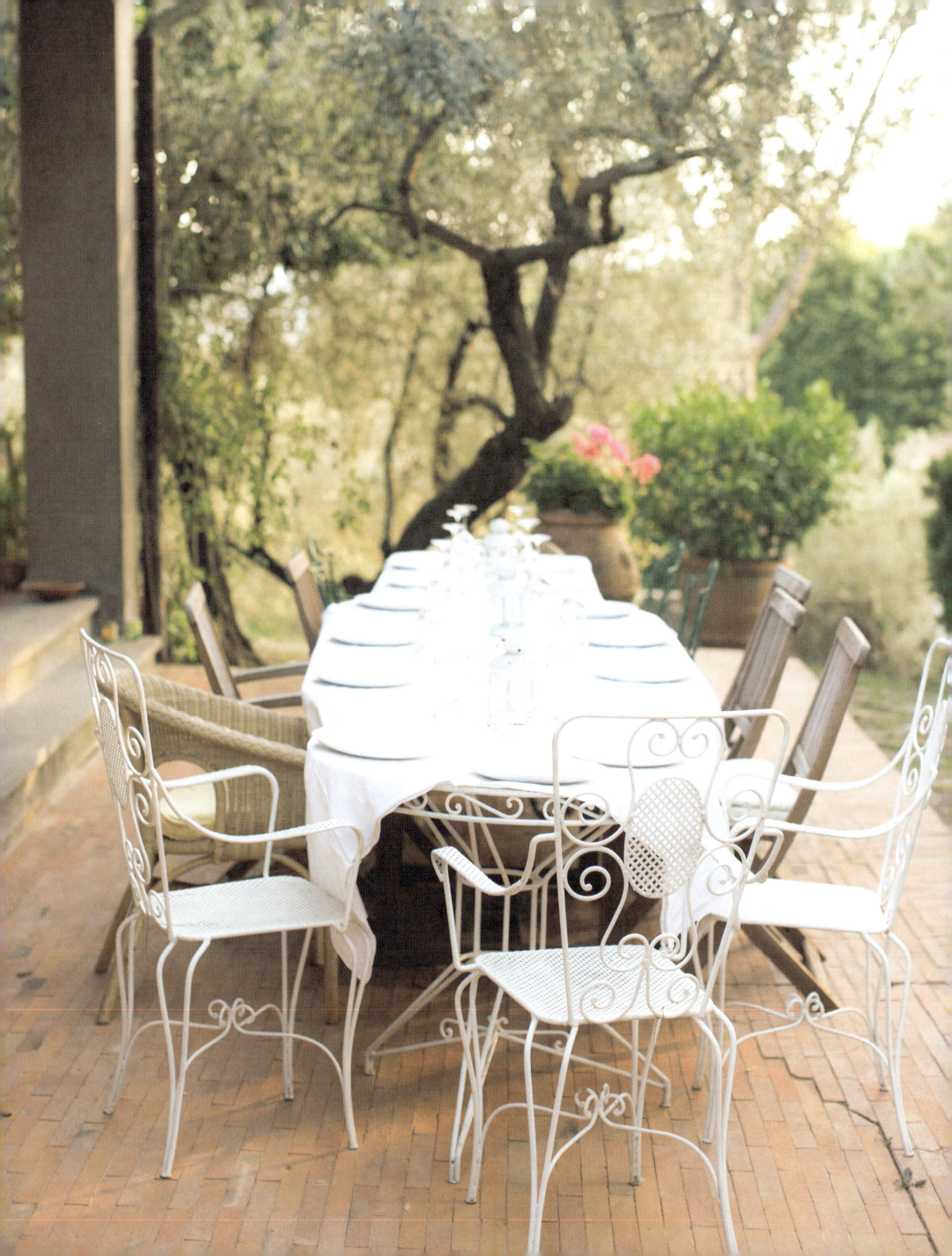

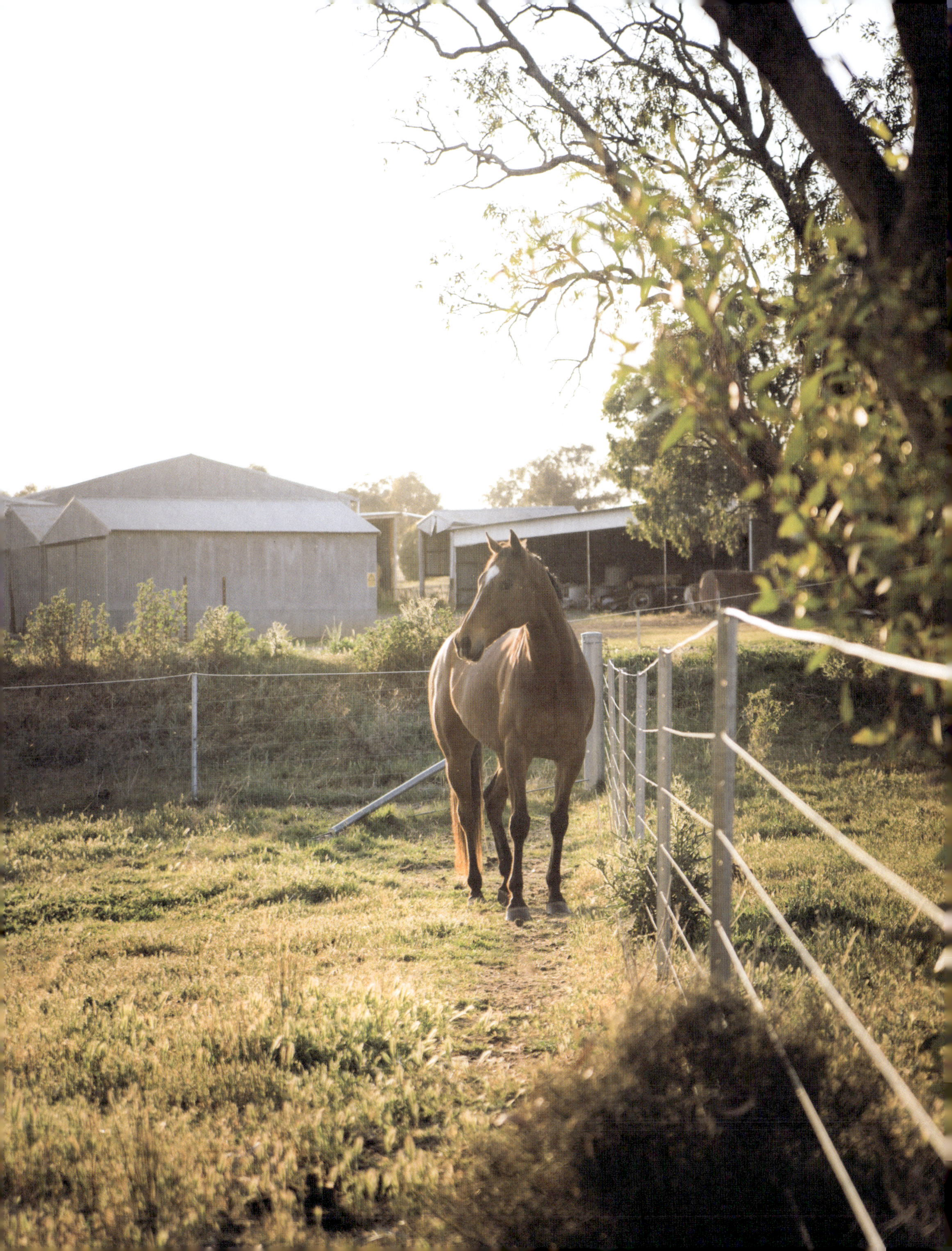

The Quick List

Dried foliage or leaves on display

Metal buckets or watering cans as styling utensils or plant pots

Fragrant herbs to suggest the aromas of country cooking

Personal touches, such as pictures or rugs

Ambient lighting for long evenings

Stylish plastic glassware for fancy picnics

An outdoor shower, bath or tap

Local stone or recycled bricks to create features

In-built sound systems for outdoor areas

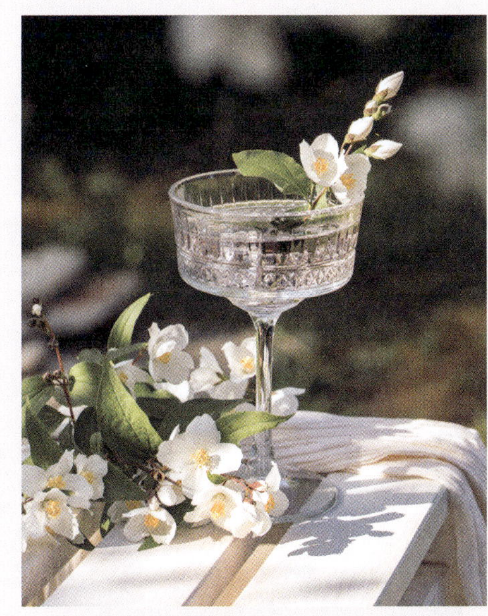

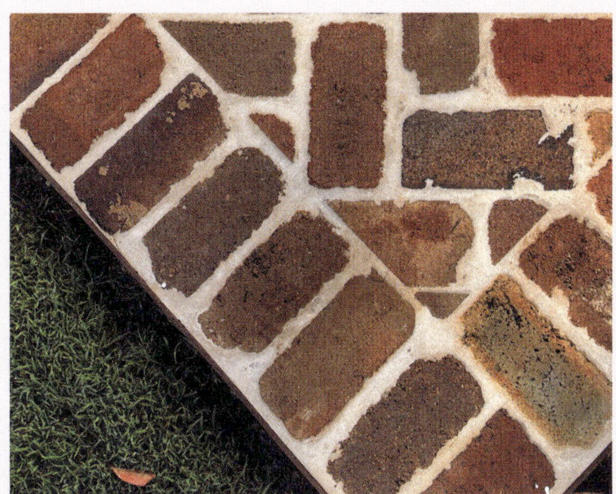

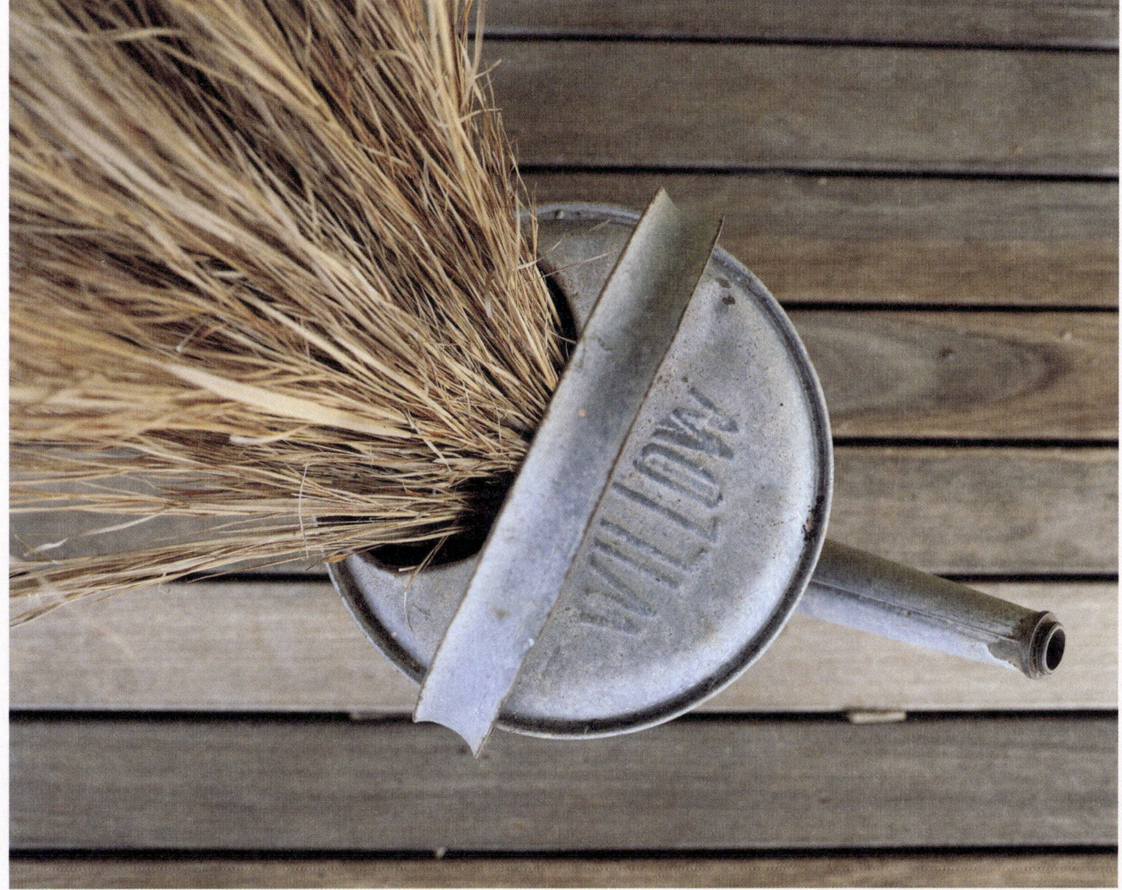
WILLOW

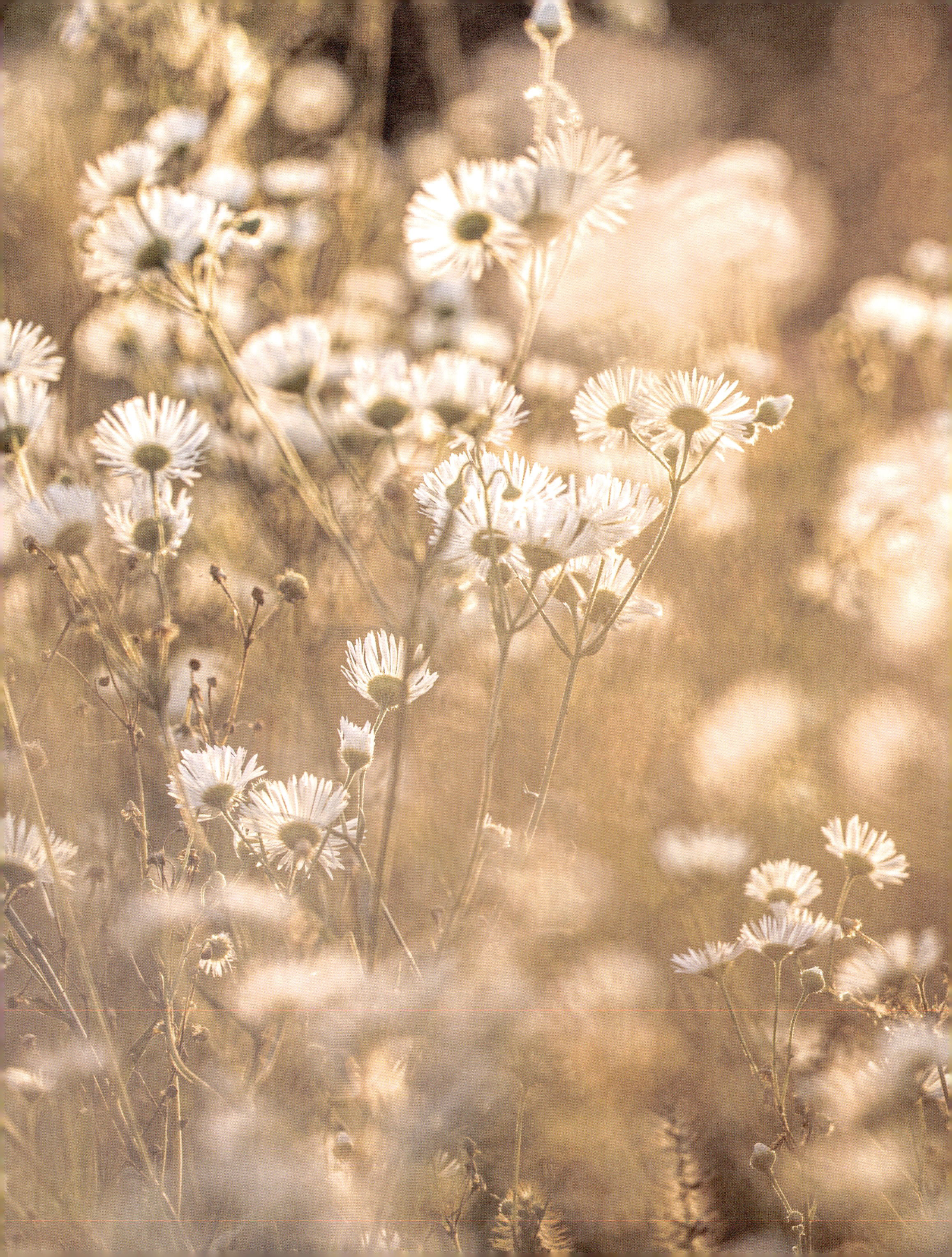

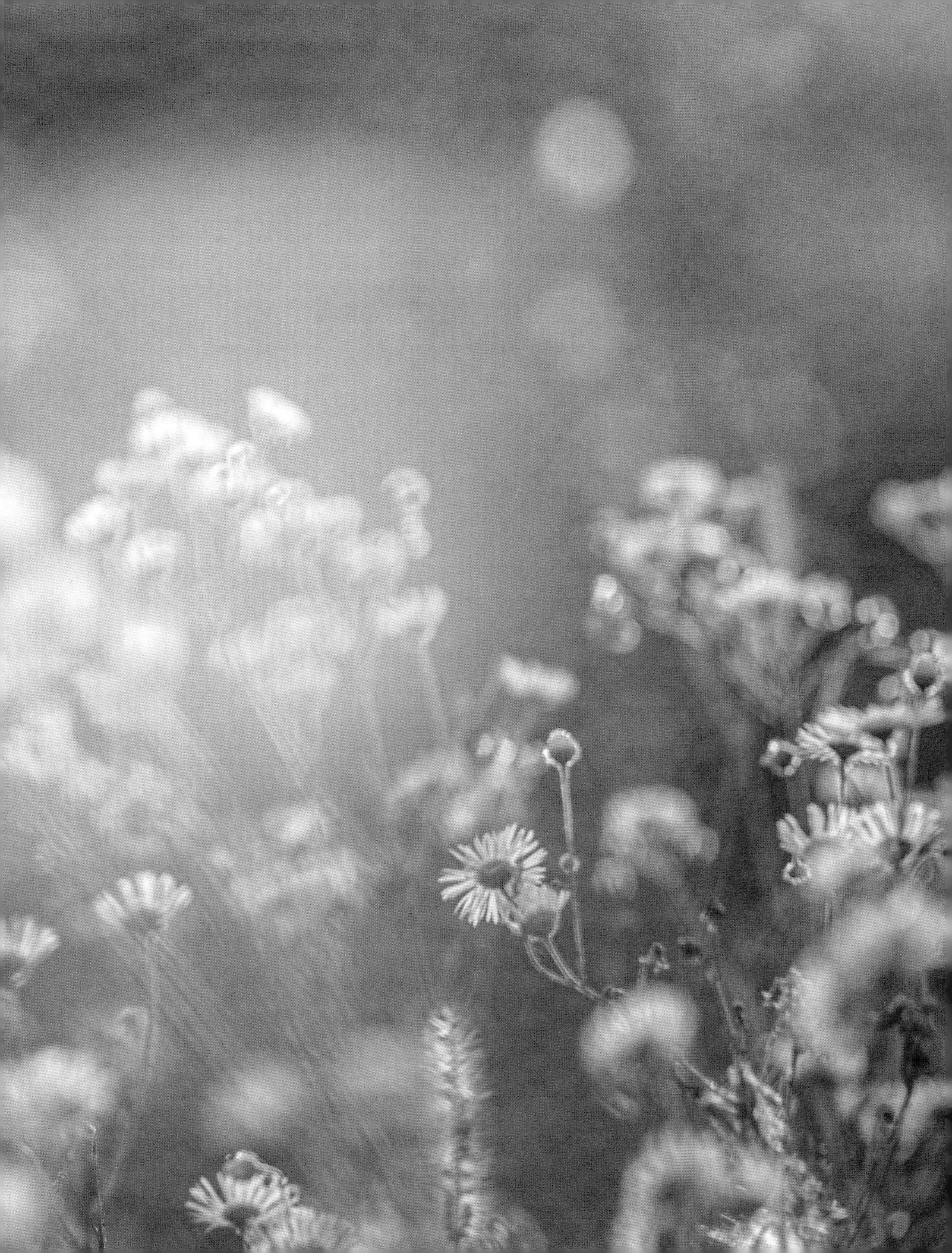

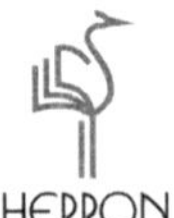

HERRON

First Published in 2024 by Herron Book Distributors Pty Ltd
14 Manton St
Morningside
QLD 4170
www.herronbooks.com

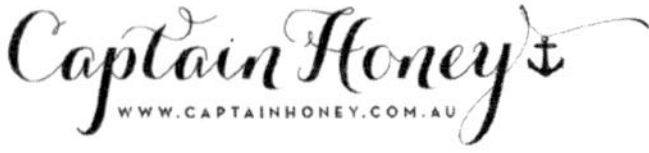

Custom book production by Captain Honey Pty Ltd
12 Station Street
Bangalow
NSW 2479
www.captainhoney.com.au

Cataloguing-in-Publication. A catalogue record for this book is available from the National Library of Australia

ISBN 978-1-922944-76-4

Printed and bound in China

This book was created on the land of the Arakwal people of the Bundjalung Nation. We acknowledge the traditional custodians of the land and pay our respects to their elders both past and present.

PHOTO CREDITS, with thanks

Front cover:
Property: The Wensley, Wensleydale
Instagram: @TheWensley
Photography: Lisa Cohen
Styling: Tess Newman Morris

Back cover: Top right
Design: Cadence and Co
Photography: The Palm Co

Back cover: Left
Design: Cadence and Co
Photography: The Palm Co

Pages: 4, 68-69, 201
Property: airbnb - The Ridge House, Gippsland
Photography: Marnie Hawson

Pages: 10-11, 17, 26, 49, 62-63, 72-75, 102-103, 106, 118, 161, 169, 177, 207-209
Design: Sherinah Peck - airbnb - Farmhouse on Oxley
Photography: The Palm Co

Pages: 12, 30, 74, 75, 152-153
Design: Cadence and Co
Photography: The Palm Co

Pages: 16 (top left), 24, 47 (top left), 94-95, 107, 120 (bottom), 124-125, 126, 127, 128 (top right), 165, 184-185, 209, 221 (bottom)
Property: The Grange, Clunes
Photography: Natalie Winter

Pages: 16 (top right), 32-33, 90, 100
Design: Cinder Design
Photography: The Palm Co

Page: 34-35
© Austock
Photography: Hannah Puechmarin

Page: 42-43
Design: Branch Designs
Photography: The Palm Co

Page: 48
Austock
Photographer: Danielle Monique

Page: 56, 58, 64-65, 78, 132-133, 144, 162 (bottom right) 167, 182,
Property: airbnb - The Milker's Cottage, Nanneella
Photography: Claira Jade

Page: 66
Design: Hemma Interiors
Photography: The Palm Co

Page: 150
Design: The Stables
Photography: The Palm Co

Page: 178
Design: Folk Studios
Photography: The Palm Co

Page: 188
Design: The Palm Co
Photography: The Palm Co

Pages: 131, 202, 212, 218 © Stocksy

The above images are reproduced with permission. Copyright remains with the photographers.

All other photos © Shutterstock